COMPLEMENTARY & INTEGRATIVE THERAPIES FOR NURSING PRACTICE

Fifth Edition

COMPLEMENTARY & INTEGRATIVE THERAPIES FOR NURSING PRACTICE

Karen Lee Fontaine

*Professor Emeritus, College of Nursing,
Purdue University Northwest,
Hammond, Indiana*

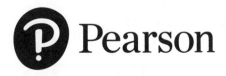 Pearson

330 Hudson Street, NY, NY 10013

Vice President, Health Science and TED: Julie Levin Alexander
Director of Portfolio Management and Portfolio Manager: Katrin Beacom
Editor in Chief: Ashley Dodge
Portfolio Management Assistant: Erin Sullivan
Associate Sponsoring Editor: Zoya Zaman
Product Marketing Manager: Christopher Barry
Field Marketing Manager: Brittany Hammond
Vice President, Digital Studio and Content Production: Paul DeLuca
Director, Digital Studio and Content Production: Brian Hyland

Managing Producer: Jennifer Sargunar
Content Producer (Team Lead): Faraz Sharique Ali
Content Producer: Neha Sharma
Manager, Rights Management: Gina Cheselka
Operations Specialist: Maura Zaldivar-Garcia
Cover Design: iEnergizer Aptara®, Ltd.
Cover Photo: Olga Lyubkina/Shutterstock
Full-Service Management and Composition: iEnergizer Aptara®, Ltd.
Printer/Binder: LSC Communications
Cover Printer: Phoenix Color
Text Font: 10/12 Palatino LT Pro

Library of Congress Cataloging-in-Publication Data

Names: Fontaine, Karen Lee, 1943- author.
Title: Complementary & integrative therapies for nursing practice / Karen Lee Fontaine.
Other titles: Complementary and alternative therapies for nursing practice
Description: Fifth edition. | Boston : Pearson, [2019] | Preceded by Complementary and alternative therapies for nursing practice / Karen Lee Fontaine. Fourth edition. 2015. | Includes bibliographical references and index.
Identifiers: LCCN 2017035719| ISBN 9780134754062 | ISBN 0134754069
Subjects: | MESH: Complementary Therapies—nursing | Nursing Care—methods | Integrative Medicine
Classification: LCC RT42 | NLM WY 86.5 | DDC 610.73—dc23 LC record available at https://lccn.loc.gov/2017035719

1   17

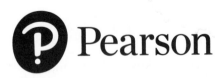 **Pearson**

ISBN-10:   0-13-475406-9
ISBN-13: 978-0-13-475406-2

This book is dedicated to:

Patti Cleary, Editorial Consultant extraordinaire. I could not have completed this edition without her wisdom and guidance.

Al Renslow, husband extraordinaire, whose patience, sense of humor, and faith in me made it all worthwhile.

CONTENTS

TRY THIS*

---

*"Try This" features throughout the chapters, provides you with examples of how you can integrate these practices into your own life, and also gives you ideas for client education. A list of resources is also included in every chapter.

PREFACE

The profession of nursing has advanced beyond the Western biomedical model to incorporate many healing tools used by our Asian, Latino, Native American, African, and European ancestors. We are rapidly rediscovering that these ancient principles and practices have significant therapeutic value. Some see this movement as a "return to our roots." Others believe it is a response to runaway health-care costs, growing dissatisfaction with high-tech medicines, and increasing concern over the adverse effects and misuse of medications and other treatments. The growth of consumer empowerment also fuels this movement.

As nurses, how do you begin to assimilate thousands of years of healing knowledge? How do you begin this journey of integrating practices into your own lives? In your professional practice, how do you model healthful living? How do you help clients choose their own healing journeys? How do you break down the barriers between conventional and complementary and integrative therapies? Learning about these practices, like anything else, is a slow process involving a steady accumulation of bits of information and skills that eventually form a coherent pattern called knowledge. Although it is possible to learn a great deal about healing practices from reading, thinking, and asking questions, you must in the long run learn about healing through participation. Without hands-on experience, you can be a good student, but you can never be a great nursing practitioner of the healing arts. I trust this book will be one step in a lifelong exploration of and experiences with healing practices.

Consumers do not wish to abandon conventional medicines, but they do want to have a range of options available to them including herbs and nutritional supplements, manual healing methods, mind–body techniques, and spiritual approaches. Some practices, such as exercise, proper nutrition, meditation, and massage, promote health and prevent diseases. Others, such as herbs and homeopathic remedies, address specific illnesses. Many other practices do both. The rise of chronic disease rates in Western society is increasingly motivating consumers to consider self-care approaches. As recently as the 1950s, only 30% of all diseases were chronic, and curable—largely infectious—diseases dominated, for which medical interventions were both appropriate and effective. Now, 80% of all diseases are chronic. Western medicine, with its focus on acute disorders, trauma, and surgery, is considered to be the best high-tech medical care in the world. Unfortunately, it is not responding adequately to the current epidemic of chronic illnesses.

Ethnocentrism, the assumption that one's own cultural or ethnic group is superior to others, has often prevented Western health-care practitioners from learning "new" ways to promote health and prevent chronic illness. With consumer demand for a broader range of options, we must open our minds to the idea that other cultures and countries have valid ways of preventing and curing diseases that could be good for Western societies. Although the information may be new to us, many of these traditions are hundreds or even thousands of years old and have long been part of the medical mainstream in other cultures.

I have titled this book *Complementary & Integrative Therapies for Nursing Practice* because I believe we need to merge complementary approaches with Western-based nursing practices resulting in integrative therapies. I have tried to provide enough information about these therapies to help guide practice decisions. This text, as an overview and practical guide for nurses, does not pretend to be an exhaustive collection of all the facts and related research, nor does it offer meticulous documentation for all claims made by the various therapies. The goal of the text is to motivate you, the reader, to explore these approaches, increase your knowledge about factors that contribute to health and illness, and expand your professional practice appropriately.

It is possible to classify alternative practices in any number of ways. I have chosen to present more than 40 approaches categorized into seven units. In Unit 1, I introduce the philosophical approaches to both Western biomedicine and complementary and integrative medicine, as well as evidence-based health care in these therapies. Concepts common to many approaches are defined and discussed, such as energy, breath, spirituality, and healing. Unit 2 presents a number of health-care practices that have been systematized throughout the centuries worldwide. These typically include an entire set of values, attitudes, and beliefs that generate a philosophy of life, not simply a group of remedies. The chapters cover Traditional Chinese medicine, Ayurvedic medicine, and Native American healing and curanderismo. Unit 3 comprises chapters relating to botanical healings used by 80% of the world's population. Chapters cover herbs and nutritional supplements, aromatherapy, homeopathy, and naturopathy. Unit 4 presents manual healing methods—some from ancient times and some developed in the latter half of the 20th century. The chapters discuss chiropractic, massage, pressure point therapies, hand-mediated biofield therapies, and combined physical and biofield therapies. The chapters in Unit 5 cover types of mind–body techniques for healing and include yoga, meditation, hypnotherapy and guided imagery, dreams, intuition, music as a therapeutic tool, biofeedback, and movement-oriented therapies. Unit 6 presents two spiritual approaches to therapeutic intervention: working with shamans and the use of faith and prayer. Unit 7 includes two chapters on miscellaneous practices: bioelectromagnetics and animal-facilitated therapy.

The appendix provides specific information on managing the types of common health problems that respond well to alternative therapies and lifestyle modification.

This book does not recommend treatments but, rather, describes alternative practices, their backgrounds and claims, preparation of practitioners, concepts, diagnostic methods, treatments, and evidence from research studies. "Integrated Nursing Practice" is an important section of every chapter designed to help you, the nurse, expand your practice by providing you with specific information and suggestions.

In this fifth edition, I have continued the "Considering the Evidence" feature with all new research relating to the chapter topic. Seven of these features present a systematic review of randomized control trials, while three present primary research. "Considering the Evidence" boxes not only present current studies but also are designed to further critical thinking and perhaps inspire you to design studies to answer your own questions. Each study answers the following questions: What was the approach of the research? What was the aim/purpose/objective of the research? How was the study done? What were the significant findings of the research? What additional questions might I have? What is the clinical significance of this study?

NEW TO THIS EDITION

- Updated all research sections and increased the number of systematic reviews of randomized controlled trials
- Increased emphasis on integrative nursing practice
- Expanded the lists of resources to include more international resources
- Expanded the appendix by including nine additional common health-care problems
- Added material on:
  - African healing
  - Forest bathing
  - Health disparities
  - Health literacy
  - Native American sacred land
  - Precision Medicine Initiative
  - Low-level laser therapy
  - Watsu®

Nurses are in a unique position to take a leadership role in integrating complementary healing methods into Western health-care systems. Nurses have historically used their hands, heart, and head in more natural and traditional healing interactions. By virtue of their education and relationships with clients, nurses can help consumers assert their right to choose their own healing journey and the quality of their life and death experiences.

My dear friend and colleague has written the following letter to you about her lived experience uniting biomedicine with complementary and integrative approaches.

Dear Reader,

It is both a pleasurable and enlightening experience for me to contribute to your text, *Complementary & Integrative Therapies for Nursing Practice*, through the development of the "Considering the Evidence" feature. I approach this work hopeful that it may inspire you, the reader, to engage in critical thinking, assist in your understanding of the significance of research to inform your nursing practice, and, perhaps, propose future studies to answer your own researchable questions. While I am very committed to the importance of nursing research, I have asked Karen Lee

Fontaine to allow me the privilege of sharing my anecdotal experience with you as it relates to my personal journey with complementary and integrative therapies. I hope my story and insight can inspire you to reflect on and embrace the important content of this text in your nursing practice. After learning of my diagnosis of bilateral breast cancer, I actively participated in a myriad of Western medicine therapies while integrating complementary and integrative therapies. Although the chemotherapy experience was both emotionally and physically taxing, I considered the massage therapist as part of "my team," and I looked forward to this dimension of comfort during this challenging time. Engaging in yoga enhanced "restful sleep" as a response to the overwhelming fatigue that frequently accompanies Western therapies such as chemotherapy and radiation and just the daily awareness that "you have cancer." Acupressure relieved uncomfortable postoperative symptoms. T'ai chi continues to be an opportunity to focus on myself and reflect on the positives associated with this journey. Reiki and reflexology is my specified "me time." As I continue to engage in the associated deep breathing exercises, it stimulates my mind to drift to affirmative thoughts and so many positive memories from my life. For me, "living with cancer" is more of an "inconvenience" in my life's journey. I can appreciate this may not be the experience for everyone, but I can personally assure you that integrating many of the therapies discussed in this text allows me a "quality of life" while simultaneously working with conventional medicine's goal for a "quantity of life." With the combination of both, even after some time, I feel I have been given the power to survive and, perhaps, make a difference in the lives of those currently living this journey!

While it has been several years since my original diagnosis and initiating the "cancer treatment path," I am unwavering in my belief of the **POWER** of complementary and integrative therapies in enhancing one's quality of life. I frequently share my story with women recently diagnosed with cancer and just embarking on their "new reality" and encourage them to integrate these therapies in their treatment plan. I hope my story gives you a sense of hope and empowerment in caring for persons both professionally and personally who are partaking on a strenuous journey related to their health. I can recall in my own nursing practice experiencing feelings of helplessness when caring for persons undergoing complex treatments with so many uncertainties related to their health outcome. I can attest that your understanding, knowledge, and support in the implementation of complementary and integrative therapies can significantly affect their "quality of life" and allow you the privilege of making a difference in their health journey.

Dolores M. Huffman, RN, PhD
Professor Emeritus, College of Nursing
Purdue University Northwest, IN

ACKNOWLEDGMENTS

I would like to express thanks to the many people who have inspired, commented on, and in other ways assisted in the writing and publication of the fifth edition of this book. On the publishing and production side at Pearson, I was most fortunate to have an exceptional team of editors and support staff. My thanks go to Julie Levin Alexander, Publisher, and Neha Sharma, Content Producer, who provided support and guidance throughout this project. Sadika Rehman, Project Manager, kept this book on schedule and dedicated her time and skills to its completion.

Previous Edition Contributors

Dolores M. Huffman, PhD, RN
Professor Emeritus
College of Nursing
Purdue University Northwest
Hammond, IN

Sheila Lewis, BScN, MHSc
Associate Lecturer
Department of Nursing, Faculty of Health
York University
Toronto, ON, Canada

Leslie Rittenmeyer, PsyD, CNS, CNE, RN
Professor
College of Nursing
Purdue University Northwest
Research Associate: Northwest Indiana Center for Evidence Based Practice:
A Joanna Briggs Institute Collaborating Centre
Hammond, IN

REVIEWERS

Carol Athey, MA, MSN,RN, CNOR, CCAP
Clinical Instructor
Stephen F. Austin State University
DeWitt School of Nursing
Nacogdoches, Texas

Karen Avino, EdD, MSN, RN, AHN-BC, HWNC-BC
Assistant Professor
University of Delaware
School of Nursing
Newark, Delaware

Lori A. Edwards, DrPH, MPH, RN, PHCNS-BC
Assistant Professor
University of Maryland
School of Nursing
Baltimore, Maryland

Teresa Johnson, DCN, RD, LD
Associate Professor
Troy University
School of Nursing
Troy, Alabama

Dr. Kim Link, DNP, PMHNP
Assistant Professor
Western Kentucky University
School of Nursing
Bowling Green, Kentucky

Dr. Dawn Garrett Wright, PhD, CNE
Associate Professor
Western Kentucky University
School of Nursing
Bowling Green, Kentucky

Healing Practices: Complementary and Integrative Therapies for Nurses

Happiness, grief, gaiety, sadness are by nature contagious.
Bring your health and your strength to the weak and sickly,
and so you will be of use to them. Give them, not your
weakness, but your energy, so you will revive
and lift them up.

HENRI-FREDERIC AMIEL

1

Integrative Healing

Time is generally the best doctor.

OVID

Most of nursing education in the United States, Canada, the United Kingdom, Europe, and Australia—often referred to as Western countries—has been under the umbrella of biomedicine, and thus Western nurses are familiar and comfortable with its beliefs, theories, practices, strengths, and limitations. Fewer nurses have studied alternative medical theories and practices and as a result may lack information or even harbor misinformation about these healing practices. Unlike the profession of medicine in general, however, the profession of nursing has traditionally embraced two basic concepts embodied by alternative therapies—holism and humanism—in its approach with clients. Nurses have long believed that healing and caring must be approached holistically and that biological, psychological, emotional, spiritual, and environmental aspects of health and illness are equally important. This humanistic perspective includes propositions such as the mind and body are indivisible, people have the power to solve their own problems, people are responsible for the patterns of their lives, and well-being is a combination of personal satisfaction and contributions to the larger community. This theoretical basis gives nurses a solid foot in each camp and places them in the unique position to help create a bridge between biomedicine and alternative medicine (Buchan, Shakeel, Trinidade, Buchan, & Ah-See, 2012; Dossey & Keegan, 2016; Peplau, 1952; Quinn, 2000).

BACKGROUND

Many interesting exchanges around the world have debated the appropriate terminology of various healing practices. Some people become vested in the use of particular terms and have difficulty getting past the language limitations. For example, many

3

people view the term *alternative medicine* as being too narrow or misleading and are concerned that the term lacks a full understanding of traditional healing practices. It would be helpful for a common language to be developed without these constraints. As language evolves, the terms used today may be quite different from those that will be in use 20 years from now. For consistency, the terms chosen for this text are **conventional medicine** or **biomedicine** to describe Western medical practices, and the terms **alternative medicine** or **complementary medicine** to describe other healing practices. **Traditional medicine** refers to indigenous medical systems such as Traditional Chinese Medicine (TCM). **Integrative medicine** embodies conventional and complementary and alternative medicine. There are no universally accepted terms. The following list presents commonly used words and their counterparts:

Mainstream	Complementary/Alternative
Modern	Ancient
Western	Eastern
Allopathic	Homeopathic; holistic
Conventional	Unconventional
Orthodox	Traditional
Biomedicine	Natural medicine
Scientific	Indigenous healing methods

The line between conventional medicine and complementary and alternative medicine is imprecise and frequently changing. For example, is the use of megavitamins or diet regimens to treat a disease considered medicine, a lifestyle change, or both? Can having one's pain lessened by massage be considered a medical therapy? How should spiritual healing and prayer—some of the oldest, most widely used, and least studied traditional approaches—be classified? Although the terms *alternative* and *complementary* are frequently used, in some instances they represent the primary treatment modality for an individual. Thus, conventional medicine sometimes assumes a secondary role and becomes a complement to the primary treatment modality.

Conventional Medicine

Biomedical or Western medicine is only about 200 years old. It was founded on the philosophical beliefs of René Descartes (1596–1650)—that the mind and body are separate—and on Sir Isaac Newton's (1642–1727) principles of physics—that the universe is like a large mechanical clock in which everything operates in a linear, sequential form. This mechanistic perspective of medicine views the human body as a series of body parts. It is a *reductionist approach* that converts the person into increasingly smaller components: systems, organs, cells, and biochemicals. People are reduced to patients, patients are reduced to bodies, and bodies are reduced to machines. Health is viewed as the absence of disease or, in other words, nothing is broken at present, and sick care is focused on the symptoms of dysfunction. Physicians are trained to fix or repair broken parts through the use of drugs, radiation, surgery, or replacement of body parts. The approach is aggressive and militant—physicians are in a war against disease, with a take-no-prisoners attitude. Both consumers and practitioners of biomedicine believe it is better to

- do something rather than wait and see whether the body's natural processes resolve the problem.
- attack the disease directly by medication or surgery rather than try to build up the person's resistance and ability to overcome the disease.

Biomedicine views the person primarily as a physical body, with the mind and spirit being separate and secondary or, at times, even irrelevant. It is a powerful medicine in that it has virtually eliminated some infectious diseases, such as smallpox and polio. It is based on science and technology, personifying a highly industrialized society. As a "rescue" medicine, the biomedical approach is appropriate. It is highly effective in emergencies, traumatic injuries, bacterial infections, and some highly sophisticated surgeries. In these cases, treatment is fast, aggressive, and goal oriented, with the responsibility for cure falling on the practitioner.

The priority of intervention is on opposing and suppressing the symptoms of illness. This approach is evidenced in many medications with prefixes such as *an-* or *anti-*, as in analgesics, anesthetics, anti-inflammatories, and antipyretics. Biomedicine characterizes each disease in terms of its mechanisms of action, based on the belief that most individuals are affected in the same way. There is minimal consideration for how the disease affects the person or how the person affects the disease (Maitland, 2016). Thus, treatment is basically the same for most people. Because conventional medicine is preoccupied with parts and symptoms and not with whole working systems of matter, energy, thoughts, and feelings, it does not do well with long-term systemic illnesses such as arthritis, heart disease, and hypertension. Despite higher per capita spending on health care in the United States than in all other nations, in 2013, U.S. life expectancy ranked only 37th, and the infant mortality rate ranked 56th among the 225 nations studied (World Factbook, 2013–2014; World Health Rankings, 2016). In comparison of 19 developed countries, the United States had the highest rate of preterm births. Sadly, the United States has failed to be a world leader in providing a healthier quality of life (Raheim, 2015).

Complementary and Alternative Medicine

Complementary and alternative medicine (CAM) is an umbrella term for as many as 1,800 therapies practiced worldwide. Many forms have been handed down over thousands of years, both orally and in written records. These therapies are based on the medical systems of ancient peoples, including Egyptians, Chinese, Asian Indians, Greeks, and Native Americans. Others, such as osteopathy and naturopathy, evolved in the United States during the past two centuries. Still others, such as some of the mind–body and bioelectromagnetic approaches, are on the frontier of scientific knowledge and understanding.

The National Center for Complementary and Integrative Health (NCCIH) at the National Institutes of Health (NIH) defines CAM therapies as a broad range of healing philosophies, approaches, and therapies that conventional medicine does not commonly use, accept, study, understand, or make available (National Center for Complementary and Integrative Health, 2016).

Although they represent diverse approaches, CAM therapies share certain attributes. They are based on the paradigm of *whole systems* and the belief that people are more than physical bodies with fixable and replaceable parts. Rather, mental, emotional, spiritual, and environmental components of well-being are considered to play crucial and equal roles in a person's state of health. Interventions are individualized within the entire context of a person's life (Micozzi, 2015). Even Hippocrates, the father of Western medicine, espoused a holistic orientation when he taught physicians to observe their patients' life circumstances, emotional state, stresses, environment, inherited constitution, and their subjective experience of an illness. Socrates agreed, declaring, "Curing the soul; that is the first thing." In alternative medicine, symptoms are believed to be an expression of the body's wisdom as it reacts to cure its own imbalance or disease. Other threads or concepts common to most forms of alternative medicine include the following:

- An internal self-healing process exists within each person.
- People are responsible for making their own decisions regarding their health care.
- Nature, time, and patience are the three great healers.

When Albert Einstein (1879–1955) introduced his theory of relativity in 1905, our way of viewing the universe changed dramatically. Einstein said that mass and energy are equivalent and interconvertible, and all matter is connected at the subatomic level. No single entity could be affected without all its connecting parts being affected. In this view, the universe is not a giant clock but a living web. The human body is animated by an integrated energy called the **life force**. The life force sustains the physical body but is also a spiritual entity that is linked to a higher being or infinite source of energy. When the life force flows freely throughout the body, a person experiences optimal health and vitality. When the life force is blocked or weakened, organs, tissues, and cells are deprived of the energy they need to function at their full potential, and illness or disease results.

Alternative medicine is especially effective for people with chronic, debilitating illnesses for which conventional medicine has few, if any, answers. It has much to offer in the arena of health promotion and disease prevention. As costs of conventional medicine increase and people continue to suffer from chronic illnesses and degenerative diseases, alternative medicine is moving closer to the mainstream. A growing number of complementary and alternative therapies are eligible for reimbursement by third-party payers in the United States. The most commonly reimbursed treatments are chiropractic, biofeedback, acupuncture, hypnotherapy, and naturopathy. Box 1.1 provides an overview of the paradigms of conventional and alternative medicine.

BOX 1.1

Paradigms of Medicine

View	Conventional Medicine	Alternative Medicine
Mind/body/spirit	are separate	are one
The body is	a machine	a living microcosm of the universe
Disease results when	parts break	energy/life force becomes unbalanced
Symptoms	dysfunctional and need to be fixed	communicators about the state of the whole person
Role of medicine	to combat disease	to restore mind/body/spirit harmony
Approach	treat and suppress symptoms	search for patterns of disharmony or imbalance
Focuses on	parts/matter	whole/energy
Treatments	attempt to "fix" broken parts; specific to disease	support self-healing; personalized for the individual
Primary interventions	drugs, surgery, diet, radiation	exercise, herbs, stress management, social support
System	sick care	health care

Integrative Medicine

Integrative medicine embodies conventional and complementary and alternative medicine, making use of the best available evidence of both approaches to healing. It is a multidisciplinary, collaborative, holistic approach that encompasses mind, body, and spirit. It stresses the relationship between the client and the practitioner as well as the human capacity for healing. Integrative practitioners believe that clients have the right to make informed choices about their health-care options. The focus is on "using the least invasive, least toxic, and least costly methods to help facilitate health" (Willison, 2006, p. 255). The goal of integrative medicine is to find new solutions to prevention and treatment of health-care problems.

Dr. Andrew Weil has been the driving force for integrative medicine in the United States and hopes to reform the entire medical delivery system by changing the way we look at health and disease and by modifying the education of physicians. His program at the Arizona Center for Integrative Medicine at the University of Arizona College of Medicine was the first to adopt this new curriculum. Currently, more than 60 medical schools have adopted this integrative approach. In 2008, the World Health Organization (WHO) stressed the importance of integrative medicine and advocated the inclusion of complementary and alternative therapies in biomedical health-care education.

Nursing must also be open to change to meet the goal of true integrative care. Holistic nursing is an advanced specialty practice focusing on health and wellness, assisting with the healing process, supporting individuals, and easing suffering. Colleges of nursing must integrate the principles and skills of holistic nursing throughout all the levels of nursing curricula if we are to be a force in the changing health-care systems.

ASSUMPTIONS

In understanding conventional and alternative medicine, it is helpful to study the assumptions basic to their theories, practices, and research. These assumptions include the origin of disease, the meaning of health, the curative process, and health promotion.

Origin of Disease

Biomedicine and alternative medicine have widely divergent assumptions regarding the origin of disease. Biomedicine was shaped by the observations that bacteria were responsible for producing disease and pathological damage and that antitoxins and vaccines could improve a person's ability to ward off the effects of pathogens. Armed with this knowledge, physicians began to conquer a large number of devastating infectious diseases. As the science developed, physicians came to believe that germs and genes caused disease, and once the offending pathogen, metabolic error, or chemical imbalance was found, all diseases would eventually yield to the appropriate vaccine, antibiotic, or chemical compound.

Conventional medicine has also been influenced by Darwin's concept of survival of the fittest; that is, all life is a constant struggle, and only the most successful competitors survive. Applied to medicine, this notion means that humans live under constant attack by the thousands of microorganisms that, in the Western view, cause most diseases. People must defend themselves and counterattack with treatments that kill the enemy. Based on this assumption, symptoms are regarded as harmful manifestations and should be suppressed. For example, a headache is an annoyance that should be eliminated, and a fever should be reduced with the use of medications.

Complementary and alternative medicine is based on the belief of a life force or energy that flows through each person and sustains life. *Balance* refers to harmony among organs in the body and among body systems, and in relationships to other individuals, society, and the environment. A balanced organism presents a strong defense against external insults such as bacteria, viruses, and trauma. When the life force or energy is blocked or weakened, the vitality of organs and tissues is reduced, oxygen is diminished, waste products accumulate, and organs and tissues degenerate. Symptoms are the body's way of communicating that the life force has been blocked or weakened, resulting in a compromised immune system. Disease is not necessarily a surprise encounter with a bacterium or a virus, since these are ever present, but rather the end result of a series of events that began with a disruption of the life force. Based on this assumption, symptoms are not suppressed unless they endanger life, such as a headache from an aneurysm or a body temperature above 105°F. Rather, symptoms are cooperated with because they express the body's wisdom as it reacts to cure its own disease. For example, a headache is a signal that one's whole system needs realignment, and a fever may be the result of the breakdown of bacterial proteins or toxins. When symptoms are suppressed, they are not resolved but merely held in abeyance, gathering energy for renewed expression as soon as the outside, counteractive force is removed. Worldwide, there are multiple cultural, spiritual, and religious explanations of the cause of disease. These explanations direct the choice of treatment—be it biomedicine, traditional healing, or integrative health care.

Meaning of Health

If you were to ask a healer from the Chinese, Indian, or Native American tradition about the meaning of health, you would receive answers very different from those given by a Western physician. The biomedical view of health, in the past, was often described as the absence of disease or other abnormal conditions. That definition has been expanded to include the view that health is not a static condition; the body constantly changes and adapts to both internal and external environmental challenges. The majority of conventional medical practitioners would define health as a state of well-being. They may disagree, however, about who determines well-being—the health professional or the individual. With some exceptions, wellness and health promotion have, for the most part, been left to the initiative of the individual.

Those practicing complementary and alternative or integrative medicine describe health as a condition of wholeness, balance, and harmony of the body, mind, emotions, and spirit. Health is not a concrete goal to be achieved; rather, it is a lifelong process that represents growth toward potential, an inner feeling of aliveness. *Physical* aspects include optimal functioning of all body systems. *Emotional* aspects include the ability to feel and express the entire range of human emotions. *Mental* aspects include feelings of self-worth, a positive identity, a sense of accomplishment, and the ability to appreciate and create. *Environmental* aspects include physical, biological, economic, social, and political conditions. *Spiritual* aspects involve self, others, and society. Self-components are the development of moral values and finding a meaningful purpose in life. Spiritual factors relating to others include the search for meaning through relationships and the feeling of connectedness with others and with an external power often identified as God or the divine source. *Societal* aspects of spiritual health can be understood as a common humanity and a belief in the fundamental sacredness and unity of all life. These beliefs motivate people toward truth and a sense of fairness and justice to all members of society.

Curative Process

The curative process is another area of divergent viewpoints. Conventional medicine promotes the view that external treatments—drugs, surgery, radiation—cure people, and practitioners are trained to fix or repair broken parts. The focus is on the disease process or abnormal condition. Alternative practitioners look at conditions that block the life force and keep it from flowing freely through the body. Healing occurs when balance and harmony are restored. The focus is on the health potential of the person rather than the disease problem. The cure model and the healing model are presented with greater detail in Chapter 2.

Health Promotion

Conventional and complementary and alternative medical systems have somewhat different foci on promotion of health. The thrust of conventional medicine is disease prevention. Consumers are taught how to decrease their risk of cancer, cardiac disorders, obesity, and other life-threatening diseases that kill most people prematurely in Western society. Although these behaviors are important, disease prevention is only one piece of health promotion. From the complementary and alternative perspective, health promotion is a lifelong process that focuses on optimal development of people's physical, emotional, mental, spiritual, and environmental selves. An individual's worldviews, values, lifestyles, and health beliefs are considered to be of critical importance. Consumers are encouraged to adopt healthier lifestyles, to accept increased responsibility for their own well-being, and, through greater self-reliance, to learn how to handle common health problems on their own. As the *Healthy People 2020* report illustrates (U.S. Department of Health and Human Services, 2010a), the health care delivery system of the future must make use of all approaches that effectively promote optimal health using best available evidence and knowledge. Box 1.2 describes NCCIH 2016 strategic plan. In the United States, the Patient Protection and Affordable Care Act, a federal statute, was signed into law by President Barack Obama in 2010. One goal of this act is to provide affordable health care for every American (U.S. Department of Health and Human Services, 2010b). In 2015, President Obama announced the *Precision Medicine Initiative* funded in the 2016 budget. Most biomedical treatments have been designed for the "average" patient, which may or may not be effective for individuals. Precision medicine takes into account genes, environments, and lifestyles when predicting which treatments might be most effective. A current example of precision medicine is the molecular testing of various cancers that enables physicians to select treatments to improve health and minimize adverse effects. Potentially, precision medicine will improve individualized care and more rapid development of new treatments (Fact Sheet: President Obama's Precision Medicine Initiative, n.d.).

BOX 1.2

NCCIH Strategic Plan 2016

- Fundamental science and methods development
- Improving care for hard-to-manage symptoms
- Fostering health promotion and disease prevention

Source: National Center for Complementary and Integrative Health (2016).

RESEARCH

Scientific beliefs rest not just on facts but on paradigms (broad views of how these facts are related and organized). Differences in views among groups of nursing and medical researchers are a reflection of the different scientific paradigms—quantitative and qualitative research. Although each method results in a different type of knowledge, both provide information to researchers and consumers. Evidence-based practice is covered in Chapter 3.

Quantitative research represents the principles of the Western scientific method, which include formulating and testing hypotheses and then rejecting or accepting the hypotheses. Every question is reduced to the smallest possible part. Results can be replicated and generalized, and outcomes can be predicted and controlled. Quantitative research is said to be objective in that the observer is separate from what is being observed. Another part of this objective paradigm is that all information can be derived from physically measurable data. This type of research has been extremely effective for isolating causative factors of disease and developing cures. However, it cannot explain the whole person as an integrated unit.

Qualitative research seeks to understand events in context-specific settings. It studies the context and meaning of interactive variables as they form patterns reflective of the whole. Researchers observe, document, analyze, and qualify the interactive relationship of variables. In the science of physics, it is believed that objectivity is ultimately not possible. The Heisenberg uncertainty principle states that the act of observing phenomena necessarily influences the behavior of the phenomena being observed. Another part of the paradigm relates to the belief that interactions between living organisms and environments are transactional, multidirectional, and synergistic in ways that cannot be reduced. This holistic approach (the whole is greater than the sum of the parts) is basic to qualitative research.

Practitioners of conventional medicine believe that procedures and substances must pass blinded randomized controlled trials (RCTs) to be proven effective. As a testing method, an RCT examines a single procedure or substance in isolated, controlled conditions and measures results against another existing therapy or the best available treatment. This approach is based on the assumption that single factors cause and reverse illness, and these factors can be studied alone and out of context. In contrast, practitioners of integrative and complementary medicine believe that no single factor causes anything, nor can a magic substance single-handedly reverse illness. Multiple factors contribute to illness, and multiple interventions work together to promote healing. RCTs are incapable of reconciling this degree of complexity and variation.

Although major complementary and alternative medical systems may not have been subjected to a great deal of quantitative research, they are generally *not* experimental therapies. They rely on well-developed clinical observational skills and experience that is guided by their explanatory models. Likewise, many biomedical practices are guided by observation and experience and have *not* been tested quantitatively. New medicines must have rigorous proof of efficacy and safety before clinical use. Tests, procedures, and treatments, however, are not similarly constrained. Western physicians, like alternative practitioners, use the same well-developed clinical observational skills and experience, guided by their explanatory biomedical model. Some of these discrepancies are disappearing, and the emphasis is now on evidence-based practice and the rapid growth of CAM research.

This text does not offer meticulous documentation for all claims that are made by the various therapies. The National Center for Complementary and Integrative Health at the National Institutes of Health has been mandated to explore complementary and alternative healing practices in the context of rigorous science, to train researchers, and to provide the public with authoritative information. NCCIH has established 16 research centers to explore the safety and efficacy of a wide range of therapies. In addition, NCCIH funds hundreds of research projects and grants every year. The NIH Office of Dietary Supplements is conducting scientific studies regarding the role of dietary supplements in the improvement of health care. As a result of these and other international efforts, the evidence base for alternative therapies has grown significantly.

The results of scientific studies can be accessed at two websites. NCCIH and the National Library of Medicine (NLM) have partnered to create CAM on PubMed (nccih.nih.gov/research/camonpubmed/). This site provides access to citations from the MEDLINE database and links to many full-text articles at journal websites. The Cochrane Library (www.update-software .com/cochrane/), an international effort, consists of a regularly updated collection of evidence-based medicine databases, including the Cochrane Database of Systematic Reviews. This site lists thousands of randomized trials for various alternative therapies. This information is extremely helpful for both consumers and providers of health care. The reader is advised to access these sites for information regarding the latest research results. Chapter 3 covers evidence-based nursing practice in more detail.

CONSUMERS

Many Americans are looking beyond conventional medicine for relief from illness and improvement of health. According to a number of random surveys,

BOX 1.3

Frequently Reported Conditions of Those Seeking Alternative Therapies

Back pain
Head cold
Neck pain
Joint pain
Arthritis
Anxiety/depression
Stomach upset
Headache
Chronic pain
Insomnia

Source: National Center for Complementary and Integrative Health (2012).

two-thirds of adults in the United States use one or more types of alternative medicine, often to treat a chronic medical condition such as one of those listed in Box 1.3. Most of these consumers fail to discuss the use of alternative therapies with their primary conventional practitioner, even though the vast majority of people use both approaches simultaneously (Raheim, 2015).

The mainstream medical community can no longer ignore alternative therapies. The public interest is extensive and growing. One has only to look at the proliferation of popular health books, health food stores, and clinics offering healing therapies to realize that this interest cannot be dismissed. In March 2000, President Clinton ordered the establishment of the White House Commission on Complementary and Alternative Medicine Policy in an attempt to integrate conventional and alternative medicine. The mission of the advisory committee was to make legislative and administrative recommendations for the education and training of health-care professionals and to make suggestions for access and delivery of health care.

What are consumers seeking from alternative medicine? Some have the same goal for both types of medicine, such as control of chronic pain with pain medications and acupuncture. Other consumers may have a different expectation for each approach, such as seeing a conventional practitioner for antibiotics to eradicate an infection and using an alternative practitioner to improve natural immunity through a healthy lifestyle. A person receiving chemotherapy may use meditation and visualization to control the side effects of the chemotherapeutic agents. People who combine conventional and alternative therapies are making therapeutic choices on their own and assuming responsibility for their own health.

BOX 1.4

Reasons for Choosing Alternative Therapies

Pursue therapeutic benefit

Seek a degree of wellness not supported in biomedicine

Attend to quality-of-life issues

Prefer high personal involvement in decision making

Practitioners spend more time with clients

Believe conventional medicine treats symptoms, not the underlying cause

Find conventional medical treatments to be lacking or ineffective

Avoid toxicities and/or invasiveness of conventional interventions

Decrease use of prescribed or over-the-counter medications

Identify with a particular healing system as a part of cultural background

Sources: Alwhaibi and Sambamoorthi (2016); Ghildayal, Johnson, Evans, and Kreitzer (2016); Johnson, Jou, Rhee, Rockwood, and Upchurch (2016).

It is important for nurses to understand the reasons consumers choose alternative practitioners. Some utilize alternative healers because of financial, geographic, and cultural barriers to biomedical care. Many turn to alternative healers for a sense of hope, control, personal attention, physical contact, and regard for the whole person that seems to be overlooked in conventional medicine. Some of the common reasons for seeking alternative practitioners are listed in Box 1.4.

It may be difficult for consumers to figure out how and where to get the best health care. At times it may be problematic to find reliable information to help separate the healers from those who pretend to have medical knowledge. Consumers should *be wary* of healers who

- say they have all the answers,
- maintain that theirs is the only effective therapy,
- promise overnight success,
- refuse to include other practitioners as part of the healing team, and
- seem more interested in money than in people's well-being (Tiedje, 1998).

Some alternative specialties are more regulated and licensed than others, but none come with guarantees any more than conventional medicine comes with guarantees. Most types of alternative practices have national organizations of practitioners that are familiar with legislation, state licensing, certification, or registration laws. Many of these organizations are found in the Resources section at the end of each chapter in this text.

INTEGRATED NURSING PRACTICE

Nursing has been moving away from a biomedical orientation that has largely defined and directed it toward a nursing–caring–healing model. Watson (1997) described it as a shift from a *nursing qua medicine* paradigm (nurses helping physicians practice medicine) to a *nursing qua nursing* paradigm (practicing the distinct art and science of nursing). This movement has reconnected nurses with the finest tradition of Florence Nightingale in using their hands, heart, and head in creating healing environments. The modern nurse–healer draws on biomedical and caring–healing models by utilizing technology and focusing on caring relationships and healing processes. Dossey and Keegan (2016) have described the modern nurse–healer as having a hybrid of scientific skills and spiritual commitment. Nurses need scientific principles, methods, and skills, but they also need to teach people ways to become more self-reliant as they shift from caregivers to healers.

In 1979, Watson published her text *Nursing: The Philosophy and Science of Caring*, which evolved from her experiences of nursing within the limitations of traditional biomedical models. She sought to bring new meaning to the nursing paradigm of caring–healing and health. Her caritas process was developed to balance the "cure" stance of Western medicine. Watson's theory has since evolved into "clinical caritas processes." This perspective describes nurse–client relationships based on spirituality, love, caring, healing environments, wholeness, and unity of being (Watson, 2007).

The *art of nursing* is in being there, with another person or persons, in an atmosphere of caring. **Caring** involves compassion and sensitivity to each person within the context of her or his entire life. In the past, the biomedical model urged nurses not to care too much or get too involved. Caring, successful nurses, however, do get involved with clients as they practice nursing as an art instead of nursing as just a day-to-day job. Caring is a philosophy or context within which nurses practice nursing. Their practice is made caring not by the tools they use but by the attitude or perspective they bring. It is possible, of course, to use the tools of alternative therapies in the same reductionist way of biomedicine. For example, if one knows the pressure point for headaches and simply uses this pressure point for pain relief without any further assessment, it can hardly be considered holistic or healing. The symptom of headache has been addressed, but the meaning of the headache and the person's experience of the pain has been totally ignored.

The plurality of the sick care, health-care system may be one of its greatest strengths. It enables us to meet the diverse needs of diverse populations. The question is, how can we combine the best ideas of conventional nursing practice and complementary and alternative healing practices? First, we must have education. At the basic level, our nursing curricula must include courses in caring and alternative therapies. All nurses could learn Therapeutic Touch (TT), healthy dietary plans, the use of basic herbs, and the use of visualization in the healing process. Since 2004, basic alternative therapies content is included in the NCLEX-RN examination. Because state boards of nursing vary in their detail of criteria for alternative therapies and nursing practice, it is critical that you check the Nurse Practice Act of your state.

The White House Commission on Complementary and Alternative Medicine Policy states "since the public utilizes both conventional health care and complementary and alternative medicine, the Commission believes that this reality should be reflected in the education and training of all health practitioners" (National Institutes of Health, 2002, p. 51). The Commission goes on to say that "although there has been notable progress in introducing CAM into medical, nursing, and other fields of conventional health-care education in recent years, more needs to be done" (p. 51). We must also participate in continuing education courses to expand our knowledge beyond the basic level. With additional education, we can learn such therapies as basic massage and reflexology, meditation, and yoga. Some nurses will choose to continue their education through master of science in nursing degrees with a holistic nursing concentration or through certificate programs for nurse practitioners. Other nurses will choose to complete formal programs in alternative medicine such as naturopathy, Ayurveda, homeopathy, chiropractic medicine, or hypnotherapy. Advanced practice nurses should provide leadership in research and education in alternative therapies.

Health disparities continue to exist in the United States. Differences in the quality of health care are based on race, ethnicity, sex, gender identity, age, disability, linguistic difficulties, socioeconomic status, geographical location, and infrastructure. As nurses, we must address these barriers to health care on the local and national level.

Next, we must provide community education to help people become health literate. We must provide people with information, tools, skills, and support to enable them to make healthy decisions about life and negotiate their way through the health-care systems. As nurses, we have the opportunity to initiate conversations about alternative therapies. Growing immigrant populations call for more attention to a variety of health expectations, needs, and preferences. We must also become familiar with the alternative practices immigrants bring with them. An important consideration in evidence-based practice is patient preference. We must also attempt to keep ourselves healthy and to exemplify good health because teaching by example is a powerful influence. We can teach wherever our practice is located: acute care, long-term care, community nurse-managed centers, and in areas of advanced practice nursing. And, finally, we must document our findings, utilize and participate in nursing research, keep current with evidence-based practice, and design new studies to measure the effectiveness of various healing practices.

Self-Care

Before we nurses can care for clients, we must first learn to value and care for ourselves. One of your goals in reading this text might be to discover how to care for yourself more effectively, because only then will you have the energy to care for your clients. Caring for yourself means reducing unnecessary stress, managing conflict effectively, communicating clearly with family and friends, and taking time out for yourself. Caring for yourself may include developing a daily routine in practices such as relaxation, meditation, prayer, yoga, communion with nature, and other such forms of contemplation. In Watson's words, "If one is to work from a caring–healing paradigm, one must live it out in daily life" (Watson, 1997, p. 51). The following guidelines will help you maintain your self-care practices (Jahnke, 1997):

- Choose self-care activities that appeal to you and fit into your lifestyle.
- Do one or more of these practices every day. Consider them as important as food and sleep.
- Seek guidance and support from teachers/practitioners, if appropriate.
- Find a good spot for your practice that is physically and mentally comfortable.
- Build up your practice slowly. Success is not gained by aggressive or compulsive practice.
- Look for opportunities to practice with others.
- Focus on relaxing. The foundation of all self-healing, health enhancement, stress mastery, and personal empowerment is deep relaxation.

References

Alwhaibi, M., & Sambamoorthi, U. (2016). Sex differences in the use of complementary and alternative medicine among adults with multiple chronic conditions. *Evidence-Based Complementary and Alternative Medicine.* doi:10.1155/2016/2067095

Amiel, H.-F. (1882, December). *Amiel's Journal.*

Buchan, S., Shakeel, M., Trinidade, A., Buchan, D., & Ah-See, K. (2012). The use of complementary and alternative medicine by nurses. *British Journal of Nursing,* 21(11): 672–675.

Conklin, J. M. (1883). *Bek's first corner and how she turned it.* John F. Shaw & Company.

Dossey, B. M., & Keegan, L. (2016). *Holistic Nursing: A Handbook for Practice* (7th ed.). Burlington, MA: Jones & Bartlett.

Fact Sheet: President Obama's Precision Medicine Initiative. (n.d.). Retrieved from www.whitehouse.gov/the-press-office/2015/01/30/fact-sheet-president-obama-s-precision-medicine-initiative

Ghildayal, N., Johnson, P. J., Evans, R. L., & Kreitzer, M. J. (2016). Complementary and alternative medicine use in the US adult low back pain population. *Global Advances in Health and Medicine.* doi:10.7453/gahmj.2015.104

Jahnke, R. (1997). *The Healer Within.* San Francisco, CA: Harper.

Johnson, P. J., Jou, J., Rhee, T. G., Rockwood, T. H., & Upchurch, D. M. (2016). Complementary health approaches for health and wellness in midlife and older US adults. *Maturitas.* doi:10.1016/j.maturitas.2016.04.012

Jowett, B. (Trans.) (1875). *The Dialogues of Plato: Charmides. Lysis. Laches. Protagoras. Euthydemus. Cratylus. Phaedrus. Ion. Symposium.* Macmillan.

Maitland, J. (2016). *Embodied Being.* Berkeley, CA: North Atlantic Books.

Micozzi, M. S. (2015). Translation from conventional medicine. In M. S. Micozzi

(Ed.), *Fundamentals of Complementary and Alternative Medicine* (5th ed., pp. 3–21). St. Louis, MO: Saunders.

National Center for Complementary and Integrative Health. (2012). What complementary and integrative approaches do Americans use? Retrieved from http://nccih.nih.gov/research/statistics/NHIS/2012/key-findings

National Center for Complementary and Integrative Health. (2016). The 2016 strategic plan. Retrieved from www.nccih.nih.gov/about/strategic-plans/2016

National Institutes of Health. (2002). *White House Commission on Complementary and Alternative Medicine Policy, Final Report*. Washington, DC: U.S. Government Printing Office. Retrieved from www.whccamp.hhs.gov

Peplau, H. E. (1952). *Interpersonal Relations in Nursing*. New York, NY: Putnam.

Quinn, J. F. (2000). The self as healer: Reflections from a nurse's journey. *AACN Clinical Issues*, 11(1): 17–26.

Raheim, S. (2015). CAM and the community. In M. S. Micozzi (Ed.), *Fundamentals of Complementary and Alternative Medicine* (5th ed., pp. 35–40). St. Louis, MO: Saunders.

Tiedje, L. B. (1998). Alternative health care: An overview. *Journal of Obstetric, Gynecologic, and Neonatal Nursing,* 27(5): 557–562.

U.S. Department of Health and Human Services. (2010a). *Healthy People 2020*. Washington, DC: U.S. Government Printing Office.

U.S. Department of Health and Human Services. (2010b). Patient Protection and Affordable Care Act. Retrieved from http://www.hhs.gov/healthcare/rights/law/index.html

Watson, J. (1997). The theory of human caring: Retrospective and prospective. *Nursing Science Quarterly*, 10(1): 49–52.

Watson, J. (2007). Caring theory defined. University of Colorado Denver, College of Nursing. Retrieved from www.nursing.ucdenver.edu/faculty/theory_caring.htm

Willison, K. D. (2006). Integrating Swedish massage therapy with primary health care initiatives as part of a holistic nursing approach. *Complementary Therapies in Medicine*, 14: 254–260.

World Factbook. (2013–2014). Washington, DC: Central Intelligence Agency.

World Health Rankings. (2016). Retrieved from www.worldlifeexpectancy.com

Resources

American Holistic Health Association
P.O. Box 17400
Anaheim, CA 92817-7400
714.779.6152
www.ahha.org

American Association of Integrative
Medicine
2750 E. Sunshine St.
Springfield, MO 65804
877.718.3053
www.aaimedicine.com

Australian National Institute of
Complementary Medicine
www.nicm.edu.au

National Center for Complementary and
Integrative Health
National Institutes of Health
9000 Rockville Pike
Bethesda, MD 20892
888.644.6226
www.nccih.nih.gov

2

Basic Concepts Guiding Integrative Therapies

For breath is life, and if you breathe well,
you will live long on earth.

SANSKRIT PROVERB

There is some kiss we want with our whole
lives, the touch of spirit upon the body.

RUMI

In this book, separate chapters are devoted to each of the most widely used methods in complementary and alternative medicine. Because the methods share many principles, there is overlap in the various types of complementary and alternative practices. Although practices are grouped in units, many of the practices could be placed in several units. Thus, before examining the specifics of each practice, it may be helpful to introduce several concepts common to most healing practices, namely, balance, spirituality, energy, and breath.

BALANCE

An expression in the Native American culture, "walking in balance," describes the philosophy of a peaceful coexistence and harmony with all aspects of life. This concept of balance is found in all cultures throughout time. Balance is viewed as a path rather than a steady state, and it is believed that each of us has a unique path as we move through life. In terms of optimal wellness, the concept of balance consists of mental, physical, emotional, spiritual, and environmental components. Not only does each component have to be balanced, but equilibrium is necessary among the components. *Physical* aspects include optimal functioning of all body systems. *Emotional* aspects include the ability to feel and express the entire range of human emotions. *Mental* aspects include feelings of self-worth, a positive identity, a sense of accomplishment, and the ability to appreciate and create. *Spiritual* aspects involve moral values, a meaningful purpose in life, and a feeling of connectedness to others and to a divine source. *Environmental* aspects include physical, biological, economic, social, and political conditions. Walking in balance is a learned skill and one that must be practiced regularly to engage in the process of healthy living. This concept of balance appears repeatedly throughout the various alternative healing practices.

Cyclic Rhythms

The daily lives of all living things are filled with various changes that take place in cyclic patterns. **Circadian rhythms** are regular fluctuations of a variety of physiological factors over 24 hours. Most familiar is the 24-hour temperature and sleep patterns. These include adrenal, thyroid, and growth hormone-secreting patterns, as well as temperature, sleep, arousal, energy, appetite, and motor activity patterns. **Ultradian rhythms** are regular fluctuations repeated throughout a 24-hour day. An example of an ultradian rhythm is the 90-minute REM/non-REM sleep cycle. **Infradian rhythms** are regular fluctuations over periods longer than 24 hours, such as the menstrual cycle. The constant rhythmic processes bring about a dynamic, healthy balance in the body.

Rhythms may be desynchronized by external or internal factors. An example of external desynchronization is jet lag, in which rapid time zone changes result in a decreased energy level and ability to concentrate, as well as mood variations. In some individuals, internal desynchronization may result in depression. The tendency toward internal desynchronization is probably inherited, but stress, lifestyle, and normal aging influence it. Attention to the rhythmic nature of one's own being reveals an intimate relationship with the rhythms of the surrounding natural world.

Musical Rhythms

Health is about balance or harmony of body, mind, and spirit. In a state of optimal health, all frequencies are in harmony, like a finely tuned piano. In fact, music is often employed in healing, from the ancient use of the drum, rattle, bone flute, and other primitive instruments to the current use of music as a prescription for health. Several nursing research studies have demonstrated the effectiveness of music therapy for persons with mental disorders, autism, dementia, cancer, cognition disorders, and neurological problems. Chapter 21 covers music and its research in greater detail.

Dr. Andrew Weil, the leader in the field of integrative medicine, has created the *Mindbody Tool Kit* (2005) to help people utilize self-healing techniques. *Sound therapy* consists of classical music combined with healing sound frequencies. The combination of sounds entrains the brain to theta and delta brain waves, the state of deep relaxation in which the body and mind can heal themselves. The benefits of sound therapy are far reaching. People who may benefit from sound therapy include those

- experiencing an illness.
- who are having or have had surgical procedures.
- who are having or have had chemotherapy infusions.
- in intensive care.
- in labor and delivery.
- experiencing anxiety, depression, or insomnia.
- who wish to maintain a high level of wellness.

Drumming and chanting are powerful ways to bring oneself in balance with self, others, and the world. The drumbeat serves as a focus for concentration and quiets the chattering mind. The pace of the drumbeat enhances theta brain wave production. In one study, middle-aged people who participated in drumming sessions experienced significantly decreased Stress–Anxiety Index scores (Smith, Viljoen, & McGeachie, 2014).

SPIRITUALITY

Spiritual healing techniques and spiritually based health-care systems are among the most ancient healing practices. Spirit is the liveliness, richness, and beauty of one's life. It is who one is and how one exists in the world. Spirituality is the drive to become all that one can be, and it is bound to intuition, creativity, and motivation. It is the dimension that involves relationship with oneself, with others, and with a higher power. Spirituality is that which gives people meaning and purpose in their lives. It involves finding significant meaning in the entirety of life, including illness and death (Dossey & Keegan, 2016; Kreitzer & Wagner, 2014).

Many people are searching for wholeness in their lives and a way to allow their innermost selves to grow and expand. Spiritual healing practices guide individuals to places within themselves they did not know existed, through techniques as ancient as prayer, contemplation, meditation, drumming, storytelling, and mythology. In consciously awakening the energies of the spirit, people are able to move toward healing places and sacred moments in their lives.

During periods of stress, illness, or crisis, people search for meaning and purpose in their pain and suffering. They ask questions such as Why am I sick? or Why did this bad thing happen? This spiritual quest for meaning can lead to insight and healing or to fear and isolation. In the words of Ken Wilber:

> A person who is beginning to sense the suffering of life is, at the same time, beginning to awaken to deeper realities, truer realities. For suffering smashes to pieces the complacency of our normal

fictions about reality, and forces us to become alive in a special sense—to see carefully, to feel deeply, to touch ourselves and our world in ways we have heretofore avoided. It has been said, and truly I think, that suffering is the first grace. (quoted in Borysenko & Borysenko, 1994, p. 191)

Spirituality is often confused with religiosity, which is not surprising, because the two constructs are closely related. **Religion** involves a search for the sacred, a group identity, and a sense of belonging. **Spirituality**, a much broader concept, is the search for wholeness and purpose that underlies the world's religions. Removing the dogma, the politics, and the cultural influence from any of the world's religions uncovers the same questions, the same seeking, and the same answers. The concept of spirituality does not undermine any religion but rather enhances all religions by illuminating their commonalities and the unity of all people. Spirituality reveals far more similarities than differences among individuals. Chapter 25 covers faith and prayer as it relates to health and well-being.

Many traditions also speak of spiritual guides. Some individuals think of them as guardian angels, and others, as Beings of Light who guide people through near-death experiences. Buddhists think of them as *devas*. Cherokees call them *Adawees*, the great protectors of the Four Directions. *Malakh*, or "messenger," is the Hebrew word for angel. There are the cherubim and the seraphim and the four great archangels: Uriel, Raphael, Michael, and Gabriel. The Iranian angel Vohu Manah is believed to have revealed the message of God to Zoroaster some 2,500 years ago. Similarly, the archangel Gabriel is credited for revealing the Quran to Muhammad a thousand years later. Gabriel, honored by Jews, Christians, and Muslims, has a special role as a mediator between human consciousness and the higher realms from which spirit descends into the body. Although no Western scientific evidence supports the existence of angels, one can find phenomenological evidence. Many first-person accounts of near-death occurrences involve angels and similar experiences from people of different ages, from diverse cultures, and with different personal and religious beliefs (Borysenko & Dveirin, 2007).

ENERGY

The concept of energy has been recognized for centuries and in most cultures. Many ancient and current cultures have great respect for the subtle and unseen forces in life. Most spiritual traditions share the belief that energy is the bridge between spirit and physical being. Meditation and prayer are believed to be subtle energy phenomena that represent contact with the spiritual dimension.

Chinese Taoist scholars believed that energy, not matter, was the basic building material of the universe. Albert Einstein and other physicists proved that matter and energy are equivalent and that energy is not only the raw material of the cosmos but the glue that holds it together. Modern scientists now view the universe in terms of forces instead of tiny particles of matter. Their experimental findings are similar to the intuitive observations of China's ancient scholars. Everything in the world—animate and inanimate—is made of energy. People are beings of energy, living in a universe composed of energy.

Although Western scientists agree on this theory, they do not yet fully agree that a distinct energy system exists within the human body. For energy to be "real," it must be measurable by scientific instruments. By this logic, of course, brain waves did not exist prior to the invention of electroencephalographs! Because technology is not yet capable of measuring all the energy fields in the body, references to energy are not often found in conventional medicine.

For more than 2,000 years, various practitioners worldwide have insisted that a person is more than the physical body. According to these healers, a "life force" of subtle energy surrounds and permeates every person. Energy is viewed as the force that integrates the body, mind, and spirit; it is that which connects everything. The Japanese call this energy *ki* (pronounced "key"); the Tibetans refer to it as *lung* (pronounced "loong"); the Polynesians call it *mana*; Native Americans call it *oki, orenda,* or *ton*; Americans call it *subtle energy* or bioenergy; the Greeks call it *pneuma*; and the Hindus give it the name *prana*. Prana is sometimes translated from the Sanskrit as "primary energy," "breath," or "vital force." The Chinese refer to this energy as *qi* or *chi* (pronounced "chee") and believe that it takes the form of two opposite but complementary phases, yin and yang. *Yin* is the earth, moon, night, fall and winter, cold, wetness, darkness, the feet, the left side, the female gender, and passivity. Yin is involved in tissue growth. *Yang* is the sun, day, spring and summer, heat, dryness, light, the head, the right side, the male gender, and aggressiveness. Yang is involved in tissue breakdown. It is believed that each person is a unique combination of the complementary energies yin and yang. This union of opposites constitutes wholeness. Figure 2.1 shows the t'ai chi symbol, which illustrates the yin and yang of Chinese thought. The white dot on the black portion of the symbol and the black dot on the white section are reminders that each quality contains some of its opposite. Further descriptions of yin and yang are found in Chapter 4.

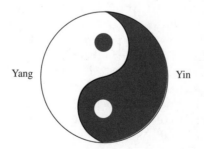

FIGURE 2.1   T'ai Chi Symbol

It is believed that qi creates qi. In other words, physical activities such as eating, work, and rest, as well as nonphysical aspects of life such as will, motivation, feelings, desires, and a sense of purpose in life, are all made possible by qi. Those same activities and aspects also create more qi. Most schools of thought basically agree on the following points regarding energy:

• Energy comes from one universal source.
• Movement of energy is the basis of all life.
• Matter is an expression of energy and vice versa.
• All things are manifestations of energy.
• The entire earth has energetic and metabolic qualities.
• People are composed of multiple, interacting energy fields that extend out into the environment.
• People's relationships with one another are shaped by the interactions of their energies.
• Qi, ki, and prana have no exact counterpart in conventional medicine, though the concept of a physical bioenergy system is under research. It is described as a weak but complex electromagnetic field that is hypothesized to involve electromagnetic bioinformation for regulating homeodynamics (Dossey & Keegan, 2016; McRae, 2015).

Chakras

The Hindu concept of *chakras* (a Sanskrit word for "spinning wheel") describes seven major energy centers within the physical body. Chakras have been described by most Eastern cultures and several South American cultures (such as Mayan) for thousands of years. **Chakras** are major centers of both electromagnetic activity and circulation of vital energy. They are usually thought of as funnels of perpetually rotating energy and are considered the gateways through which energy enters and leaves the body. Each chakra in the body is recognized as a focal point of the life force relating to physical, emotional, mental, and spiritual aspects of people and is the network through which the body, mind, and spirit interact as one holistic system. Figure 2.2 illustrates the sites of the chakras in the body.

The concept of chakras may be foreign to the Western scientific mind, but chakras are not completely unknown to those familiar with Judeo-Christian culture, particularly in the artwork and sculptures passed down through the ages. For centuries, the crown chakra, which signifies a conscious awareness of the divine, has been painted as a halo over those who are consciously aware of a divine presence in their lives.

The seven main chakras are vertically aligned up the center of the body, from the base of the pelvis to the top of the head. Each has its own individual characteristics and functions, and each has a corresponding relationship to various organs and structures of the body, to one of the endocrine glands, and to one of the seven spectral colors of the rainbow. The characteristics of the

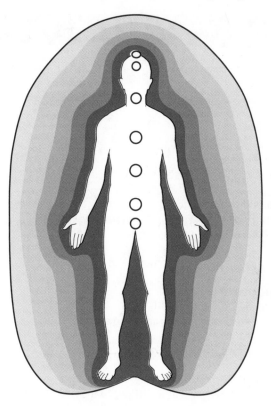

FIGURE 2.2   The Chakras and the Auric Field

seven major chakras are described in Box 2.1. Of the many smaller chakras throughout the body, the most significant are in the palms of the hands. The hand chakras are considered extensions of the heart chakra and, as such, radiate healing and soothing energies. Spiritual healers who practice the laying on of hands concentrate energy in their hand chakras. Each chakra has a purpose and a function that

- regulates the human energy system and maintains an equilibrium of health (purpose); and
- links body, mind, and spirit and exchanges energy (function).

Each chakra also operates at its own optimum frequency; generally, the lower the chakra on the body, the lower its frequency. If one frequency is out of sync, all others will be also.

The main purpose in working with and understanding the chakras is to create integration and wholeness within people. The chakras are the "doorways" through which the energy is attracted into the body and then

BOX 2.1

The Chakras

1. **Root chakra**
   Location: base of the spine
   Center of: physical vitality, urge to survive
   Gland: adrenal glands
   Organs/structures: kidneys, bladder, spine
   Color: red
2. **Sexual or navel chakra**
   Location: slightly below the navel, in front of the sacrum
   Center of: sexual energy, ego, extrasensory perception
   Gland: gonads
   Organs/structures: reproductive organs, legs
   Color: orange
3. **Solar plexus chakra**
   Location: slightly above the navel
   Center of: unrefined emotions, urge for power
   Gland: pancreas
   Organs/structures: stomach, liver, gallbladder
   Color: yellow
4. **Heart chakra**
   Location: middle of the chest at the height of the heart
   Center of: unconditional affection, compassion, devotion, love, spiritual growth
   Gland: thymus
   Organs/structures: heart, liver, lungs, circulatory system
   Color: emerald
5. **Throat chakra**
   Location: throat area
   Center of: communication, self-expression, creativity
   Gland: thyroid
   Organs/structures: throat, upper lungs, digestive tract, arms
   Color: blue
6. **Third-eye chakra**
   Location: middle of the forehead, a little higher than the eyebrows
   Center of: the will, intellect, spirit, spiritual awakening, visualization
   Gland: pituitary
   Organs/structures: spine, lower brain, left eye, nose
   Color: purple
7. **Crown chakra**
   Location: at the top of the head at the fontanel
   Center of: highest level of consciousness or enlightenment, intuition, direct spiritual vision
   Gland: pineal
   Organs/structures: upper brain, right eye
   Color: golden white

distributed to cells, tissues, and organs. If chakras stop functioning properly, the intake of energy will be disturbed, and the body organs served by that chakra will not get their needed supply of energy. Eventually, organ functioning will be disrupted, leading to weakened organs with a diminished immune defense. If this process continues, the end result will be dysfunction and disease. Dr. Dean Ornish (1999), well known for his program to reverse coronary artery disease through diet, exercise, support groups, and meditation, without surgery or drugs, believes that a closed heart chakra (unresolved anger and fear) is related to blocked coronary arteries. Consequently, the meditation technique he incorporates into his program involves opening the heart chakra. His holistic approach has now become a recognized program practiced nationwide.

Aura

Closely related to the notion of chakras is the concept of aura. The **aura** is the energy field surrounding each person as far as the outstretched arms and from head to toe. This energy field is both an information center and a highly sensitive perceptual system that transmits and receives messages from the internal and external environments. Each of the seven layers of the auric field is associated with a chakra; the first layer is related to the first chakra, and so on. Each layer has physical, mental, emotional, and spiritual dimensions and purposes, and the layers function together through the transmission of energy. Box 2.2 lists characteristics of the auric field, and Figure 2.2 shows a diagrammatic view of the auric field. Virtually every alternative healing therapy has a way of interpreting the body's subtle energy, which will be discussed throughout this text.

Meridians

A person's vital energy is not simply radiated outward but has patterns of circulation within the body, referred to as the meridian system. **Meridians** are a network of energy circuits or lines of force that run vertically through the body, connecting all parts. Meridians may be understood more clearly if they are compared to a major city's highway system with entrance and exit ramps, merging roads, and connecting surface streets. If a flood blocks an exit ramp, the streets served by this ramp become inaccessible, which, in turn, affects the people who live and work on those streets. Also, the traffic may back up on the highway, as cars wait for the ramp to reopen, creating a traffic jam. Meridians operate similarly in a person's body. If some type of blockage affects one's hip, for example, the pathways of energy leading to that hip get "backed up." Pain or discomfort restricts the motion of the hip, which may affect the position of the foot, which creates a strain on other sets of muscles. These changes in the body's general posture affect the positions of the internal organs, which, in turn, restrict the nutrition to the organs, alter organ function, and thereby change the body's balance. As the body and mind are affected, the person will think and feel differently, leading to more tension and more changes (Cohen, 2015).

BOX 2.2
Seven Layers of the Auric Field

Level 1. Etheric body
Location: 1/4 to 2 inches beyond the physical body
Center of: physical functioning and physical sensation
Color: light blue to gray

Level 2. Emotional body
Location: 1 to 3 inches beyond the physical body; roughly follows the outline of the physical body
Center of: emotional aspects of person
Color: all colors of the rainbow

Level 3. Mental body
Location: 3 to 8 inches beyond the physical body
Center of: instinct, intellect, intuition
Color: bright yellow with additional colors superimposed

Level 4. Astral body
Location: 6 to 16 inches beyond the physical body
Center of: love
Color: same colors as in level 3 but infused with the rose light of love

Level 5. Etheric template body
Location: 18 to 24 inches beyond the physical body
Center of: higher will connected with divine will, speaking, listening, working, taking responsibility for our actions
Color: clear lines on cobalt blue background

Level 6. Celestial body
Location: 24 to 33 inches beyond the physical body
Center of: celestial love, spiritual ecstasy, protection, and nurturance of all life
Color: shimmering pastel colors

Level 7. Causal body
Location: 30 to 42 inches, forming an egg shape around the body
Center of: higher mind; integration of spiritual and physical body
Color: shimmering gold threads

Each meridian passes close to the skin's surface at places called *hsueh*, which means "cave" or "hollow" and is translated as point or acupuncture point. Because each meridian is associated with an internal organ, the acupuncture points offer surface access to the internal organ systems. The flow of qi can be strengthened or weakened by manipulating specific points.

The California Institute for Human Science (www.cihs.edu) is the U.S. center for research on a device called the Apparatus for Meridian Identification (AMI). The AMI measures the flow of ions through the body and in 10 minutes can completely evaluate the condition of a person's meridian system and the corresponding internal organs related to those meridians. This stream of ions is not vital energy or qi itself. Rather, it is a secondary electromagnetic effect of qi—in a sense, its imprint in the physical domain. The AMI is now available for distribution as a diagnostic tool in complementary and alternative therapies and in conventional medicine. The AMI is used as a diagnostic tool in alternative and integrative therapies.

Energy Concentration

The mind's energy, or willpower, can be developed by individuals to control their body's energy system to an extraordinary degree. Healers can concentrate and manipulate energy in remarkable ways using their energy to align and balance the electromagnetic field of the patient. In attempting to trace the source of healers' energy, studies demonstrate that it seems to come from the central body in the area between the solar plexus and the lower abdomen. The Chinese refer to this spot as the *tan dien* or the home of qi, and the Hindus refer to it as the *solar plexus chakra* or the seat of prana (Cohen, 2015).

Grounding and Centering

Two terms common in various healing practices and related to energy and balance are *grounding* and *centering*. **Grounding,** as its name suggests, relates to one's connection with the ground and, in a broader sense, to one's whole contact with reality. Being grounded suggests stability, security, independence, having a solid foundation, and living in the present rather than escaping into dreams. It means having a mature sense of responsibility for oneself. Much of the sense of grounding comes from identification with the lower half of one's body—the parts of being that are less conscious and have more instinctive functions of movement. Learning to breathe into the belly, for example, is vital for grounding, for if the breath is shallow, contact with feelings and reality is limited. Many of the practices in this text, such as biofield therapies, mind–body techniques, and spiritual therapies, help increase one's groundedness.

Centering refers to the process of bringing oneself to the center or middle. When people are centered, they are fully connected to the part of their body where all their energies meet. Centering is the process of focusing one's mind on the center of energy, usually in the navel or solar plexus chakra. All movement in the body originates from this center, providing the meeting point for body and mind. It is commonly considered the "earth" center, for it

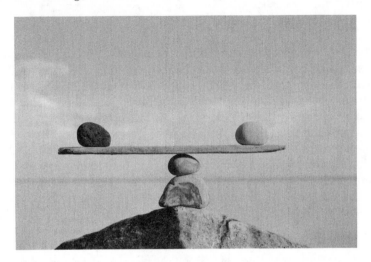

FIGURE 2.3   A State of Balance Supports Health and Well-Being

Source: Anatoli Styf/Shutterstock.

gathers energy from the earth rising up through the legs. Centering can be done through movement, as in t'ai chi, or can be found in stillness, as in meditation. Being centered allows one to operate intuitively, with awareness, and to channel energy throughout the body. See Figure 2.3 as an illustration of balance and well-being.

BREATH

Breath is at the center of all spiritual and religious traditions. In many languages, the words for *spirit* and *breath* are one and the same—Sanskrit *prana*, Hebrew *ruach*, Greek *pneuma*, and Latin *spiritus*. In Christianity, the Holy Spirit is referred to as "the breath of life." To *inspire*, or take in spirit, means not only to inhale but to encourage, motivate, and give hope. To *expire*, or lose spirit, means not only to exhale but to die, cease to exist, to end, or be destroyed.

In Eastern cultures, when air is inhaled, so is vital energy, which flows into the body to nourish and enliven. In Traditional Chinese Medicine, the exhalation is considered the yin part of the breath, and the inhalation is yang. It is impossible only to breathe in without breathing out or to breathe out without breathing in. It is the continuous dynamic balance of yin and yang that contributes to health and well-being. Most of the healing traditions worldwide believe that breath is the most important function of life, and restrictions in breathing lead to dysfunction and disease.

In Western culture, the breath has been considered simply a mechanical, metabolic function of the body. Scientists are now beginning to recognize that breath can be used for healing, improving the body's self-repair processes, and reducing vulnerability to illness. Oxygen is toxic to viruses, bacteria, yeasts, and parasites in the body, and cancer cells find it more difficult to survive in an oxygen-rich environment. Andrew Weil (1995a) believes that "breath is the master key to health and wellness, a function we can learn to regulate and develop in order to improve our physical, mental, and spiritual well-being" (p. 86).

The breath is constantly adapting to accommodate the needs of the situation at hand. When people eat heavy meals or exercise rapidly, when their noses are congested or dry, or when their environment is filled with pleasant or unpleasant smells, their breathing changes. Every change in posture has an effect on the combination of muscles used to breathe. Breath does not feel the same standing or sitting as when one is lying down. Breathing also changes under stress. For example, anxious people take shallow "chest" breaths, using only their chest muscles to inhale rather than their diaphragm. As a result, only the top part of their lungs fills with air, depriving the body of the optimal amount of oxygen.

Many people, even when feeling relaxed, breathe in a shallow way that keeps them in a constant state of underoxygenation that contributes to a decreased level of energy and increased vulnerability to illness. The typical shallow chest breath moves about half a pint of air, whereas a full abdominal breath can move 8 to 10 times that amount. Forming healthy breathing habits can produce dramatic results. Probably no other single step that people can take will so profoundly and positively affect body, mind, and spirit. Deep breathing can counter stress. Just three deep, full belly breaths can move individuals from panic to calmness by increasing their oxygen intake. Much of perceived stress is worrying about the future or the past, and deep breathing is a great way to return to the present. Twenty minutes of deep breathing exercises a day can lower blood pressure by increasing oxygen intake, which decreases workload on the cardiovascular system (Dossey & Keegan, 2016).

INTEGRATED NURSING PRACTICE

In complementary and alternative medicine, the focus of restoring health is within each person and cannot be "given" to a client by any health-care practitioner. Drugs, herbs, procedures, surgeries, or mind–body techniques may be helpful or necessary but by themselves do not cure disease. People must, and do, rebalance and repair themselves. The profession of nursing was founded on this philosophy and view of life as noted by Florence Nightingale's (1860) basic premise that healing is a function of nature that comes from within the individual. She saw the role of the nurse as putting the "patient in the best condition for nature to act on him."

In contrast, biomedicine has taught people to listen to external authorities and to view themselves as helpless victims of disease. Conventional medicine is based on the idea of cure, which usually refers to the elimination of the signs and symptoms of disease. "Curing," however, is effective for only about 15% to 20% of the sick population. In 80% to 85% of acute disruptions of health, one of three things happens with or without medical intervention: The person gets well, develops a chronic disorder for which there is no cure, or

BOX 2.3

The Cure Versus Heal Models

Medical–Curing Model	Nursing–Healing Model
Diseases are cured	People are healed
Focus on diagnosis	Focus on meaning
Patient is dependent	Person is autonomous
Effective for 15–20% of population; cure may or may not be possible	Effective for everyone; healing is always possible
Body is viewed as a machine; disease results when parts break	Body is a living microcosm of the universe; disease results through imbalance
Role of medicine is to combat disease; practitioners are soldiers in a war	Role of medicine is to restore harmony; practitioners are the Peace Corps, fostering learning and growth
Body is passive recipient of treatments to fix it	Body is capable of self-healing
Primary treatments are drugs, surgery, radiation	Primary treatments are diet, herbs, stress management, social support
Focus on pain	Focus on the human experience of pain, which is suffering
Caring is seen as a means to an end	Caring is the end in itself

Sources: Dossey and Keegan (2005, 2016); Quinn (1989); Watson (2007).

dies. When the focus is on cure, death is seen as a failure. Certainly, the curative aspects of Western medicine have allowed many people to live healthy, productive lives. But for many others, fixing the body is not enough. As individuals search for meaning in their illness and their life, as well as a sense of connectedness with others, they begin the healing process. Box 2.3 compares the philosophy and beliefs of the medical–curing model with the nursing–healing model.

Many sick people eventually get better no matter what treatment is given or even if no treatment is given. If the person is given "something," recovery is even more likely because of the **placebo effect.** The concept of the placebo effect follows directly from biomedicine's denial of the power of self-healing. In Western research studies, the placebo is a simulated biomedical treatment with no inherent medical value. The placebo response complicates researchers' experiments. In study after study, the placebo has been found effective in at least 30% to 35% of the cases. In fact, the rate is as high as 70%; typically, 40% of individuals report excellent results, and another 30% report good results (Benson, 1997; Bishop, Adams, Kaptchuk, & Lewith, 2012; Carlino, Piedimonte, & Benedetti, 2017). Norman Cousins, author of *Anatomy of an Illness* (1991) and *The Healing Heart* (1985), described the placebo as the "doctor who resides within." In fact, the placebo response in Western scientific literature demonstrates the unity of mind–body and provides great evidence of humans' self-curing capacity. Janet Quinn (1989), a leader in holistic nursing, believes that because the site of all curing is within the individual, "there are no longer any 'real' or 'placebo' treatments and effects. There are only stimuli for healing processes" (p. 554). Andrew Weil (1995b) regards the placebo response as a "pure example of healing elicited by the mind; far from being a nuisance, it is, potentially, the greatest therapeutic ally doctors can find in their efforts to mitigate disease" (p. 52).

Beliefs can also work against people. The **nocebo** is the placebo's negative counterpart. It is destructive thinking that contributes to sickness and even death. The body is good at healing, but at times individuals inhibit this process by worrying or doubting their ability to overcome the illness. Nurses must routinely assess clients' beliefs and expectations for health and use them systematically in the healing process. The goal is not to deny reality but to help people project healthy images. When a person acts "as if" the preferred reality were true, the body responds, and improved health can emerge (Frisaldi, Piedimonte, & Benedetti, 2015).

The word *heal* comes from the Greek word *halos* and the Anglo-Saxon word *haelan*, which mean "to be or to become whole." (Interestingly, the word *holy* is derived from the same source.) Thus, "healing" means "making whole"—that is, restoring balance and harmony. It is a movement toward a sense of wholeness and completion. Healing comes from surrendering to life as it is, including all feelings, from anger and despair through joy and peacefulness. The irony is that in the process of accepting life as it is, most people feel more alive and live more fully, even when facing death. When the focus is on healing, success does not depend on whether the person lives. Healing can take place even as the body weakens. Through healing, people allow themselves to be everything they already are and move toward a greater sense of the meaning of their experiences. Even when nothing can be done physically to alter the course of disease, still much can be done in a caring sense to make the human experience more meaningful and understandable (Dossey & Keegan, 2016; Quinn, 1997). As JoEllen Goertz Koerner (2011) stated: "The 'being' dimension of the role of the nurse is less about what nurses do and more about the how. . . . 'Being' is what slows down the nurse so that space is created for an authentic, deep connection with the patient and healing" (p. xiv).

Nursing has always focused on creating **healing environments** for those who have been entrusted to our care. We create healing environments when we use our hands, heart, and mind to provide holistic nursing care. We create healing environments when we empower others by providing the knowledge, skills, and support that allow them to tap into their inner wisdom and make healthy decisions for themselves. Healing environments are a synthesis of the medical–curing approach and the nursing–healing approach. We need a healthy balance between technology and compassion. We create healing environments when we take the time to be with clients in deeply caring ways. It is when we stop, become still, and enter the other's subjective world that we are able to be wholly present for that person. This moment of spiritual connection is uplifting for both client and nurse. Karilee Shames (1993) described sacred healing moments that occurred when her "goal became to inspire, to share tenderness, and to help instill a will to live, or to surrender to the call of death peacefully, if that was most appropriate. In my highest vision, this is what nursing was all about" (p. 131).

Patients come to us at the most vulnerable times of their lives. Many suffer deeply as they try to make sense of serious illness, huge losses, and unanswerable questions. Healing of spiritual suffering is as important as technical treatment of physical illness. Spirituality is also very important to the dying person's ability to complete the end-of-life task of transcending the self. Until recently, many of us gave the spiritual health of our patients very little attention. In the area of spiritual assessment, we nurses often simply wrote in the patient's religious affiliation. We must ask our patients about their spiritual beliefs if we are to know who they are and how they cope with their illnesses. There are a number of tools for assessing spirituality, such as the following. Howden's *Spirituality Assessment Scale* (*SAS*; Burkhardt & Nagai-Jacobson, 2002), the *JAREL Spiritual Well-Being Scale* (Hunglemann, Kenkel-Rossi, Klassen, & Strollenwerk, 1997), the *Spiritual Involvement and Beliefs Scale* (*SIBS*; Hatch, Burg, Naberhaus, & Hellmich, 1998), and the *Spiritual Assessment Tool* (Dossey & Keegan, 2016) are available to help us gain proficiency in the area of spiritual assessment. The tools ask questions regarding relationships, sense of balance and peace, sense of meaning and purpose in life, strengths and limitations, God or a higher power, and meditation or prayer.

We must also create healing environments for ourselves. Working with people can be draining work. As nurses, we need to learn how to restore our energy and replenish ourselves. We might compare our ability to care for others to a well of fresh, healing water. If the well is never dipped into, the water becomes stagnant and brackish. If the water is constantly drawn out and given away, with no source of replenishment, the well will soon run dry. What happens to nurses who don't sincerely care for others or take the time to replenish themselves? It soon becomes obvious by their behavior that they are stagnant or depleted; they are less patient, less tolerant, more irritable, and unhappy. Their state of "burnout" contaminates all aspects of their professional and personal lives.

When we care for others, care for ourselves, and allow others to care for us, the well of healing is constantly replenished. There are many techniques in this book that can be incorporated into daily life. It is important that we take time for ourselves, even if for only 10 minutes a day. Learning to take care of ourselves means letting go of self-defeating behaviors and attitudes. We must teach ourselves to relax without feeling guilty or selfish for taking time out. Self-renewal is a continuous process. To be there for others and care for them in their times of need, we must first look after our own well-being. It is only when we walk in balance that we can help others learn how to balance their lives.

TRY THIS
Energy

See the Aura

Find a room with a plain white background that has natural lighting or lights other than fluorescent. The lights should not be too bright and should not be shining directly on the person/subject. If you wear glasses, try the experiment with glasses on and glasses off. Ask the person to stand 18 inches in front of the white background and relax and breathe deeply. Stand 10 feet away from the person and focus on the wall, past the person's head and shoulders. You may notice a fuzzy white or gray field around the body, looking almost like a light behind the person. Continue to stare at the wall—DO NOT focus on the person. You may begin to see colors or sharp rays. This may take some time. Try different people as subjects.

You may want to try using your own hands. With the same background, hold your hands out at arm's length, in front of your face, with your palms facing each other. Point the fingertips of each hand until they are 1 inch apart. Soften your gaze and look past your fingers. Look for a gray, white, or other-colored aura.

References

Benson, H. (1997). *Timeless Healing.* New York, NY: Fireside Books.

Bishop, F. L., Adams, A. E., Kaptchuk, T. J., & Lewith, G. T. (2012). Informed consent and placebo effects. *PLoS One.* doi: 10.1371/journal.pone.0039661

Borysenko, J., & Borysenko, M. (1994). *The Power of the Mind to Heal.* Carlsbad, CA: Hay House.

Borysenko, J., & Dveirin, G. (2007). *Your Soul's Compass: What Is Spiritual Guidance?* Carlsbad, CA: Hay House.

Brule, D. (2017). *Just Breathe: Mastering Breathwork for Success in Life, Love, Business, and Beyond.* Simon & Schuster.

Burkhardt, M. A., & Nagai-Jacobson, M. (2002). *Spirituality: Living Our Connectedness.* Albany, NY: Delmar.

Carlino, E., Piedimonte, A., & Benedetti, F. (2017). Nature of the placebo and nocebo effect in relation to functional neurologic disorders. *Handbook of Clinical Neurology.* doi: 10.1016/B978-0-12-801772-2.00048-5

Cohen, M. R. (2015). *The New Chinese Medicine Handbook.* Beverly, MA: Quarto Publishing Group.

Coleman, B. (2010). *The Soul of Rumi: A New Collection of Ecstatic Poems.* Harper Collins.

Cousins, N. (1985). *The Healing Heart.* New York, NY: W.W. Norton.

Cousins, N. (1991). *Anatomy of an Illness.* New York, NY: Bantam.

Dossey, B. M., & Keegan, L. G. (2005). *Holistic Nursing: A Handbook for Practice* (4th ed.). Rockville, MD: Aspen.

Dossey, B. M., & Keegan, L. G. (2016). *Holistic Nursing: A Handbook for Practice* (7th ed.). Burlington, MA: Jones & Bartlett Learning.

Frisaldi, E., Piedimonte, A., & Benedetti, F. (2015). Placebo and nocebo effects: A complex interplay between psychological factors and neurochemical networks. *The American Journal of Clinical Hypnosis.* doi: 10.1080/00029157. 2014.976785

Hatch, R. L., Burg, M. A., Naberhaus, D. S., & Hellmich, L. K. (1998). The spiritual involvement and beliefs scale. *Journal of Family Practice, 46*: 476–486.

Hunglemann, J., Kenkel-Rossi, E., Klassen, L., & Strollenwerk, R. (1997). Focus on spiritual well-being: Harmonious interconnectedness of mind-body-spirit—Use of the JAREL spiritual well-being scale. *Geriatric Nursing, 17*: 262–266.

Koerner, J. G. (2011). *Healing Presence: The Essence of Nursing* (2nd ed.). New York, NY: Springer.

Kreitzer, M. J., & Wagner, J. E. (2014). The role of spirituality. In D. I. Abrams and A. T. Weil (Eds.), *Integrative Oncology* (2nd ed., pp. 487–503). New York, NY: Oxford University Press.

McRae, S. (2015). *The Healing Effects of Energy Medicine*. Wheaton, IL: Quest Books.

Nightingale, F. (1860). *Notes on Nursing: What It Is, and what It Is Not*. New York, NY: D. Appleton.

Ornish, D. (1999). *Love and Survival: The Scientific Basis for the Healing Power of Intimacy*. New York, NY: HarperCollins.

Quinn, J. F. (1989). On healing, wholeness, and the haelan effect. *Nursing and Health Care, 10*(10): 553–556.

Quinn, J. F. (1997). Healing: A model for an integrative health care system. *Advanced Practice Nursing Quarterly, 3*(1): 1–7.

Shames, K. H. (1993). *The Nightingale Conspiracy*. Montclair, NJ: Enlightenment Press.

Smith, C., Viljoen, J. T., & McGeachie, L. (2014). African drumming: A holistic approach to reducing stress and improving health? *Journal of Cardiovascular Medicine*. doi:10.2459/JCM.0000000000000046

Watson, J. (2007). Theoretical questions and concerns: Response from a caring science framework. *Nursing Science Quarterly, 20*(1): 13–15.

Weil, A. (1995a). *Natural Health, Natural Medicine*. Boston, MA: Houghton Mifflin.

Weil, A. (1995b). *Spontaneous Healing*. New York, NY: Knopf.

Weil, A. (2005). *Mindbody Tool Kit*. Boulder, CO: Sounds True.

Resources

American Holistic Medical Association
27629 Chagrin Blvd, Suite 213
Woodmore, OH 44122
www.holisticmedicine.org

American Holistic Nurses Association
323 N. San Francisco St., Suite 201
Flagstaff, AZ 86001
800.278.2462
www.ahna.org

British Complementary Medical
Association
P.O. Box 5122
Bournemouth BH8 OWG
0845.345.5977
www.bcma.co.uk

Canadian Holistic Nurses Association
www.chna.ca

3

The Role of Evidence-Based Health Care in Complementary and Integrative Therapies

Leslie Rittenmeyer, PsyD, CNS, CNE, RN

Evidence-based practice means doing what works and doing it the right way to achieve the best possible patient outcomes.

MUIR-GRAY (1997, 18)

BACKGROUND

Evidence-based health care encompasses all the health professions, including medicine, nursing, and allied health (Joanna Briggs Institute, n.d.). Evidence-based medicine was influenced by scholars such as David Sackett and A. L. Cochrane, and preceded evidence-based nursing. The Cochrane Collaboration, which has played a leading role in promoting evidence-based practice, arose from a concern by its founder, A. L. Cochrane, that there was little information about the outcomes of health-care practices. The emphasis of the Cochrane Collaboration was, and for the most part continues to be, the systematic review of randomized clinical trials (RCTs). This is pointed out because later in the chapter the relationship of complementary and integrative medicine to the Cochrane Collaboration will be discussed. The Joanna Briggs Institute (JBI), an interdisciplinary, not-for-profit, international research and development agency, has likewise been influential in the design and implementation of systematic review research methodologies, but has taken a more pluralistic approach to include the synthesis of research conducted in diverse methodologies believing that there is value in different types of evidence to inform clinical decision making. Philosophically, evidence-based practice means doing what works and doing it the right way to achieve the best possible patient outcomes (Muir-Gray, 1997, 18).

Definitions

Sackett, Rosenberg, Gray, Haynes, and Richardson (1996) provided the classic definition of **evidence-based medicine**. They described it as an explicit use of the best evidence available in making decisions about the care delivered to individual clients. Evidence-based medicine involves integrating individual clinical expertise with the best available external clinical evidence from systematic review. This definition caused some tensions in the discipline of nursing because it did not make the holistic paradigm clear but the science has evolved over the last two decades leading to expanded understanding of evidence-based practice (EBP).

A number of definitions of **evidence-based nursing** are found in the literature. Generally, they all emphasize that evidence-based nursing is a set of tools, resources, and procedures for finding current best available evidence from various sources and applying this evidence to make clinical decisions that promote positive health outcomes or to inform policy. This process takes into account the situation, cultural context, resources, preferences of patients, clinical expertise and judgment, and common sense. The Honor Society of Nursing, Sigma Theta Tau International (n.d.), defines evidence-based nursing as the integration of the best available evidence, nursing expertise, and the values and preferences of individuals, families, and communities who are served. DiCenso, Guyatt, and Ciliska (2005) defined evidence-based nursing as "the integration of best evidence with clinical expertise, and patient values to facilitate clinical decision making" (p. 4).

The Joanna Briggs Institute (JBI) provides a comprehensive description of evidence-based practice and its relationship to evidence-based nursing:

> Simply defined, evidence-based practice is the melding of individual clinical judgment and expertise with the best available external evidence to generate the kind of practice that is most likely to lead to a positive outcome for a client or patient.

Evidence-based nursing is nursing practice that is character-ized by these attributes. Evidence-based clinical practice takes into account the context in which care takes place; the prefer-ences of the client; and the clinical judgment of the health pro-fessional, as well as the best available evidence. (Joanna Briggs Institute, n.d.)

As you can see, all of the definitions share some similarities, namely, best available evidence, clinical expertise, patient preference, and context of the situation. All parts of the definition are equally important, although dis-cussing them in depth is beyond the scope of this chapter. For a closer analy-sis, refer to *Introduction to Evidence-Based Practice: A Practical Guide for Nursing* by Hopp and Rittenmeyer (2012).

One of the concepts though in the definitions of EBP that is worth looking more closely at is that of "patient preference." Patient preference speaks to how involved a person is in making decisions about their health care. It is often the case that patients want to pursue the use of CAM inter-ventions but do not know how to approach this with their practitioner. Patients' perception of resistance to the idea can lead to gaps in communi-cation and therefore erode the patient–practitioner relationship. Using a **shared decision-making model** helps to assure that the therapeutic relation-ship is not affected. According to the Agency for Healthcare Research and Quality (AHRQ), shared decision making is a model of patient-centered care that enables and encourages people to play a role in the medical deci-sions that affect their health. It operates under two premises. First, consum-ers armed with good information can and will participate in the medical decision-making process by asking informed questions and expressing personal values and opinions about their condition and treatment options. Second, clinicians will respect patients' goals and preferences and use them to guide recommendations and treatments. Shared decision making is a patient-centered approach that works very well when using CAM modali-ties so that patients feel comfortable asking questions and making good decisions based on knowledge.

Systematic Review

Several authors (DiCenso et al., 2005; Ingersoll, 2000; Melnyk & Fineout-Overholt, 2005; Rycroft-Malone, 2004) differentiate evidence-based practice from research utilization. Research utilization focuses on the application of individual research findings to planning and implementing patient care, whereas evidence-based practice is an integration of factors such as clinical expertise, clinical context, and patient preferences with the best available international evidence identified by a transparent, systematic research pro-cess called *systematic review.*

BOX 3.1

Joanna Briggs Institute Steps to a Systematic Review Protocol

1. **Background:** Provide a rationale for the systematic review through initial exploration of the research literature.
2. **Review Questions/Objectives; Statement of PICO or PICo Questions:** In quantitative reviews, questions should be specific regarding the patient problem or population (P), intervention (I), comparison intervention (C), and outcomes (O) (PICO questions) to be investigated. For instance, how effective is vitamin C compared with vitamin D in reducing pain in patients with osteoarthritis? Other types of questions for systematic reviews focus on the meaning of an experience, as opposed to the effectiveness of an intervention. The focus is on the phenomena of interest (PI) and the context (Co) (PICo questions). These types of questions are sometimes called *meaningful* questions, and this research is usually qualitative in design. For example, what is the experience of receiving a massage after a chemotherapy treatment?
3. **Inclusion Criteria:** Include types of participants, interventions in quantitative reviews of phenomena of interest, outcomes, or context in qualitative reviews.
4. **Types of Studies:** Choose RCTs or other quantitative designs, or the array of qualitative designs in qualitative reviews.
5. **Search Strategies:** Strategies must be transparent; identify a search strategy and the databases to be searched.
6. **Assessment of Methodological Quality:** Identify the appraisal instruments to be employed for judging the quality of the included studies.
7. **Data Collection:** Identify the extraction tools that will be used to extract data from the studies.
8. **Data Synthesis:** State how the data will be synthesized, for example, by meta-analysis or meta-aggregation.
9. **Statement of Conflict of Interest.**

Source: Joanna Briggs Institute.

A **systematic review** is the use of explicit, scientifically rigorous, and transparent research methods to critically appraise and synthesize the data from more than one research study. A systematic review protocol provides a plan to ensure scientific rigor and to minimize potential bias in the review. See Box 3.1 for the JBI steps in a systematic review protocol.

Evidence-based nursing, although closely aligned with evidence-based medicine, has differentiated itself by the value the nursing places on holistic paradigms. This difference is partly reflected in the recognition that in addition to meta-analysis of quantitative studies, evidence-based nursing requires meta-aggregation of qualitative studies (Jensen & Allen, 1996; Sandelowski & Barroso, 2003; Walsh & Downe, 2005). The latter is particularly important to the discipline of nursing because as a human science a large amount of qualitative research informs its practice. Sometimes, there is none or sparse research on a particular topic and one has to find the "best available evidence," for example, evidence that is based on the opinion of noted experts. The most important thing to keep in mind is that good evidence is generated from a transparent *a priori* protocol and the process is systematic and can be monitored. Most importantly, it culminates in a research report that provides recommendations for practice based on synthesis of the best available evidence. The primary rationale for the use of evidence-based practice is that it increases nurses' confidence that medical care and nursing care will lead to better patient outcomes. In the case of complementary and integrative therapies, this would encompass the notion of doing no harm.

Models of Practice

Numerous models of evidence-based practice can be found in the literature. The ACE Star Model (Academic Center for Evidence-Based Nursing, n.d.) from the University of Texas, and the Iowa Model from the University of Iowa (Iowa Model of Evidence-Based Practice, n.d.) are examples of these. A discussion of all models of evidence-based practice is beyond the scope of this chapter but can readily be found on their websites. This chapter focuses on the JBI model of evidence-based practice.

The JBI model of evidence-based health care conceptualizes evidence-based practice as "clinical decision-making that considers the best available evidence, in the context in which the care is delivered, client preference and the professional judgment of the health professional" (Pearson, Wiechula, Court, & Lockwood, 2007, p. 85). Included in the model are four major components of the evidence-based health-care process, namely, health-care evidence generation, evidence synthesis, evidence (knowledge) transfer, and evidence utilization (Pearson et al., 2007).

The JBI model depicts health care as a cyclic process that derives its foci from the identification of global health-care needs by clinicians and patients or consumers, and addresses those needs by generating knowledge and evidence to effectively and appropriately meet those needs "in ways that are feasible and meaningful to specific populations, cultures and settings" (Pearson et al., 2007, p. 86). The evidence is then appraised and synthesized and transferred to health-care delivery systems and clinicians who utilize and evaluate its impact on health outcomes (Pearson et al., 2007). Figure 3.1 depicts the JBI model.

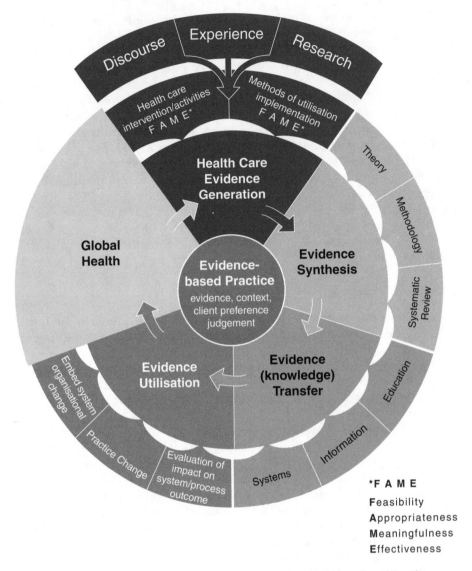

FIGURE 3.1   The JBI Model of the Joanna Briggs Institute of Evidence-Based Practice
Source: Pearson, Wiechula, Court, and Lockwood (2005).

EVIDENCE-BASED PRACTICE AND COMPLEMENTARY AND INTEGRATIVE THERAPIES

The use of complementary and integrative therapies has become increasingly prevalent. When complementary therapies are combined with biomedical care, these integrative approaches can enhance effectiveness and reduce adverse symptoms but the substitution of therapies with no evidence of safety and/or efficacy can delay or impede treatment. It is strongly recommend that medical professionals routinely inquire as to the use of these therapies during the initial evaluation.

Persons choose to pursue complementary and integrative treatment modalities for a myriad of reasons such as quality-of-life issues, holistic beliefs, unresolved pain, cultural values, or simply to avoid the invasiveness of biomedical treatments. Some have contended that the use of complementary and integrative therapies has increased because patients are dissatisfied with traditional Western health care. This may be true for some, but data from a U.S. national survey do not support this view. Adults often use and seem to value both. Of 831 respondents who saw a medical doctor and used complementary therapies in the previous 12 months, 79% perceived the combination to be superior to either one alone (Eisenberg et al., 2001).

In an update of the work of Eisenberg et al., the National Center for Complementary and Alternative Medicine (NCCAM), a part of the National Institutes of Health (NIH), released the 2007 National Health Interview Survey (NHIS) titled *Costs of Complementary and Alternative Medicine (CAM) and Frequency of Visits to CAM Practitioners: United States, 2007* (Nahin, Barnes, Stussman, & Bloom, 2009). The results of this study are found in Box 3.2. Compared with the results of the earlier survey by Eisenberg et al., the data suggest that visits to CAM providers decreased (except for acupuncture), but the use of self-care CAM strategies increased.

To relate evidence-based health care to complementary and integrative health care may seem at first glance an uncomfortable fit, but it appears this is no longer true. It is significant that the Cochrane Collaboration has a working group called the Complementary Alternative Medicine Field. The mission of this group is to facilitate the systematic review of existing RCTs to provide

---

BOX 3.2

- In 2007, adults spent $33.09 billion out of pocket on visits to CAM practitioners and purchase of CAM products.
- Nearly two-thirds of the total out-of-pocket costs were for self-care purchases of CAM products.
- Approximately one-third was spent on visits to CAM practitioners.
- Approximately 38.1 million adults made an estimated 354.2 million visits to practitioners of CAM.
- About three-quarters of both visits to CAM practitioners and total out-of-pocket costs spent on CAM practitioners were associated with manipulative and body-based therapies.
- About $14.8 billion was spent on the purchase of nonvitamin, nonmineral natural products.

information to benefit clinical decision making and the planning of future research in the field of complementary health care. The group also maintains a database of RCTs pertaining to CAM. An increasing number of systematic reviews in the field of complementary interventions can be found from other sources as well, suggesting an increasing demand by health-care practitioners for knowledge generated by systematic reviews of complementary and integrative therapies.

References

Academic Center for Evidence-Based Nursing. (n.d.). Explanation of the ACE Star Model of Knowledge Transformation. Retrieved from www.acestar.uthscsa.edu

Agency for Healthcare Research and Quality (AHRQ). (2015). Shared decision-making.

Deng, G. E., Frenkel, M., Cohen, L., Cassileth, B. R., Abrams, D. I., Capodice, J. L., ... Wardell, D. W. (2009). Evidence-based clinical practice guidelines for integrative oncology: Complementary therapies and botanicals. *Journal of the Society of Integrative Oncology*, 7(3): 85–120.

DiCenso, A., Guyatt, G., & Ciliska, D. (2005). Introduction to evidence-based nursing. In A. DiCenso, D. Ciliska, & G. Guyatt (Eds.), *Evidence-Based Nursing: A Guide to Clinical Practice* (pp. 3–19). St. Louis, MO: Elsevier.

Eisenberg, D. M., Kessler, R., Van Rompay, M. I., Kaptchuk, T. J., Wilkey, S. A., Appeal, S., & Davis, C. G. (2001). Perceptions about complementary therapies relative to conventional therapies among adults who use both: Results from a national survey. *Annals of Internal Medicine*. 135(5): 344–351.

Hopp, L., & Rittenmeyer, L. (2012). *Introduction to Evidence-Based Practice: A Practical Guide for Nursing*. Philadelphia, PA: FA Davis.

Ingersoll, G. L. (2000). Evidence-based nursing: What it is and what it isn't. *Nursing Outlook*, 48: 151–152.

Iowa Model of Evidence-Based Practice. (n.d.). Explanation of the model. Retrieved from www.uihealthcare.com/depts/nursing/rqom/evidence-basedpractice/iowamodel.html

Jensen, L., & Allen, M. (1996). Metasynthesis of qualitative findings. *Qualitative Health Research*, 6(4): 553–560.

Joanna Briggs Institute. (n.d.). Definition of evidence-based practice and nursing. Retrieved from www.joannabriggs.edu.au/

Melnyk, B. M., & Fineout-Overholt, E. (2005). Making the case for evidence-based practice. In B. M. Melnyk & E. Fineout-Overhold (Eds.), *Evidence-Based Practice in Nursing and Healthcare: A Guide to Best Practice* (pp. 3–24). Philadelphia, PA: Lippincott Williams & Wilkins.

Muir-Gray, J. A. (1997). *Evidence-Based Health Care: How to Make Health Policy and Management Decisions*. New York, NY: Churchill Livingstone.

Nahin, R., Barnes, P., Stussman, B., & Bloom, B. (2009). *Costs of Complementary and Alternative Medicine (CAM) and Frequency of Visits to CAM Practitioners: United States, 2007*. National Health Statistics Report No. 18. Hyattsville, MD: National Center for Health Statistics.

Pearson, A., Wiechula, R., Court, A., & Lockwood, C. (2005). The JBI Model of Evidence-Based Healthcare. *International Journal of Evidence-Based Healthcare*, 3(8): 209.

Pearson, A., Wiechula, R., Court, A., & Lockwood, C. (2007). A re-construction of what constitutes "evidence" in the healthcare professions. *Nursing Science Quarterly*, 20(1): 85–88.

Rycroft-Malone, J. (2004). The PARIHS framework: A framework for guiding the implementation of evidence-based practice. *Journal of Nursing Care Quarterly*, 19(4): 297–304.

Sackett, L., Rosenberg, C., Gray, M., Haynes, B., & Richardson, S. (1996). Evidence-based medicine: What it is and what it is not. *British Medical Journal*, 312: 71–72.

Sandelowski, M., & Barroso, J. (2003). Creating metasummaries of qualitative findings. *Nursing Research*, 52(4): 226–233.

Sigma Theta Tau International. (n.d.). Position statement on evidence-based nursing. Retrieved from www.nursingsociety.org

Walsh, D., & Downe, S. (2005). Meta-synthesis method for qualitative research: A literature review. *Journal of Advanced Nursing*, 50(2): 204–211.

Resources

About the Cochrane Library
www.cochrane.org

Cochrane complementary medicine field
About the Cochrane Collaboration
(fields). *Cochrane Collaboration* (2):
CE000052.

Joanna Briggs Institute
www.joannabriggs.edu

The Society for Integrative Oncology
www.integrativeoncology.gov

Agency for Healthcare Research
and Quality (AHRQ)
www.AHRQ.org

National Center for Complementary
and Integrative Health
https://nccih.nih.gov

Natural Standards
www.naturalstandard.com

Holistic Nursing and Complementary
Integrative Care: www.mass.gov

Systematized Health-Care Practices

Everything on earth has a purpose, every disease an herb to cure it, and every person a mission. This is the Indian theory of existence.

MOURNING DOVE

4

Traditional Chinese Medicine

*Love and compassion are necessities, not
luxuries. Without them humanity
cannot survive.*

DALAI LAMA

Traditional Chinese Medicine (TCM) originated in Chinese
culture more than 3,000 years ago and has spread, with
variations, throughout other Asian countries, particularly
Japan, Korea, Tibet, and Vietnam. As a comprehensive health system, it has a range of applications, from preventive health care
and maintenance to diagnosis and treatment of acute and chronic
disorders.

BACKGROUND

Traditional Chinese Medicine has a long and extensive history.
Shen Nong, the Fire Emperor, said to have lived from 2698 to
2598 B.C., is considered the founder of herbal medicine in China.
The written history itself is more than 2,500 years old, dating to
the text on internal medicine of Huang Di, the Yellow Emperor.
Written long before the birth of Hippocrates, the father of Western medicine, *Yellow Emperor's Classic of Medicine* covers such
principles as yin and yang, the five phases, the effects of the season, and treatments such as acupuncture and moxibustion.

TCM is associated with early Taoists and Buddhists, who
observed energy within themselves, in plants and animals, and
throughout the cosmos. Based on a belief in the natural order of
the universe and the direct correlation between the human body
and the cosmos, TCM philosophy stresses the constant search for

harmony and balance in an environment of constant change. By the close of the Han era (A.D. 220), the Chinese had a clear grasp of pathology, preventive medicine, first aid, and dietetics and had devised breathing practices to promote longevity. During the fourth and fifth centuries A.D., China's influence spread throughout Asia, and both Taoism and Buddhism had a marked impact on ideas about health. Sun Si Mian (A.D. 581–682), a famous physician, established himself as China's first medical ethicist. He advocated the need for rigorous scholarship, compassion toward patients, and high moral standards in physicians. In the 11th century, TCM began to focus more on social phenomena, especially human relations and ethical behavior. Initially, this orientation resulted in increased scientific medical study and publications. As TCM developed further, people began to take for granted that a breakthrough in one realm of knowledge would eventually solve all problems of human existence. (As in the West, some assume that advances in technology will solve all problems.) Eventually, sociological methods were used to solve medical problems, and clinical and empirical research reached a low point. Fortunately, the core of the scientific system was never obliterated, and the past 50 years have seen a worldwide revival of TCM (Ergil, 2015). In China today, TCM is practiced in hospitals along with Western medicine. Physicians study not only principles of anatomy, histology, biochemistry, bacteriology, and surgery but also acupuncture, acupressure, and herbal medicine. Patients can choose TCM or Western approaches or a combination of these for their particular problem. Inpatient and outpatient care is provided in large, well-equipped hospitals, as well as in private clinics and pharmacies.

PREPARATION

As of 2016, the Council of Colleges of Acupuncture and Oriental Medicine consisted of 56 schools of acupuncture in the United States that had been fully accredited or were candidates for accreditation with the Accreditation Commission for Acupuncture and Oriental Medicine (ACAOM). An accredited graduate-level program consists of 2,625 hours or 146 credits covering Oriental medicine, acupuncture theory, Chinese herbs, and biomedicine theory. Additionally, 1,330 hours of clinical practice are required. Practitioners who already have a master's degree in acupuncture are eligible for an herb certificate program of 450 hours of didactic instruction and 210 hours of clinical training in the use of Chinese herbs. Forty-three states plus the District of Columbia require passing a national board exam as a prerequisite for licensure. In addition, each state has its own eligibility requirements.

CONCEPTS

The focus of Traditional Chinese Medicine is on the patient rather than on disease, with the goal to promote health and improve the quality of life. A basic understanding of TCM requires recognition of its long-lived tradition, multiple philosophies, and varied practices. It is impossible to separate the individual concepts and the specific treatment approaches from the context of a complete theoretical system. Prevention, diagnosis, and treatment of diseases are based on the concepts of qi, yin and yang, the five phases, the five seasons, and the three treasures. Often, only isolated fragments of TCM emerge in the West.

Qi

The concept most central to TCM is *qi* or *chi* (pronounced "chee"), which is translated as energy. **Qi** represents an invisible flow of energy that circulates through plants, animals, and people, as well as through the earth and sky. It is what maintains physiological functions and the health and well-being of the individual. In TCM theory, energy is distributed throughout the body along a network of energy circuits or meridians connecting all parts of the body. The many different types of qi in the body are described according to their source, location, and function. *Yin qi* supports and nourishes the body, *wei qi* protects and warms the body, *jing qi* flows in the meridians, *zang qi* flows in the organs, and *zong qi* is responsible for respiration and circulation. Obstructed qi flow in the human body can cause problems ranging from social difficulties to illness. Its effects are specific to each individual—a person gets sick, has problems at work, or fights with family—and depend on each individual's unique qi. Certain TCM treatments such as meditation, exercise, and acupuncture are ways of enhancing or correcting the flow of qi (Cohen, 2015).

Yin and Yang

In Taoist philosophy, wholeness comprises the union of opposites—dark and light, soft and hard, female and male, slow and fast, and so on. These opposite but complementary aspects are called *yin* and *yang*. Originally, the terms designated geographic aspects such as the shady and sunny side of a mountain or the southern and northern bank of a river. Currently, the terms are used to characterize the polar opposites that exist in everything and make up the physical world.

From the health perspective, the basis of well-being is the appropriate balance of yin and yang as they interact in the body. Imbalance of yin and yang is considered to be the cause of illness. **Yin** is the general category for passivity and is like water, with a tendency to be cold and heavy. Yin uses fluids to moisten and cool the body. It provides for restfulness as people slow down and sleep. Yin is associated more with substance than with energy. Things that are close to the ground are yin or more earthy. Yin is associated with the symptoms of coldness, paleness, low blood pressure, and chronic conditions. People with excess yin tend to catch colds easily and are sedentary and sleepy. **Yang** is the general category for activity and aggressiveness. It is like fire, with its heating and circulating characteristics. Associated with things higher up or more heavenly, yang is the energy that directs movement and supports its substance. Symptoms such as redness in the face, fever, high blood pressure, and acute conditions are associated with yang. People with excess yang tend to be nervous and agitated and cannot tolerate much heat (Ergil, 2015). It must be understood that yin and yang cannot exist independently of each other. Figure 2.1 showed the t'ai chi symbol of yin and yang. Nothing is either all yin or all yang. They are complementary and depend on each other for their very existence—without night there can be no day, without moisture there can be no dryness, and without cold there can be no heat. It is the interaction of yin and yang that creates the changes that keep the world in motion; summer leads to winter, and night becomes day. Yin and yang are used in both the diagnosis and the treatment of illness. For example, if a person is experiencing too much stress—usually understood as an excess of yang—more yin activities, such as meditation and relaxation, constitute the appropriate treatment.

Five Phases

As they studied the world around them, the Chinese perceived connections between major forces in nature and particular internal organ systems. Seeing similarities between natural elements and the body, early practitioners developed a concept of health care that encompassed both natural elements and body organs. This theory is known as the **five phases theory** (*wu-hsing*). Five elements—fire, earth, metal, water, and wood—represent movement or energies that succeed one another in a dynamic relationship and in a continuous cycle of birth, life, and death. These elements do not represent static objects, since even mountains and rivers change constantly with time. In the five phases theory, it is not the substances themselves that are important but their interactions in making up the essential life force or qi (Ergil, 2015).

The rhythm of events resembles a circle known as the **creation cycle.** In this cycle, burning wood feeds fire; from its ashes, fire produces earth; earth in turn gives up its ore, creating metal; from condensation on its surface, metal brings forth water; and water nourishes and creates plants and trees, creating wood. Each element is related to a pair of internal organs. The yin organ is solid and dense, like the liver, while its yang partner is hollow or forms a pocket, like the gallbladder. The proper interaction of the organ partners influences how well the entire body functions. Fire is linked to the circulation of blood, hormones, and food. Its partner organs are the heart (yin) and small intestine (yang). Earth is linked to digestion and comprises the spleen/pancreas (yin) and the stomach (yang). Metal is linked to respiration and elimination and is made up of the lungs (yin) and large intestine (yang). Water is linked to elimination and comprises the kidneys (yin) and urinary bladder (yang). Wood is linked to toxic processing and is made up of the liver (yin) and gallbladder (yang). In addition, each organ is related to a time of day of optimal functioning. If a problem occurs during those hours when an organ is most vulnerable, the timing may alert a TCM practitioner of an imbalance in that organ system (Cohen, 2015).

Five Seasons

The four cardinal compass directions—south, west, north, and east—are affiliated with four of the five elements: fire, metal, water, and wood. The fifth element, earth, is depicted in the center. The Chinese place so much importance on the direction south that they put it at the top of their maps and navigate from it in the same way that Westerners use north. Just as south rules the top of the compass, it also represents summer, the "high noon" of the year, and is linked to fire. West, the direction of the setting sun, is associated with autumn and metal, which is used to make tools for harvesting. North is linked to winter and water, the opposite of the element fire, and is seen as a period of dormancy. East, the direction of the rising sun, is associated with spring and with wood, which represents all growing things. The fifth and central element, earth, is related to the late summer season and a time of maturity. Figure 4.1 illustrates the five directions as they correlate to the five seasons and the five elements.

The etiology of disease in TCM is linked to the five phases, five seasons, and five directions. It is believed that if one component is overbearing and excessive, then another becomes weak and debilitated. It is a complex system of checks and balances that is often not easily grasped by those with a Western perspective. Diagnosis and treatment of illness depends on understanding the five elements, seasons, and directions and how they interact.

Three Treasures

The Chinese believe that a combination of life force elements makes up the substance and functions of the body, mind, and spirit, and that these three are

SOUTH

Summer
Fire
Peak

EAST   CENTER   WEST

Spring   Late summer   Autumn
Wood   Earth   Metal
Growth   Maturity   Tools

NORTH

Winter
Water
Dormancy

FIGURE 4.1   Five Directions/Seasons/Elements

all one and the same. One way to understand this connection is to think of water and its wet, fluid nature. Compare liquid water with ice, which not only appears different but feels hard and cold. And then consider steam and its hot, gaseous nature. Despite the differences in appearance, the three different forms are the same substance. In the same way, body, mind, and spirit can be seen as different expressions of the same individual (Ergil, 2015).

The Taoists call body, mind, and spirit the three "vital treasures." They are *jing*, meaning basic essence; *qi*, meaning energy or life force; and *shen*, meaning spirit and mind. The balance of their abundance or deficiency influences the state of health. Jing is the essence with which people are born. It is similar to Western concepts of genes, DNA, and heredity. Essence is the gift from one's parents; it is the basic cellular material that allows that cell to function. It is the bodily reserve that supports life and must be restored by food and rest.

There are several types of qi: the hereditary qi, which is from the jing; the nutritive qi derived from food; and the cosmic qi from the breathed air. Wei qi is a specialized qi associated with the immune system. Wei qi circulates near the surface of the body and is the first level of protection when a bacterium or virus tries to enter the body. If the circulating wei qi is weak, it can allow a pathogen to enter the body, and illness ensues.

The vital treasure known as *shen* is the gift from heaven and represents spiritual and mental aspects of life. Shen comprises one's emotional well-being, thoughts, and beliefs. It is the radiance, or inner glow, that can be perceived by others. For people to be healthy, their physical, emotional, mental, and spiritual aspects must be balanced.

VIEW OF HEALTH AND ILLNESS

The Chinese regard the body as a system that requires a balance of yin and yang energy to enjoy good health. Each part of the body is also thought of as an individual system that requires its own balance of yin and yang to function properly. A headache is not just an event in the head, and it is more than just a pain. In Traditional Chinese Medicine, a headache is the obstruction of energy related to the overall energy patterns in the body as well as the circumstances and lifestyle of the sufferer. TCM assumes that a balanced body has a natural ability to resist or cope with agents of disease. Symptoms are caused by an imbalance of yin and yang in some part of the body, and illness can develop if the balance is disturbed for any length of time. Therefore, health is maintained by recognizing an imbalance before it becomes a disease. It is believed that everything needed to restore health already exists in nature, and it is up to the individual, with or without the aid of a health practitioner, to free up energy and restore balance using diet, herbs, acupuncture, and other yin/yang treatments (Cohen, 2015; Ergil, 2015).

The Chinese believe that all living things—people, the earth, the universe—are connected by cosmic energy. Thus, the balance of qi in an individual is connected to the balance in the environment; the forces active within the world are the same forces active within the individual body. Simply put, nothing happens without consequence to something else. The concern for balance and harmony is reflected not only in the TCM approach to the individual but also in the view that the balance and well-being of the resources of the natural world and society are vital to the overall health of all who live on the earth. Practitioners never lose sight of the multifaceted relationship between individuals, communities, societies, and nature.

Because the human body is a microcosm of the universe, extremes of climate in the body can create problems, just as extreme environmental conditions can wreak havoc on the environment. Sometimes, people experience a "cold" or yin illness caused by too much coldness in the body. For example, the symptoms of a "cold" influenza include a low-grade fever, no sweating, headache, muscle aches, stuffy nose, and a cough with clear white phlegm. Some influenzas are "hot" or yang influenzas caused by too much heat in the body. Symptoms include high fever, sweating, headache, dry or sore throat, thirst, and nasal congestion with sticky or yellow mucus. Too much cold in the body requires "warming" remedies, and too much heat in the body requires "cooling" remedies (Cohen, 2015).

DIAGNOSTIC METHODS

The Traditional Chinese Medicine practitioner has four diagnostic methods (*szu-chen*): inspection, auscultation and olfaction, inquiry, and palpation. These methods gather information about the five phases and their related body systems. The practitioner examines how the person eats, sleeps, thinks, works, relaxes, dreams, and imagines. No part of the self is considered a neutral bystander when the body is in a state of imbalance.

Inspection

Inspection refers to the visual assessment of the spirit and physical body of patients. *Spirit inspection* or observation is an assessment of the person's overall appearance, especially the eyes, the complexion, and the quality of voice. Good spirit, even in the presence of serious illness, indicates a more positive prognosis. *Tongue diagnosis* is a highly developed system of inspection of the physical body. The tongue is considered to be the visual gateway to the interior of the body. The whole body "lives" on the tongue, rather like a hologram. Different areas of the tongue correspond to the five phases and related organ systems, as depicted in Figure 4.2. The central area of the tongue is related to the spleen/pancreas and stomach. The very back of the tongue reflects the kidneys and urinary bladder. The sides of the tongue are related to the liver and gallbladder. The very tip of the tongue corresponds to the heart, and surrounding the heart are the lungs in the front third of the tongue. The practitioner inspects the color, shape, markings, and coating of the tongue to gather information about the state of balance in the person's body. For example, a moist tongue with a thin white coating may signal the presence of a

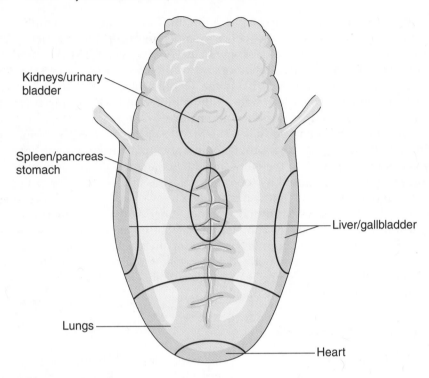

Kidneys/urinary bladder

Spleen/pancreas stomach

Liver/gallbladder

Lungs

Heart

FIGURE 4.2   Tongue Map

"cold" or yin illness, whereas a dry, yellow, or dark tongue may signal a "hot" or yang illness (Ergil, 2015).

Auscultation/Olfaction

The second part of diagnosis, auscultation and olfaction, refers to listening to the quality of speech, breath, and other sounds, as well as being aware of the odors of breath, body, and excreta. Types of sound are associated with the five phases and organ systems. How the person is breathing is a good indication of the status of the organs. Phases and organ systems are associated with specific odors such as sickly sweet, rotten, putrid, rancid, and scorched. Odors can arise from the skin itself or from the ears, nose, genitals, urine, stool, or bodily discharges. The breath may also have a distinctive odor. Usually, the stronger the odor, the more serious the imbalance has become.

Inquiry

The third part of diagnosis, inquiry, is the process of taking a comprehensive health, social, emotional, and spiritual history. The practitioner questions the person not only about the presenting complaint but also about many other factors, including sensations of hot and cold, perspiration, excreta, hearing, thirst, sleep, digestion, emotions, sexual drive, and energy level.

Palpation

Palpation is the fourth diagnostic method and includes pulse examination, general palpation of the body, and palpation of the acupuncture points. Reading the pulses, or *pulse diagnosis*, can provide key information about the person's condition. For example, a fast pulse might indicate a problem with an overactive heart or liver; a slow pulse might indicate a sluggish digestive system; pulses described as wide, flat, and soft might indicate a spleen problem; and narrow, forceful pulses might indicate a liver dysfunction. The radial pulse is felt in three positions and two layers on both the right and the left arm. The more superficial, or surface layer, belongs to the yang organs; the deeper layer belongs to the yin organs. The locations of major points used in pulse diagnosis are illustrated in Figure 4.3. The pulse allows the practitioner to feel the quality of qi and blood at the different locations in the body. Twenty-nine pulse qualities are described according to size, rate, depth, force, and volume. Examples of qualities are surging, scattered, vacuous, slippery, stringlike, and flat (Ergil, 2015).

All this diagnostic information is compiled to arrive at a "pattern of disharmony," or *bian zheng*. A single biomedical disease can be associated with a large number of Chinese diagnostic patterns. A lower urinary tract infection, for example, might be related to one of four distinct diagnostic patterns. Each of these patterns would be treated in different ways, as it is said, "one disease, different treatments." Also, many different biomedical diseases may fall into one pattern, thus the saying, "different diseases, one treatment."

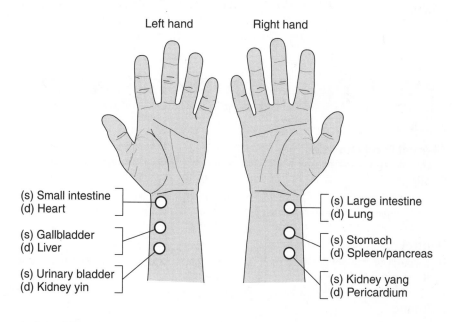

Left hand   Right hand

(s) Small intestine
(d) Heart

(s) Gallbladder
(d) Liver

(s) Urinary bladder
(d) Kidney yin

(s) Large intestine
(d) Lung

(s) Stomach
(d) Spleen/pancreas

(s) Kidney yang
(d) Pericardium

(s) = Superficial
(d) = Deep

FIGURE 4.3 Location of Major Points Used in Pulse Diagnosis

TREATMENT

Because an individual's combinations of yin and yang are unique, Traditional Chinese Medicine practitioners must tailor their treatment to each client. The goal of treatment is to reestablish a balanced flow of energy in the person through diet, herbs, massage, acupuncture, qigong, and gua sha. Feng shui, although not considered an actual treatment, is employed to improve health and well-being.

Diet

The simplest and most accessible treatment is diet. Dietary interventions are individualized on the basis of the individual's pattern of disharmony. Foods are used to rebalance the body's internal "climate" by bringing warmth to coldness or by cooling off too much heat. The thermal nature of food is described by the way a person feels after ingesting it. For example, after eating watermelon or asparagus, which are cooling foods, one feels physically and emotionally cooler. An internal feeling of warmth comes after eating warming foods such as salmon, lamb, or sweet potatoes. Neutral foods do not create a specific thermal quality and are thus good diet balancers. A diet to maintain health should be varied and include a minimum of seven different fruits and vegetables a day to avoid a cold or a hot imbalance. If a person is ill and the symptoms indicate a hot condition, then the diet should emphasize cooling foods, and vice versa. In addition to the overall daily diet, specific foods are used as medicines to correct hot and cold imbalances (Cohen, 2015). Box 4.1 lists common foods and their thermal effects on the body.

BOX 4.1

Thermal Food Qualities

Cooling

Pork, duck, eggs, clams, crab, millet, barley, wheat, lettuce, celery, broccoli, spinach, tomato, banana, watermelon, asparagus, ice cream, soy sauce

Neutral

Beef, beef liver, rabbit, sardines, yam, rice, corn, rye, potato, beet, turnip, carrot, lemon, apple

Warming

Tuna, turkey, salmon, lamb, venison, chicken, chicken liver, shrimp, trout, oats, cabbage, squash, kale, scallion, celery, ginger, sugar, garlic, pepper

Foods are categorized according to one of six tastes, each having a specific function in the body. *Sweet* foods are often used to aid digestion and qi, and influence the spleen and stomach. *Salty* foods affect the kidney and bladder and are often used to "soften" cysts or tumors and may be tried before surgery. *Sour* foods, such as lemons or tomatoes, are used to dry mucous membranes in the intestinal, urinary, reproductive, or respiratory surfaces. *Pungent* foods such as garlic and onion are used to aid digestion, stimulate circulation, and promote sweating. *Bitter* foods, such as greens or tonic water, also help in digestion and are used to regulate the bowels. *Astringent* foods, such as beans or potatoes, stop the flow of bodily secretions such as tears, saliva, and sweat.

Each food has both yin and yang energies, but often one predominates. Cooling foods and those with bitter and salty flavors are yin. Warming foods are yang, as are foods with pungent and sweet flavors. When people have an excess of yin, they may be sluggish, laid back, calm, slightly overweight, and emotionally sensitive. To balance these overly yin tendencies, yang foods are added to the diet to help activate the metabolism and provide more energy. People experiencing an excess in yang may be tense, loud, hyperactive, and aggressive. Adding yin foods to the diet cools their internal tension.

TCM practitioners recommend certain foods for balancing and improving a variety of conditions. Foods can be potent healers, especially when dealing with temporary illnesses, but they are never used as a lone treatment for serious or chronic conditions.

Herbs

Herbal medicine (*ahong yao*) is an integral part of TCM. In terms of the complexity of diagnosis and treatment, it resembles the practice of Western internal medicine. Herbs may be taken in the form of tea, or the substances may be powdered and made into pills, pastes, or tinctures for internal or external use. Just as with food, some herbs are warming (cinnamon) and some are cooling (mint).

With the exception of conditions that require surgery, herbs can be used to treat almost any condition in the practice of TCM. Herbs are often prescribed in complex mixtures and tend not to be used as isolated components, for example, as extractions from the parent plant. TCM practitioners believe that the healing benefits of herbs result from the synergistic interactions of all the components of the plant. The same herb can be used for many different disorders. Likewise, the same disorder in different people will be treated with different herbs, depending on the assessment of the individual. Herbs are used in the following ways: antiviral, antibacterial, antifungal, and anticancer. Herbs are also used to treat pain, aid digestion, lower cholesterol, treat colds and flus, increase resistance to disease, enhance immune function, improve circulation, regulate menstruation, and increase energy (Cohen, 2015). Box 4.2 lists herbs commonly used as tonics in TCM. Chapter 7 covers the use of herbs in greater detail.

BOX 4.2

Tonic Herbs Frequently Used in Traditional Chinese Medicine

Herb	Use
Astragalus	Enhances immune function by increasing activity of WBCs; increases production of antibodies and interferon
Dong quai	Blood-building tonic that improves circulation, tones the uterus, balances female hormones
Garlic	Lowers blood pressure, lowers cholesterol and triglycerides; antiseptic, antifungal
Ginger	Warming effect; stimulates digestion, decreases nausea, relieves aches and pains
Gingko	Mediates the allergic and inflammatory reaction in asthma; not to be taken with aspirin or other anticoagulants; discontinue before surgery
Ginseng	Increases appetite and digestion, tones skin and muscles, restores depleted sexual energy
Siberian ginseng	Enhances immune function, increases energy
Green tea	Lowers cholesterol; anticancer effects, antibacterial effects
Ho shou wu	Cleans the blood, nourishes hair and teeth, increases energy; powerful sexual tonic
Licorice	Used as an expectorant in bronchitis and asthma; anti-inflammatory, antitussive
Ligusticum	Inhibits bronchospasm through bronchodilation
Ma huang	Effective for mild asthma; because it contains ephedrine, in excess it can cause hypertension, tachycardia, palpitations, headache, nervousness, and insomnia. Ephedrine products are banned in many countries because of their use in producing methamphetamines.
Onion (quercetin)	Inhibits the platelet-activating factor in asthma

Massage

Traditional Chinese massage methods were described in texts as early as 200 B.C. *Tui na* is the forerunner of all forms of massage therapy that exist today. It differs from other forms of massage in that it is used to treat not only musculoskeletal problems but also internal diseases. Tui na practitioners must know Traditional Chinese Medicine to make a diagnosis before beginning treatment. Tui na is often combined with qigong exercises for building up general health, strength, and stamina. Both energizing and sedating techniques are used to treat and relieve many medical conditions. The following major techniques are in use (Pritchard, 2015):

- *Ma*—rubbing with palm or fingertips
- *Pai*—tapping with palm or fingertips

- *Tao*—strong pinching with thumb and fingertip
- *An*—rapid and rhythmical pressing with thumb, palm, or back of the clenched hand
- *Nie*—twisting, with both thumbs and tips of the index fingers grasping and twisting the area being treated
- *Ning*—pinching and lifting in a stationary position
- *Na*—rhythmic compression along energy channels
- *Tui*—pushing, often with slight vibratory effect

Massage increases circulation of blood and lymph to the skin and underlying muscles, bringing added nutrients and pain relief. Massage can help restore proper movement to injured limbs and joints and help restore a sense of balance. Massage is an effective method of reducing stress and tension that usually leads to a feeling of relaxation. Massage is the treatment modality of first choice for children. Chapter 12 covers massage in greater detail.

Acupuncture

Acupuncture involves stimulating specific anatomic points called *hsueh* where each meridian passes close to the skin surface. Puncturing the skin with very fine needles is the usual method, but practitioners may also use pressure (shiatsu), friction, suction, heat, or electromagnetic energy to stimulate points. The primary goal of acupuncture is the manipulation of energy flow throughout the body following a thorough assessment by a TCM practitioner. Treatment is offered in the context of the total person and with the goal of correcting the flow of qi to restore health. Some Western health-care practitioners who have learned the techniques of acupuncture miss the broader context and limit their focus to an injured or painful body part.

Acupuncture is effective in the treatment of acute and chronic pain and motion disabilities. In addition, it is used in respiratory and cardiovascular conditions (asthma, COPD, palpitations, hypertension); eye, ear, nose, and throat disorders (conjunctivitis, tinnitus, Ménière's disease, rhinitis, sore throat); gastrointestinal problems (gastritis, ulcers, colitis, constipation, irritable bowel syndrome); urogenital conditions (premenstrual syndrome, endometriosis, menopausal symptoms, prostatitis, incontinence, erectile problems); skin disorders (eczema, shingles, urticaria); psychiatric problems (anxiety, depression, schizophrenia); and in addictive disorders and withdrawal syndromes. Auricular acupuncture is a complete system on its own and is quite powerful for balancing the hormones and overall energy of the body. Contraindications to acupuncture are childhood, pregnancy, hemophilia, and acute cardiovascular disorders (Ergil & Ergil, 2015). Chapter 13 covers acupuncture in more detail.

Moxibustion is an application of heat from certain burning substances at acupuncture points on the body. A systematic review of moxibustion to correct breech birth presentation found it to be effective at 33 to 35 weeks of gestation. The Health Ministry of Spain has begun a multicenter, randomized controlled trial of moxibustion and breech birth (Ergil & Ergil, 2015).

Cupping is the application of suction cups on the skin. The cups create a vacuum on the skin and break up accumulated toxins. The first few applications result in painless circular areas of erythema or ecchymosis. When the toxins are successfully removed from the body, cupping no longer creates these marks (Ergil & Ergil, 2015).

Qigong

Qigong (pronounced "chee-gong") is the art and science of using breath, movement, self-massage, and meditation to cleanse, strengthen, and circulate vital life energy and blood. In India, the comparable practice is called yoga. Both these traditions of self-healing have been called "moving meditation" or "meditation in motion." T'ai chi, which is familiar to many Americans, is a more physical form of qigong. In China, millions of people from children, to workers, to elders, to patients in the hospital practice qigong daily. The techniques are easy to learn and simple to apply for all people, well or sick. Qigong decreases fatigue and forgetfulness and generates energy by enhancing bodily functions. Chapter 23 presents movement therapies in more detail.

It is inevitable that taking a deep breath triggers a sense of relaxation. By adding the intention to relax with the breath, the effect is even greater. Adding gentle movements or self-massage to the deep breathing and relaxation generates increased self-healing abilities. The focus on deep and intentional relaxation allows for release of emotional stress, for a sense of tranquility, and for one's natural spirituality to arise.

Gua Sha

Gua sha (pronounced "gwaw saw") is a TCM technique of smearing oil on the skin and then rubbing it with a flat jade stone, spoon, or other round-edged tool to bring out impurities in the body (see Figure 4.4). *Gua* means "to rub or

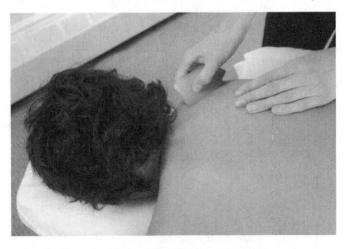

FIGURE 4.4   Gua Sha Treatment Using a Flat Stone
Source: Tyler Olson/Shutterstock.

scrape." *Sha* is the red rash that appears afterward, signifying that the impurities have been expelled through the skin. Most practitioners do gua sha on the arms, back, and chest, where many of the meridians are located. Gua sha is used to treat such problems as fibromyalgia, hypertension, arthritis, muscle aches, and early onset of colds and flu.

Feng Shui

Feng shui (pronounced "fung shway") is the ancient Chinese system of arranging the environment for living in harmony with one's surroundings. It began thousands of years ago in China and India as a process of decorating graves and has now gained popularity in many parts of the world. For modern practitioners, feng shui is a design system based on the flow of energy through one's home and environment. The primary objective is to control and balance surroundings in a way that brings happiness, prosperity, and health. Feng shui is based on the principles of qi, yin and yang, five phases, five seasons, and numbers and as such is an adjunct to other healing methods.

Many people are aware of the impact their surroundings have on them and use feng shui principles to improve their lives. Practitioners assess the interaction between the home's energy field and those of the people who reside there. These combined energy forces are significant factors in why and how we develop certain diseases and can be altered to improve our health status. Feng shui practitioners help people determine placement of furniture, colors, and designs that are comfortable, healthy, and supportive. For example, the entrance to the home should draw people into its nurturing space. The front door is seen as an opening for qi, and obstructions near the door can block good qi, prosperity, and luck from entering the home. Feng shui describes stairway placement; front and back door alignment; bedroom arrangement; placement of electronic equipment; living room, dining room, kitchen, and bathroom arrangement; use of a fireplace; and the choice of art. Mirrors have many curative uses, such as lighting up dark corners, slowing down the flow of qi, and deflecting unwanted influences.

Color is a vibration to which people respond both consciously and unconsciously. *Red* is stimulating and dominant and is associated with warmth and prosperity. *Yellow* is associated with intellect, decisiveness, and optimism. *Green* symbolizes growth, fertility, and harmony, while *blue* is peaceful and soothing. *Purple* is dignified and spiritual, *brown* suggests stability and safety, *pink* is linked to happiness and romance, and *orange* encourages communication. *White* symbolizes new beginnings and purity. *Black* is mysterious and independent. The aim of feng shui is to ensure good qi flow, balance, and harmony with one's surroundings. Feng shui music is designed to help people improve their physical and mental health through naturally balancing the energy in the physical and etheric bodies (Liang, 2016).

RESEARCH

Although extensive research has been done in China through the institutions of Traditional Chinese Medicine, much clinical research has been in the form of reports of observed results of various treatments. Many of these reports have been difficult to translate into Western languages and into the causal and analytic type of research modalities typical of the biomedical model. Research standards throughout the world are subject to cultural influences. Not all cultures require their medical practitioners to conduct randomized, double-blind clinical trials. Consequently, the research data are influenced by the location of the study. Research that is meaningful to the scientific communities of China and Japan may not have the same impact on European and North American biomedical communities.

Extensive research has been published on the pharmacology and toxicity of many traditional herbs. Researchers in China and Japan have studied the therapeutic value of herbs in the following areas: chronic hepatitis, rheumatoid arthritis, hypertension, atopic eczema, various immunologic disorders including AIDS, and certain cancers. Herbs are also given to control the side effects of chemotherapy and radiation. It would be useful to repeat these studies using biomedical research criteria. Research on the medical effects of qigong has been continuing since the mid-1980s and is now focusing on qigong as a biophysical rather than a mystical force. Acupuncture is one of the most thoroughly researched and documented TCM practices. Research studies are covered in more detail in the chapters devoted to these specific practices. Research opportunities in the future might include studies regarding manual healing therapies, bioelectricity, magnetic physical interventions, and the use of mind–body interactions for health purposes.

A small sampling of studies included the following findings:

- A systematic review and meta-analysis of TCM found that acupuncture, acupressure, and cupping demonstrated significant improvement in subjects with neck pain and low back pain (Yuan, Guo, Liu, Sun, & Zhang, 2015).
- A randomized controlled trial of cupping therapy demonstrated significant improvement in subjects with chronic neck and shoulder pain (Chi et al., 2016).

RELATED SYSTEMS

Tibet

In Tibetan Buddhism, religion and medicine are never separated from each other. The spiritual goal of Buddhism is to understand the nature of oneself and suffering and to develop compassion and compassionate action in one's life. Tibetan medicine, a sophisticated system, is based on general medical and philosophical assumptions as well as on each individual's emotions, attitudes, lifestyles, and spiritual beliefs. It is believed that one's positive actions produce happiness, and one's negative actions produce suffering. This belief in cause and effect is referred to as **karma**.

In Tibetan medicine, disease results from two causes. The first cause is spiritual, something brought from past-life karma. Spiritual diseases are mediated by a qualified teacher who uses meditation and yoga to balance body, mind, and spirit. The process of learning how to control one's mind to function in a balanced mode with one's body is called **dharma**.

The second cause of disease involves factors from this life, including seasonal changes, personal habits and behaviors, poisons, and negative spirits. Illness is considered to be a lack of internal harmony or balance or a lack of harmony with the larger external environment. The process of diagnosis is similar to that of Traditional Chinese Medicine. Essential components in helping people mobilize their resources for self-healing are caring and compassion. As Forde (2008) stated, "The most revered healing method in Tibetan medicine is compassion" (p. 14). We in the biomedical field should take careful note of that philosophy.

Other treatments include dietary changes, massage, exercise, yoga, meditation, breath work, moxibustion, and acupuncture. Surgery is used only when absolutely necessary. Herbal medicines are made from a variety of herbs, minerals, fruits, twigs, roots, and animals. As in the Native American tradition, the state of the practitioner's mind and the method of gathering are important to the medication's therapeutic outcome. All preparation of medicines begins with prayer (Rinpoche & Shlim, 2015).

Korea

Chinese medicine arrived in Korea in approximately 200 B.C. The close relationship between China and Korea facilitated the exchange of ideas for hundreds of years. In the 10th century A.D., Korea established its political independence from China, but cultural and medical exchange continued. A contemporary innovative system developed in Korea in 1971 involves hand and finger acupuncture. Energy channels of the entire body are mapped onto the hands, where they are stimulated using short, fine needles and magnets. This system is rapidly gaining in popularity throughout the world (Ergil & Ergil, 2015).

Japan

The history of medical information exchange dates to the first century A.D. By the eighth century, many Chinese medical texts were translated for use in Japan. Several factors contributed to the unique adaptation of Chinese medicine. The scarcity of herbs led to an emphasis on lower prescription doses in Japan. Palpation, as a part of the diagnostic process, includes palpation of the abdominal energy pathways. An area of specialization in Japanese medicine relegates acupuncture, massage, and herbs to separately licensed practitioners. In Japanese medicine, acupuncture involves the use of somewhat finer gauge needles than those used for Chinese acupuncture and shallower insertion. Shiatsu is a holistic health-care model using energy techniques to support well-being and to prevent illness. Treatment is based on the relationship between the client and practitioner, who uses gentle pressure along the meridians to correct energy imbalances.

Forest bathing, or shinrin-yoku, is a recent intervention in Japanese medicine. People are encouraged to go to the forest and walk for 80 minutes at a time. It has been found that the clean, fresh air and quiet atmosphere increases relaxation, enhances human natural killer (NK) action, reduces sympathetic activity and negative emotions, and increases parasympathetic activity. Forest bathing is encouraged as a method of promoting health and preventing disease (Li et al., 2016).

Europe

The history of Chinese medicine in Europe dates to the middle of the 16th century A.D., when European physicians who traveled and studied in China and Japan wrote texts on acupuncture. In the 1950s and 1960s, two notable English acupuncturists, Dr. Felix Mann and Dr. Sidney Rose-Neil, influenced the development of acupuncture in English-speaking countries (Ergil, 2015).

United States

In 1826, Dr. Franklin Bache became one of the first U.S. physicians to use acupuncture in his practice. When large numbers of Chinese laborers arrived in the United States, they were accompanied by TCM physicians and herbal merchants. Ah Fong Chuck became the first licensed practitioner of TCM in the United States in 1901 when he was awarded a medical license in Idaho. With the advent of World War II and the interruption of the herb supply from China, these practices disappeared or retreated into Chinatowns nationwide. In the 1970s, President Nixon reopened communication with China, and the practice of TCM began to gain visibility once again throughout the United States. Now, a clear interest in acupuncture, herbs, and qigong can be found among many North Americans (Ergil, 2015).

INTEGRATED NURSING PRACTICE

For Chinese immigrants, Western medicine is used for acute or life-threatening situations. Traditional Chinese Medicine is their usual health practice. Managing one's health and illness in the immigrant culture is a family affair rather than an individual process. Family and friends provide health information and share in the decision-making process. This understanding helps nurses provide culturally sensitive care (Kong & Hsieh, 2012).

Although nurses are not educated as TCM practitioners, some principles are common to both nursing and TCM. Nursing and TCM practitioners believe that people are at once mind, body, emotions, and spirit; energy fields become unbalanced as a response to stress; energy fields are constantly interacting; people heal themselves; and the client–practitioner relationship is one of partnership.

Caring and compassion are considered to be essential components in helping people mobilize their resources for self-healing in both the practice of nursing and TCM. A critical attitude on the part of the compassionate nurse is one of *intent* to help and comfort. Even though outcomes of illness are not primarily in the hands of health-care practitioners, nurses must still be willing to do their best. In addition to using their valuable technical skills, they must be present in the moment for each client. It means grounding and centering oneself before entering into a healing relationship with another person. It means keeping the focus on the other person rather than being distracted by personal internal dialogue. All levels of nursing practice incorporate principles of caring as a guiding focus for nursing intervention. Some nurses will want to continue their education through in-depth study of the principles and practices of TCM. Requirements and programs of study can be obtained from the Council of Colleges of Acupuncture and Oriental Medicine, the address of which is found in the Resources section.

Before we can care for our clients, we must first learn to value and care for ourselves. Drawing from TCM, self-care means seeking ways to establish and maintain balance and harmony in our lives. Exercise programs might include vigorous exercise such as aerobics, running, or swimming; moderate exercise such as dancing or walking; or gentle movement exercise such as qigong, t'ai chi, or yoga. Touching and being touched are important to our sense of well-being. Self-massage, partner massage, and professional therapeutic massage contribute to a sense of balance and connection with others. Meditation, prayer, and worship are spiritual aspects of self-care. Breath work is both a physical way to increase relaxation and decrease stress and a spiritual way to connect with the universe.

Diet is another area in which TCM can provide some practical guidelines. North Americans seem to fluctuate in their eating habits between overindulgence in food and starvation diets that neglect the principle of balance. Limiting the diet to a few fruits and vegetables may be as harmful as a steady diet of hamburgers. In TCM, it is believed that illness can be avoided by eating a varied diet as much as possible. For example, a cold or hot imbalance is avoided by eating a minimum of seven different fruits and vegetables each day.

For mild, temporary illnesses one might use a number of diet remedies. The cold type of the common cold and flu previously described as characterized by low-grade fever, no sweating, headache, muscle aches, stuffy nose, and a cough with clear white phlegm is treated with warming foods such as garlic, ginger, chives, pepper, pumpkin, apple, onion, and lamb. The hot type of the common cold and flu with its symptoms of high fever, sweating, headache, dry or sore throat, thirst, nasal congestion, and sticky or yellow mucus responds to cooling foods such as watermelon, eggplant, banana, plums, tomato, and tofu. The cold type of low back pain that is characterized by coldness and severe pain in the lower back that gradually worsens over time, is not relieved by lying down, and is aggravated by rainy days is treated with hot foods including garlic, chicken, apple, yam, celery, onion, peach, and mustard greens. The hot type of back pain that includes symptoms such as soreness of the lower back that is relieved by lying down, weakness of the legs, and frequent relapses is treated with cooling foods such as peanuts, sesame, soybeans, beef, pineapple, and grapes.

Like many other forms of alternative therapies, TCM regards breath as an important function of life. Restrictions in breathing lead to dysfunction and disease. Forming healthy breathing habits can counter stress and help balance body, mind, emotions, and spirit.

References

Chi, L. M., Lin, L. M., Chen, C. L., Wang, S. F., Lai, H. L., & Peng, T. C. (2016). The effectiveness of cupping therapy on relieving chronic neck and shoulder pain: A randomized controlled trial. *Evidence-Based Complementary and Alternative Medicine.* doi: 10.1155/2016/7358918

Cohen, M. R. (2015). *The New Chinese Medicine Handbook.* Beverly, MA: Quarto Publishing.

Ergil, K. V. (2015). China's traditional medicine. In M. S. Micozzi (Ed.), *Fundamentals of Complementary and Alternative Medicine* (5th ed., pp. 477–507). St. Louis, MO: Elsevier Saunders.

Ergil, K. V., & Ergil, M. C. (2015). Classical acupuncture. In M. S. Micozzi (Ed.), *Fundamentals of Complementary and Alternative Medicine* (5th ed., pp. 508–543). St. Louis, MO: Elsevier Saunders.

Forde, R. Q. (2008). *The Book of Tibetan Medicine.* New York, NY: Sterling.

Kong, H., & Hsieh, E. (2012). The social meaning of Traditional Chinese Medicine: Elderly Chinese immigrants' health practice in the United States. *Journal of Immigrant Minority Health,* 14(5): 841–849. doi:10.1007/s10903-011-9558-2

Li, Q., Kobayashi, M., Kumeda, S., Ochiai, T., Miura, T., Kagawa, T., . . . Kawada, T. (2016). Effects of forest bathing on cardiovascular and metabolic parameters in middle-aged males. *Evidence-Based Complementary and Alternative Medicine.* doi: 10.1155/2016/2587381

Liang, S. (2016). *Feng Shui On a Dime.* Los Angeles, CA: Transformind Books.

Pritchard, S. (2015). *Tui Na: A Manual of Chinese Massage Therapy* (2nd ed.). London: Jessica Kingsley Publishers.

Quintasket, C. (1990). The dutiful wife. *The Salishan Autobiography* by Mourning Dove.

Rinpoche, C. N., & Shlim, D. R. (2015). *Medicine & Compassion.* Somerville, MA: Wisdom Publications, Inc.

Silver, T. (2011). *Outrageous Openness: Letting the Divine Take the Lead.* Urban Kali Production.

Yuan, Q. L., Guo, T. M., Liu, L., Sun, F., & Zhang, Y. G. (2015). Traditional Chinese Medicine for neck pain and low back pain: A systematic review and meta-analysis. *Public Library of Science.* doi: 10.1371/journal.pone.0117146

Resources

Academy of Chinese Culture and Health
Sciences
1601 Clay Street
Oakland, CA 94612
510.763.7787
www.acchs.edu

American Academy of Medical
Acupuncture
1970 E. Grand Ave., Suite 330
El Segundo, CA 90245
310.364.0193
www.medicalacupuncture.org

American Association of Acupuncture
and Oriental Medicine
P.O. Box 162340
Sacramento, CA 95816
866.455.7999
www.aaaomonline.org

Australian Chinese Medical Association
P.O. Box 2328
Carlingford Court
NSW 2118
61.2.9873.6222
www.acma.org.au

Chinese Medicine and Acupuncture
Association of Canada
154 Wellington Street
London, ON N6B 2K8
519.642.1970
www.cmaac.ca

Council of Colleges of Acupuncture and
Oriental Medicine
600 Wyndhurst Ave, Suite 112
Baltimore, MD 21210
410.464.6040
www.ccaom.org

5

Ayurvedic Medicine

The secret of health for both mind and body is not to mourn for the past, not to worry about the future . . . but to live the present moment wisely and earnestly.

SIDDHARTHA GAUTAMA BUDDHA

BACKGROUND

Ayurveda, one of the oldest medical systems in the world, has been practiced for more than 5,000 years in India. It is a holistic and sophisticated system encompassing balance of body, mind, and spirit, as well as balance between people, their environments, and the larger cosmos. *Ayurveda* is a Sanskrit word derived from two roots—*ayur*, which means "life," and *veda*, or "knowledge"—and translates literally to the science of life. Ayurveda has been adapted by Hindu, Buddhist, and other religious groups and is undergoing a renaissance both in India and throughout the West. Similar systems of medicine are Siddha medicine of South India and Unani medicine of India and Asia.

Ayurveda is an intricate system with a tradition of integrating that which is useful for other systems. This ancient system has adapted to modern science and technology, including biomedical science and quantum physics. This blending of Ayurveda and conventional medicine has proved very compatible (Micozzi, 2015).

CONCEPTS

Ayurveda asserts a fundamental connection between the microcosm and macrocosm. People are a creation of the cosmos and as such are minute representations of the universe, containing within them everything that makes up the surrounding world. One must understand the world to understand people and, conversely, must understand people to understand the world. Ayurveda emphasizes the interdependence of the health of the individual and the quality of societal life. Therefore, measures to ensure the collective health of society, such as pollution control and appropriate living conditions, are supported. Much like in Traditional Chinese Medicine, the focus is on the person rather than on disease (Shunya, 2017).

Five Elements

Ayurveda views nature and people as made up of five elements or qualities. These elements are earth, water, fire, air, and space and contain both matter and energy. As they interact, these elements give rise to all that exists. The *earth* element is dense, heavy, and hard. In the human body, all solid structures and compact tissues are derived from the earth element. The *water* element is liquid and soft and exists in many forms in the body, such as plasma, cytoplasm, saliva, nasal secretions, eye secretions, and cerebrospinal fluid. The *fire* element is hot and light and is believed to regulate body temperature as well as being responsible for digestion, absorption, and assimilation. The solar plexus is the seat of fire in the body. Fire manifests in the brain as the gray matter that allows one to recognize, appreciate, and comprehend the world. The *air* element is cold, mobile, and rough and in the cosmos is the magnetic field responsible for the movement of the earth, wind, and water. In the body, the air element governs cellular function, the movement of breath, and movements of the intestines. Thought, desire, and will are also governed by the air principle. The *space* element is clear and subtle and makes up most of the body. Space plays a unique role because it allows the existence of sound, which needs space to travel. Sound includes not only audible sound like music but subtler vibrations that resonate in the body (Fondin, 2015; Rhyner, 2017).

People are a composite of these five elements, which combine in various ways to govern mind, body, and spirit. Ayurveda sees the body as *doshas* (vital energies), *dhatus* (tissues), and *malas* (waste products). It is the dosha's job to assist with the creation of all the various tissues of the body and to remove any unnecessary waste products from the body.

Doshas

Doshas, or tridosha, are both structures and energy and are the mediators between body tissues, wastes, and the environment and are responsible for all physiological and psychological processes. The Sanskrit names for the three doshas are *Vata, Pitta,* and *Kapha.* As the driver or mover of the entire body, the Vata dosha is the most important. It is composed of the elements of air and space and is involved with all elimination, physical and mental movement, and nervous function. If Vata becomes imbalanced, it can cause the other two doshas to become imbalanced. The Pitta dosha is composed of the elements

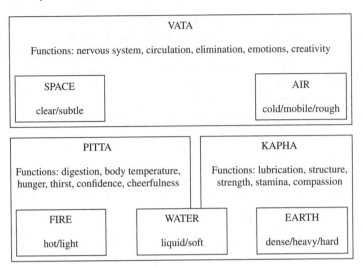

FIGURE 5.1 The Elements and the Doshas

fire and water, governs enzymes and hormones, and is responsible for digestion, body temperature, hunger, thirst, sight, complexion, courage, and mental activity. The Kapha dosha, composed of the elements of earth and water, is the heaviest of the three doshas. It provides the structure, strength, and stability that the body needs. It is also responsible for lubrication, sexual power, and fertility. Figure 5.1 illustrates the connections between the elements and the doshas.

Body Types

Vata, Pitta, and Kapha are present in every cell, tissue, and organ, but each person is made up of unique ratios of the three doshas. This individual constitution is determined by genetics, diet, lifestyle, and emotions. Each dosha gives an indication of physical strengths and limitations. According to Ayurveda, there are 10 body types:

- *Single-dosha types.* One dosha is predominant:
  Vata
  Pitta
  Kapha
- *Two-dosha types.* One dosha is predominant, and there is a strong secondary dosha:
  Vata–Pitta, Pitta–Vata
  Pitta–Kapha, Kapha–Pitta
  Kapha–Vata, Vata–Kapha
- *Three-dosha types.* All three doshas are in equal proportions:
  Vata–Pitta–Kapha

Knowing one's body type is the key to balancing one's life in the way that nature intended. This balance goes beyond physical and mental health and includes personal relationships, work satisfaction, spiritual growth, and social harmony. As a general rule, the strongest dosha in one's constitution has the greatest tendency to increase, making people most susceptible to illnesses associated with an increase of that dosha (Rhyner, 2017).

Vatas are connected to the air and space, so they are similar to the wind—dry, cool, and capable of fast, variable movement and thought. The basic pattern of the Vata type is "changeable." Vata people are unpredictable and often start things without finishing them. Stress usually leads to anxiety or fear. They are responsive to sound and touch and dislike loud noise. Balanced Vata people are happy, enthusiastic, and energetic. When out of balance, they have a tendency to be impulsive. See Box 5.1 for characteristics of the Vata body type.

BOX 5.1
Learn Your Dosha

Vata Type
- Light, thin build
- Thin, dry skin
- Dark, coarse, curly hair
- Irregular hunger and digestion
- Difficulty putting on weight
- Light, interrupted sleep
- Tendency toward constipation
- Aversion to cold weather, craving for warmth
- Bursts of mental and physical energy
- Performs activity quickly
- Quick to grasp new information but quick to forget
- Tendency for worry, anxiety, fearfulness
- Excitability, changing moods
- Enthusiasm, vivaciousness
- Fast talking

Pitta Type
- Medium build
- Fair, soft, warm skin
- Fine, soft, blond, light brown, or red hair
- Sharp hunger and thirst, strong digestion
- Cannot skip meals
- No problem gaining or losing weight
- Aversion to hot weather, craving for coolness
- Moderate strength and endurance

(continued)

- Sound but short sleep
- Sharp, clear, precise speech
- Sharp intellect and good, quick memory
- Enterprising character, likes challenges
- Busy lifestyle, achiever
- Tendency toward anger, irritability under stress, judgmental

Kapha Type
- Solid, powerful build
- Thick, pale, cold skin
- Thick, wavy, lustrous hair
- Tendency to obesity, hard to lose weight
- Slow digestion, mild hunger
- Heavy sleep and for a long period of time
- Oily, smooth skin
- Aversion to cold, damp weather
- Steady energy, great strength and endurance
- Graceful in action
- Slow to grasp new information but good retentive memory
- Good organizer
- Affectionate, tolerant, forgiving
- Tendency to be greedy and possessive
- Tendency to be complacent
- Slow speech that may be labored

Pittas are aligned with fire and act with fervent determination. The basic pattern of the Pitta type is "intense." Pitta people are ambitious, outspoken, bold, orderly, and efficient. They tend to respond to the world visually and enjoy being surrounded by fine objects. Balanced Pitta people are sweet, joyous, and confident. Box 5.1 lists the characteristics of the Pitta body type.

Kaphas are a combination of earth and water and, therefore, move slowly and gracefully. The basic pattern of the Kapha type is "relaxed." Kapha people are stable, steady people who have a happy, tranquil view of the world. They are graceful people who wake up slowly, eat slowly, and speak slowly. They respond to the world through taste and smell and tend to place a great deal of importance on food. See Box 5.1 for characteristics of the Kapha body type.

Few people are single-dosha types. Most are two-dosha types, with one dosha predominant but not extreme. The dominant dosha gives people their primary reactions to the world, which are then moderated by the second dosha. Those with the two doshas of Vata–Pitta type are quick moving, friendly, and talkative with a sharp intellect. They are not as unpredictable or irregular as the single Vata type. They enjoy challenges, but stress makes them tense and hard driven. People who have a combination of Pitta and Kapha types are stable personalities but have a tendency toward anger and criticism. They have steady energy and good stamina but are less motivated to be active. Those whose doshas are the Kapha–Vata type may have a hard time identifying themselves, since the Vata and Kapha tend to be opposites. Usually, they have a thin body type but with a relaxed, easygoing manner. They tend to procrastinate but can be quick and efficient when necessary. People who are three-dosha types tend to have good immunity, lifelong good health, and longevity (Rhyner, 2017).

Tissues/Dhatus

The seven **dhatus** or tissues are the structures of the body, are responsible for nourishment, and must be retained for health. They are *rasa* (plasma), *rakta* (blood cells), *mamsa* (muscle), *meda* (adipose), *asthi* (bone), *majja* (bone marrow), and *shukra* (reproductive tissue). In general, Ayurveda practitioners work to keep these tissues intact and healthy (Shunya, 2017).

Waste Products/Malas

The **malas**, or wastes, are the nonretainable substances within the body. Urine, feces, and sweat, for example, need to be released and eliminated as the body rids itself of toxins. Excretion of the malas cleanses; thus, people are cautioned against inhibiting the body's natural functions, including sneezing, yawning, burping, urinating, defecating, and passing gases. Vata is the dosha that causes these urges, and suppression of them disturbs Vata. Ayurveda encourages expression of these urges in a way that is not offensive to other people (Micozzi, 2015).

Energy/Prana

Prana, which the Chinese call qi, in Sanskrit means "primary energy," sometimes translated as "breath" or "vital force." Prana is not only the basic life force but also the original creative power. Prana has many levels of meaning, from the physical breath to the energy of consciousness. The five pranas are categorized according to movement, direction, and body region. The navel is considered the pranic center of the physical body. *Prana vayu*, forward-moving air, moves inward and regulates the intake of substances into the body. This prana moves energy from the head down to the navel. It is the basic energy that drives the person in life. *Apana vayu*, air that moves away, moves downward and directs all forms of elimination and reproduction. It controls the movement of energy from the navel down to the root chakra at the base of the spine. *Udana vayu*, upward-moving air, brings about the transformations of life energy. It governs the growth of the body and the release of positive energy. This prana moves energy from the navel up to the head. *Samana vayu*, balancing air, moves from the periphery to the center and moves energy from the entire body back to the navel. It aids in all types of processing—food, oxygen, and emotional and mental experiences. *Vyana vayu*, outward-moving air, moves from the center to the periphery and regulates energy out from the navel through the entire body. It directs the circulation of nutrients throughout the body (Fondin, 2015).

VIEW OF HEALTH AND ILLNESS

When the doshas are balanced, individuals experience health on all levels: mental, emotional, physical, spiritual, and environmental. Health is much more than the mere absence of disease. *Mentally* healthy people have good memory, comprehension, intelligence, and reasoning ability. *Emotionally* healthy people experience evenly balanced emotional states and a sense of well-being or happiness. *Physically* healthy people have abundant energy with properly functioning senses, digestion, and elimination. From a *spiritual* perspective, healthy people have a sense of aliveness and richness in life, are developing in the direction of their full potential, and are in good relationships with themselves, with other people, and with the cosmos. *Environmentally* healthy individuals have minimal economic, social, and political stress.

Balancing one's doshas does not mean trying to achieve an equal portion of Vata, Pitta, and Kapha. One cannot change the ratio of doshas that are present from conception. Health is the balance of each dosha that is right for that particular individual. Doshas, however, are responsive to people's habits, such as diet, exercise, and daily routines, which can either deplete or increase the doshas. Although both states of imbalance lead to ill health or disease, increased doshas are more problematic than decreased doshas.

Imbalance in the doshas is the first sign that mind, body, and spirit are not perfectly coordinated. One type, called *natural imbalance*, is due to time and age. Natural imbalances are typically mild and normally do not cause problems. Each dosha becomes more predominant during certain times of day as energy moves through six cycles in each 24-hour period: Vata predominates from 2 to 6, day and night; Kapha during the hours of 6 to 10; and Pitta from 10 until 2. Each dosha also predominates during particular seasons and stages of life. Kapha dominates during childhood and during the spring season, Pitta during summer and middle age, and Vata during fall and the latter part of one's life.

Unnatural imbalances of the doshas can be caused by a variety of factors, each of which falls into one of three broad categories of disease. *Adhyatmika* diseases originate *within* the body and include hereditary and congenital diseases. *Adhibhautika* diseases originate *outside* the body and include trauma, bacteria, and viruses. *Adhidaivika* diseases originate from *supernatural sources*, including those diseases that are otherwise unexplainable, such as illnesses originating from seasonal changes, divine sources, planetary influences, and curses. While some of these causes are beyond individual control, lifestyle and diet are within one's control. Preventing disease and improving overall health depends on the recognition of dosha imbalance and an understanding of the factors that increase and decrease each of the doshas (Payyappallimana & Venkatasubramanian, 2016).

Imbalanced Vata shows up as rough skin, weight loss, anxiety, restlessness, insomnia, decreased strength, constipation, arthritis, hypertension, rheumatic disorder, and cardiac arrhythmia. Pitta imbalance includes a yellowish complexion, excessive body heat, insufficient sleep, weak digestion, inflammation, inflammatory bowel disease, skin disease, heartburn, and peptic ulcer. Kapha imbalance presents as a pale complexion, coldness, lethargy, excessive sleep, depression, sinusitis, respiratory disease, asthma, and excessive weight gain (Fondin, 2015).

Several factors aggravate or increase each of the doshas. Factors that increase Vata are excessive exercise; wakefulness; falling; cold; late autumn and winter; fear or grief; agitation or anger; fasting; and pungent, astringent, or bitter foods. Factors that increase Pitta are anger; fasting; strong sunshine; midsummer and early autumn; and pungent, sour, or salty foods. Factors that increase Kapha are sleeping during the daytime; spring and early summer; heavy food; milk products; sugar; and sweet, sour, or salty foods (Rhyner, 2017).

DIAGNOSTIC METHODS

The first question asked is not "What disease does this person have?" but "Who is this person?" The complete process of diagnosis takes into account physical, mental, and spiritual components integrated with the social and environmental worlds in which the person lives. In addition to using X-rays or other biomedical diagnostic tools, Ayurvedic practitioners diagnose by observing people, touching them, taking pulses, and interviewing them.

Pulse Diagnosis

Pulse diagnosis is a highly specialized skill that requires great sensitivity. The process, as illustrated in Figure 5.2, involves placing the index, middle, and

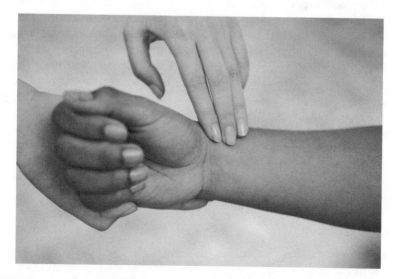

FIGURE 5.2 An Ayurvedic practitioner uses the index, middle, and ring fingers to locate three pulse points that are related to the flow of prana in the body and the three doshas.

Source: Gerard Brown/DK Images.

ring fingers of the right hand on the radial arteries of the right hand of men and the left hand of women. The general feel of the pulse is related to body type. A Vata pulse, felt by the index finger, is irregular or wavering, resembling the movement of a snake. A Pitta pulse, felt at the middle finger, feels forceful and throbbing, resembling the movement of a frog. A Kapha pulse, felt at the ring finger, is said to be gliding, resembling the movement of a swan. A three-dosha pulse resembles the movement of a woodpecker. Ayurvedic doctors may also take pulse readings at other points on the body as well. These points include the brachial artery above the elbow, the femoral artery, and pulse points at the temples, ankles, and top of the feet. This basic form of pulse reading gives the practitioner a vital clue to the person's body type. Pulse diagnosis is remarkably comprehensive. Experienced physicians not only can diagnose present diseases but also can tell what diseases the person has experienced in the past and which they are likely to develop in the future (Micozzi, 2015).

Tongue Diagnosis

Tongue diagnosis can also reveal the functional status of internal organs. A healthy tongue should be pink, clear, and shiny. A discoloration and sensitivity of a particular area of the tongue, or both, indicate dosha dysfunction. Kapha imbalance is evidenced by a whitish tongue, Pitta imbalance by a yellow-green tongue, and Vata imbalance by a brown to black tongue (Fondin, 2015).

Urine Diagnosis

Ayurvedic practitioners do urine examinations as another way to understand dosha imbalances. A midstream specimen is collected first thing in the morning. Healthy urine should be clear without much foam. Kapha imbalance gives the urine a cloudy appearance, Pitta imbalance imparts a dark yellow color, and a Vata imbalance presents as pale yellow and oily urine. The practitioner also puts a few drops of sesame oil in the urine and examines it in the sunlight. The shape of the drops signifies which dosha is imbalanced: A snakelike shape with wave movement indicates Vata; an umbrella shape with multiple colors, Pitta; and a pearl shape, Kapha. The movement of the oil in the urine indicates the prognosis of the disease. If the drop spreads immediately, the illness is probably easy to cure. If the oil drops to the middle of the urine sample, the illness is more difficult to cure. If the oil sinks to the bottom, the illness may be impossible to cure (Micozzi, 2015).

Body Observation

The practitioner carefully examines the skin, nails, and lips. Cool, hot, rough, or dry skin indicates imbalance. Imbalance can be visualized in the nails by longitudinal striations, bumps, or a parrot beak at the end of the nail. Dry, rough lips or inflammatory patches on the lips are another sign of imbalance. Coldness, dryness, roughness, and cracking indicate Vata imbalance. Hotness and redness indicate Pitta imbalance. Wetness, whiteness, and coldness indicate a Kapha imbalance (Micozzi, 2015).

TREATMENT

Specific lifestyle interventions are a major preventive and therapeutic approach in Ayurveda. Each person is prescribed an individualized diet and exercise program depending on dosha type and the nature of the underlying dosha imbalance. Care is taken to not cause new symptoms by suppressing the presenting symptoms. Herbal preparations are added to the diet for preventive or regenerative purposes, as well as for the treatment of specific disorders. Yoga, breathing exercises, and meditative techniques are also prescribed by the practitioner (Murray, 2012).

Nutrition

In Ayurveda, a balanced diet is different from the Western balanced diet derived from the basic food groups of meat, dairy, fruit, grains, and vegetables. Ayurveda recognizes six tastes: sweet, sour, salty, pungent, bitter, and astringent. A balanced Ayurveda diet must contain all six tastes at every meal but in different proportions depending on dosha type. The word *taste* includes not only the perceptions on the tongue but also the immediate effect of the substances within the body. Each of the six tastes is derived from two of the five elements. Sour, salty, and pungent have the fire element and so increase body temperature, dilate body channels, and allow energy and toxins to flow out from the body. Sweet, bitter, and astringent have no fire and thus are cooling, promoting relaxation. Sweet, sour, and salty have the water element and soften tissues, lubricate mucous membranes, and increase water retention (Payyappallimana & Venkatasubramanian, 2016).

Ayurveda describes the actions of each of the six tastes. *Sweet* promotes the vitality of body tissues, soothes the five senses, and adds bulk and firmness. Used in excess, sweet creates obesity, weak digestion, and a tendency to excessive sleep and heaviness. *Sour* improves the taste of food, increases digestion, and awakens the mind. In excess, sour wastes muscles and causes a buildup of toxins in the blood. *Salty* promotes digestion, moisturizes the body, softens all organs, and acts as a laxative and sedative. In excess, salty causes stagnation of blood, wasting of the muscles, wrinkling of the skin, and digestive hyperacidity. *Pungent* cleanses the mouth, opens the vessels, improves blood flow, and cures disorders of excess fluid in the body. In excess, pungent causes fatigue, emaciation, dizziness, and thirst. *Bitter*, though it does not taste good in itself, restores the sense of taste, detoxifies, relieves thirst, and is antibacterial, germicidal, and antipyretic. In excess, bitter causes wasting of the tissues, weakness, and dryness. *Astringent* is drying, firming, and sedating. It stops bleeding and aids in healing of wounds. In excess, astringent causes premature aging, constipation, retention of wastes, spasms, and convulsions and weakens vitality (Payyappallimana & Venkatasubramanian, 2016).

Three pairs of *gunas,* or qualities, are inherent in food: heavy or light, oily or dry, and heating or cooling. The following are examples:

- *Heavy:* wheat, beef, cheese
- *Light:* barley, chicken, skim milk
- *Oily:* milk, soybeans, coconut
- *Dry:* honey, lentils, cabbage
- *Heating:* pepper, honey, eggs
- *Cooling:* mint, sugar, milk

It is not necessary to memorize which foods reduce which doshas because any number of books offer long lists of foods matched to the dosha, taste, and guna. Many people seem to know naturally what their bodies need for balance. See Box 5.2 for the relationship between the doshas, tastes, and gunas. To counter an excess of Vata, diet recommendations consist of warm food with moderately heavy textures; salt, sour, and sweet tastes; and added

BOX 5.2

Foods in Relation to Doshas

Vata			
Balances		*Aggravates*	
Salty	Hot	Pungent	Light
Sour	Oily	Bitter	Dry
Sweet	Heavy	Astringent	Cold

Pitta			
Balances		*Aggravates*	
Bitter	Heavy	Pungent	Hot
Sweet	Cold	Sour	Light
Astringent	Dry	Salty	Oily

Kapha			
Balances		*Aggravates*	
Pungent	Light	Sweet	Heavy
Bitter	Dry	Sour	Oily
Astringent	Hot	Salty	Cold

Sources: McIntyre (2012); Murray (2012); Pole (2012).

oil. Examples of foods to include are asparagus, carrots, green beans, avocados, bananas, melons, rice, wheat, chicken, seafood, chickpeas, and tofu. To counter an excess of Pitta, diet recommendations are for cool or warm (but not hot) foods with moderately heavy textures and bitter, sweet, and astringent tastes. Examples of foods to include are broccoli, cabbage, lettuce, apples, grapes, raisins, barley, oats, ice cream, chicken, shrimp, chickpeas, and tofu. Coconut, olive, and soy oils are acceptable. For an excess of Kapha, diet recommendations include warm, light food, cooked without much water; pungent, bitter, and astringent tastes; and a minimum of butter and oil. Examples of foods to include are cauliflower, celery, leafy green vegetables, apricots, pears, dried fruits in general, barley, corn, rye, skim milk, chicken, shrimp, sunflower seeds, and raw honey (Payyappallimana & Venkatasubramanian, 2016).

Every food can be characterized by taste and guna. In addition to a diet balanced in terms of fats, carbohydrates, and proteins, people need variety in salty, sour, sweet, pungent, bitter, and astringent foods. The goal of diet management is to avoid aggravating any of the doshas and keep them calm and balanced.

Herbs

In Ayurveda, natural medicines are primarily herbal but may include animal and mineral ingredients, and even powdered gemstones. Practitioners prescribe many thousands of herbs. Like food, herbs are classified according to the six tastes. Herbs, however, are more potent and specific in their action than is food. Some herbs used for preventive and regenerative purposes are readily available. The use of herbs for treating disease must be medically supervised. As in Traditional Chinese Medicine, the entire plant is used. It is believed that the plant contains other chemicals that buffer the active ingredient, thus reducing possible side effects.

Like foods, herbs balance doshas. Vata-balancing herbs include ginseng, licorice, Indian pennywort, bala, and sitopaladi. Aloe vera, comfrey root, Indian gooseberry, and saffron are used to balance Pitta; and elecampane, honey, and sitopaladi balance Kapha. Herbs usually take longer to work than Western medications prescribed by practitioners. Historically, Ayurvedic herbs have had little exposure outside India but are now becoming more familiar with the rapid explosion of interest in herbal medicines in North America. The following are a few of the more common herbs found in health food stores. Sitopaladi is a very good herbal formula for colds and flu. Indian pennywort (brahmi) enhances a person's ability to focus mentally and learn new material. Guggulu is a powerful purifying agent, well known for lowering of blood cholesterol levels. Shilajit, with its antispasmodic qualities, is effective in acute and chronic respiratory illnesses. Bala, or Indian country mallow, is helpful in all types of nervous system disorders and certain types of heart disease. These few examples of herbs give one an idea of how they are used as natural body medicines (Shukla, Bhatnagar, & Khurana, 2012). In some instances, heavy metals such as lead, mercury, and arsenic have been found in Ayurvedic herbal medicines. Thus, people have been cautioned about ordering these herbs from overseas or through the Internet (Meiman, Thiboldeaux, & Anderson, 2015). Chapter 7 presents herbs in more detail.

Exercise

According to Ayurveda, exercise should conform to one's dosha type. Kapha people can perform moderately heavy exercise such as aerobics, running, dancing, and weight training. Because of their physical strength, Kaphas excel at endurance sports. Pitta people, who have more drive than endurance and an intense competitive spirit, should engage in a moderate amount of exercise. Brisk walking or jogging, hiking, swimming, and skiing are appropriate. People with a Vata dosha might enjoy jogging, but exercises like stretching, yoga, and t'ai chi are better choices. Such individuals have bursts of energy but tire quickly and may push themselves past their limits. Walking is probably the best exercise for all people, because it calms all dosha types. Ayurveda recommends a brisk half-hour walk every day (Shunya, 2017).

For people over the age of 80 or under 10, as well as those who have serious Vata and Pitta imbalances, exercise should be very gentle. Exercise should always leave a person ready for work as opposed to being work itself. Several other exercise precautions must be noted. One should not engage in exercise sooner than half an hour before and 1 to 2 hours after a meal. Exercising in the evening is discouraged because it is better for the body to slow down and prepare for sleep. Exercise is discouraged in wind or cold, since heavy breathing of cold, damp air is unhealthy for the respiratory tract. Also discouraged is exercise during the intense heat of the day, since environmental heat causes an even greater rise in body temperature.

The key to exercise is moderation and regularity. Ayurveda suggests that all exercise should be done at half of one's capacity. That means working out just until sweat appears on the forehead, under the arms, and along the spinal column. This amount of exercise improves digestion, prevents constipation, improves circulation, stimulates metabolism, regulates body temperature, and maintains body weight. Exercise keeps one's senses and mind alert and attentive as well as being effective in inducing relaxation and sleep. Overexercise, as indicated by panting and heavy sweating, may cause dehydration, muscle aches, breathlessness, and even chest pain. It is believed that overexercise eventually contributes to arthritis, sciatica, or heart conditions (Shunya, 2017).

Yoga

Yoga, developed in the Ayurvedic tradition, is one of the most effective forms of exercise for the body as well as nourishment for the mind and spirit. Hatha yoga, the most familiar form of yoga in North America, is a combination of body positions, breathing exercises, and mental focus on the present. Stretching helps relax and tone the muscles, improves circulation, improves concentration, and helps one regain energy. Yoga is increasingly being recognized for maintaining general health as well as helping people manage chronic disorders such as headaches, insomnia, hypertension, and depression. Further information about yoga is found in Chapter 16.

Breathing

Practicing controlled breathing is a valuable technique that leads to a healthier lifestyle. Several techniques can be utilized to relax the mind and body. Simple breathing helps people become aware of their breath and often relieves tension. Simple breathing involves closing the eyes and observing the breath, becoming more aware of its pattern and changes. Slow, easy breathing is continued for several minutes until a sense of relaxation is achieved. Alternate nostril breathing, *pranayama*, is another technique that can ease difficulty in breathing by making the respiratory rhythm more regular, which in turn soothes the entire nervous system. Pranayama is helpful prior to meditation because it focuses attention inward. Pranayama is performed while seated with the eyes closed. Figure 5.3 illustrates the position. The index and middle fingers of the right hand are placed on either side of the nose. The thumb closes the right nostril while the person breathes in through the left nostril. The left nostril is then closed with the ring finger, and the right nostril is opened for the out-breath and the next in-breath. The right nostril is then closed, and the out-breath occurs through the left nostril. After several cycles, breathing naturally gets deeper and smoother.

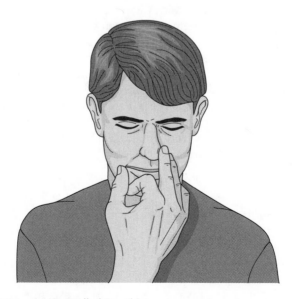

FIGURE 5.3 Pranayama/Controlled Breathing

Meditation

An important part of daily life in Ayurveda, meditation is considered a powerful tool to help maintain health. Meditation is a moment-to-moment awareness that cleanses the body, mind, and spirit. It is finding the quiet in the mind. As the mind is brought into a silent and receptive state, new energy comes into being, which is conducive to a state of health and peace. Further information about meditation is found in Chapter 17.

Massage

Marma therapy is a massage technique focusing on 107 sensitive points, called *marmas*, located on the skin. These points are similar to the acupuncture points called *hsueh* in Traditional Chinese Medicine. Marma therapy predates the Chinese approach and is likely the parent to acupuncture and acupressure. Marmas are activated through various methods. One is through yoga movements that gently stretch specific marma points. Warm oil dripped on the center of the forehead (shirodhara) on a major marma point can be profoundly soothing. A daily self-massage with oil can reach all the marmas on the skin. Once taught, these techniques can be practiced at home. Massage is covered in more detail in Chapter 12.

Aromatherapy

Aromatherapy is based on olfactory stimuli used to help balance the doshas as each responds to specific signals. Specialized olfactory cells provide instant connection of odors with the brain. The hypothalamus responds through regulation of body functions, the limbic system responds with emotions, and the hippocampus responds with memories, which explains how smells can elicit memories so vividly. In general, Vata is balanced by warm, sweet, and sour aromas such as basil, orange, rose geranium, clove, and other spices. Pitta is balanced by sweet, cool aromas like rose, mint, cinnamon, sandalwood, and jasmine. Kapha is balanced by warm aromas with spicy overtones such as juniper, eucalyptus, camphor, and clove. People whose doshas are out of balance are given specific oils to restore dosha balance. Aromatherapy may be used at any time but is often prescribed at night because it helps induce sleep. Aromatherapy is discussed further in Chapter 8.

Music

India has a long tradition of merging music and medicine. Unlike the distinct tones of most Western music, the tones in Indian music tend to blend together, creating a soothing, unifying sound. As with taste and smell, doshas can be balanced with certain tones and rhythms. The three doshas peak at different times of the day, and traditional Indian music smooths the process of these transitions. Ten minutes of music can be used as a gentle wake-up in the morning, after a meal to settle digestion, just before bedtime to aid sleep, and during the recovery period from an illness. Music therapy is discussed further in Chapter 21.

Purification

Panchakarma, or purification therapy, involves five procedures, any or all of which can be chosen based on the person's general condition, the season, and the nature of the disease. The five therapies of panchakarma are experienced over a period of a week and involve purifying the body through the use of sweating, emetics, purgatives, enemas, and nasal inhalations. Commonly administered by an Ayurvedic physician with the help of a number of assistants, the benefits of panchakarma are relief from long-standing symptoms, renewed health, and extended longevity (Fondin, 2015).

RESEARCH

Many Western researchers believe that they look at reality in an objective way. In contrast, Ayurvedic researchers believe that nothing happens in a vacuum. Everything that happens does so in relationship to what is occurring around it. The principle of research is that knowledge cannot be separated from its context.

As with Traditional Chinese Medicine, many studies have been difficult to translate into Western languages and into the causal and analytic type of research modalities typical of the biomedical model. Research standards throughout the world are subject to cultural influences. Not all cultures require their medical practitioners to conduct randomized, double-blind clinical trials. Consequently, the research data are influenced by the location of the study. Research that is meaningful to the scientific Ayurvedic communities may not have the same impact on Western biomedical communities.

The following is a small sample of recent research results:

- A randomized controlled trial of Ayurvedic massage found that it was effective in the short term for individuals with chronic low back pain (Kumar et al., 2016).
- A systematic review and meta-analysis of Ayurvedic drugs Rumalaya and Shunthi-Guduchi found that these were significantly effective in reducing pain levels in individuals with osteoarthritis (Kessler, Pinders, Michalsen, & Cramer, 2015).
- A randomized, single-blinded pilot study found that Ayurvedic oil dripping therapy (shirodhara) improved the quality of sleep for individuals with sleep problems (Tokinobu, Yorifuji, Tsuda, & Doi, 2016).

INTEGRATED NURSING PRACTICE

Although most nurses have not been educated in Ayurvedic medicine, they can integrate a number of principles into their professional practice. Ayurveda teaches self-discovery and self-understanding; it encourages people to learn how they can maintain their health and how and when they become sick, and it advocates lifestyle changes to maximize one's well-being.

The designation of doshas and dosha imbalance is a highly sophisticated process performed by professional practitioners. Using Box 5.1 as a checklist, individuals can begin to learn their dosha or body type, as follows:

- Make a check mark next to the description that best fits how you have been most of your life. If two descriptions apply to you, check both.
- Consider the qualities carefully. There are no right or wrong answers. Be honest and check how you really are, not how you would like to be.
- Look for lasting trends. For example, if your sleep has been heavy and prolonged most of your life but is now light and fitful, the change is likely due to imbalance rather than dosha type. Check your usual pattern.
- Note whether each dosha has some checks, because everyone's body type has Vata, Pitta, and Kapha components.
- Total the number of checks for each dosha. The dosha with the greatest number should be your body type. If the highest two dosha scores are close, you are probably a two-dosha type. If all three dosha scores are close, you are a three-dosha type.

Determining their unique blend of doshas allows people to begin to understand how their health is affected by internal and external influences. As people become more familiar with their body, they can observe and experience the effect of what they eat and do each day; how they think and feel; the state of their metabolism, digestion, and elimination; the relationships they engage in; their jobs; and the environment in which they find themselves. Because all these factors are interdependent, problems in one area can cause problems in other areas.

People's dosha balance can be disrupted in a number of ways. An inappropriate diet and lifestyle for one's dosha type will cause a slowly developing excess or deficiency in doshas. If people suffer significant trauma, however, the dosha levels can change immediately and dramatically. Dosha imbalance can also result from an accumulation of toxins or from too many experiences of a particular dosha without enough experiences from the other doshas. Once people understand their baseline dosha type, they can assess imbalances that may contribute to disease. Nurses can remind people that the strongest dosha in their constitution has the greatest tendency to increase. For example, Kapha-type clients have a natural tendency toward those things with Kapha qualities, and thus they increase their Kapha energy. Those individuals whose lifestyle includes a desk job, overeating, not exercising, and sleeping excessively may experience an excess in their Kapha dosha. They may need to consciously add opposite qualities to pacify or balance their Kapha energy, such as decreasing food intake, eating more pungent and bitter vegetables and astringent fruits, and increasing exercise.

Achieving balance of the doshas does not happen quickly—people need to work at it consciously. In some cases, lifestyle changes may be difficult, such as the nature of one's job, while others may be easier, such as a change in leisure activities. Typically, people find that diet, exercise, and leisure activities are the most amenable to change. For example, watching television and using computers increase Vata by stimulating the eyes and ears, and the passive nature of these activities increases Kapha. If a television program makes people angry, or their computer programs will not do what they wish, their Pitta may be stimulated. Limiting the time spent watching television and being selective with programs may help them balance their doshas and move toward a healthier state. Likewise, if people spend a lot of time at their computer, they need to take frequent breaks, move and stretch their bodies, and rest their eyes.

Individuals whose strongest dosha is Vata need to develop more regularity in their daily routines, such as eating regular meals, having an established bedtime, and slowing down and taking time to think. Because these persons have a tendency to dry skin, they should oil their skin regularly. People with Vata doshas are drawn to sensory experiences involving movement, speed, and action, and they may enjoy loud music and computer games. To maintain a healthy balance, Vata-type individuals should make an effort to balance those activities with quiet, creative pursuits such as writing, photography, or painting. Similarly, because they are attracted to vigorous exercise, they should try to engage in gentle exercise every day. Ayurveda suggests that all exercise be done at half of one's capacity. If people know they are exhausted after a 40-minute aerobics class, then they should do only 20 minutes of the class. People with Vata doshas enjoy spending their vacations sightseeing, touring, and filling their days and nights with many activities and returning home exhausted. A more beneficial vacation would be in a beautiful, sunny, and warm environment where they rest and limit their activities. Vata-type people wear clothes that are mostly dark shades, reflecting their mood.

Pitta-type individuals need to loosen up on setting and achieving goals and learn to enjoy the present moment. They can learn to achieve their ambitions without pressuring themselves. They also need to control their tendency to organize themselves and everyone else, because they become easily frustrated when things do not go as planned. Pitta-type people are stimulated by competitive, mentally challenging situations that may increase aggression or determination to win. They should learn to use constructive criticism rather than confrontation. Engaging in noncompetitive leisure activities such as gardening may help prevent an excess of Pitta. Vacations in cooler climates, and water and winter sports will cool their tendency to be warm. Pitta types should avoid overly organizing their vacations and try to enjoy whatever happens. Red clothing overstimulates Pitta and may contribute to a more aggressive approach to others. Cool, soft, pale colors help balance the Pitta dosha.

Kapha-type individuals need to vary their daily experiences to avoid becoming stuck in a rut, for example, by making small changes in the daily routine, and getting up early and going to bed late to limit the tendency to sleep too long. Because such people may prefer to sit and do nothing, they should find mentally and physically stimulating activities. Kapha is balanced by vigorous exercise, and Kapha types have good stamina, so they can exercise longer than Vata or Pitta types, but they will have to force themselves to do so. Kapha types prefer a vacation lying on a beach doing nothing but soaking up the sun. They will find, however, that sightseeing and touring will be more stimulating and balancing. All colors, except greens and dark blues, balance Kapha. Bright, strong colors are exciting and balancing.

Helping people understand their doshas is an ongoing process. As people observe their mind, body, spirit, and relationships, they learn how they respond to different qualities in everyday activities. After helping clients

TRY THIS

Massage

Sesame Oil Massage

Use the refined sesame oil sold in health food stores, not the heavy Chinese sesame oil. If you wish, you may use olive oil instead. Warm a quarter cup of oil in the microwave for 10 to 15 seconds, being careful not to overheat it.

Mini-Massage (1–2 minutes)

Use 1 tablespoon of warm oil and rub it into your scalp. Use small, circular motions with the flat of your hand. Using your palm, massage the forehead from side to side, and gently massage your temples using circular motions. Gently rub the outside of the ears. Massage both the front and the back of the neck.

Use a second tablespoon of warm oil and massage both feet using the flat of the hand. Massage each toe with your fingertips. Vigorously massage the soles of your feet. Sit quietly for a few seconds to relax, and then shower or bathe as usual.

Full-Body Massage (5–10 minutes)

Massage the scalp, ears, and neck with 1 tablespoon of warm oil as already described.

Using more oil, vigorously massage your arms using long strokes on the long parts, and circular motions at the joints.

Adding oil as necessary, massage the chest, stomach, and lower abdomen using gentle circular strokes in a clockwise direction. Massage as much of your back and spine as you can reach.

Massage the legs as you did the arms using vigorous movements.

With the remaining bit of oil, massage the feet as described earlier. Bathe with warm water and mild soap.

Source: Chopra (1991).

determine their dosha type, have them review their lifestyles in terms of diet, work, leisure activities, exercise, daily routines, quiet times, sleep, and relationships. By applying the principles of Ayurveda, people can begin making choices about the qualities they wish to incorporate into their lives. Rather than focusing on negatives (what they want to stop doing), have them focus on positives (what they want to start doing). Suggest that they limit their exposure to those qualities they do not want and enjoy those that will aid their well-being. Change begins with small steps and is a gradual process. Some people will want to seek the advice of an Ayurvedic practitioner to individualize a lifestyle change program. Remind clients that their mind and body always strive toward health and that every individual needs time, nurturing, routine, and gentle discipline to achieve a more complete level of well-being.

Considering the Evidence

Pratte, M. A., Nanavati, K. B., Young, V., & Morley, C. P. (2014). An alternative treatment for anxiety: A systematic review of human trial results reported for the ayurvedic herb ashwagandha (*Withania somnifera*). *Journal of Alternative and Complementary Medicine*, 20(2): 901–908.

What Was the Approach of the Research?
Systematic review of randomized human controlled trials.

What Was the Aim/Purpose/Objective(s) of the Research as Related to Complementary and Integrative Therapies?
To assess existing reported human trials of *Withania somnifera* (WS; common name, ashwagandha) for the treatment of anxiety.

How Was the Study Done?
A comprehensive search was conducted using the following databases: PubMed, SCOPUS, CINAHL, and Google Scholar. Additionally, the reference lists of studies identified in these databases were searched. Five international human controlled trials studies met the specified inclusion criteria.

What Were the Significant Findings of the Research?
All five studies suggested that WS intervention resulted in greater score improvements in outcomes than the placebo and psychotherapy on established anxiety and stress measures. However, the researchers indicated that the evidence should be received with caution because of the variety of the study designs and identified cases of potential bias in the review of included studies.

(continued)

What Additional Questions Might I Have?

Would additional good quality studies with a larger sample size have supported these findings? Are there adverse effects to ayurvedic herb ashwagandha? What are potential "herb–herb" interactions that may happen in persons taking ayurvedic herb ashwagandha and other herbs? What is the cost factor in taking this herb?

What Is the Clinical Significance of This Study?

This systematic review has clinical value for nurses caring for persons living with anxiety and desiring not to engage in traditional Western medicine therapies. Nurses may recognize that the ayurvedic herb ashwagandha may be an appropriate intervention for those persons living with anxiety. However, further studies of good quality involving human subjects are needed to strengthen the evidence related to this herb and enhance confidence regarding this intervention.

References

Bukkyo Dendo Kyokai. (1900). *The Teachings of Buddha*.

Chopra, D. (1991). *Perfect Health*. New York, NY: Harmony Books.

Fondin, M. S. (2015). *The Wheel of Healing with Ayurveda*. Novato, CA: New World Library.

Kessler, C. S., Pinders, L., Michalsen, A., & Cramer, H. (2015). Ayurvedic interventions for osteoarthritis: A systematic review and meta-analysis. *Rheumatology International*. doi: 10.1007/s00296-014-3095-y

Kumar, S., Rampp, T., Kessler, C. S., Jeitler, M., Dobos, G. J., Ludtke, R., . . . Michalsen, A. (2016). Effectiveness of Ayurvedic massage (*Sahacharadi Taila*) in patients with chronic low back pain: A randomized controlled trial. *Journal of Alternative and Complementary Medicine*. doi: 10.1089/acm.2015.0272

McIntyre, A. (2012). *The Ayurveda Bible*. Richmond Hill, Ontario, Canada: Firefly Books.

Meiman, J., Thiboldeaux, R., & Anderson, H. (2015). Notes from the field: Lead Poisoning and Anemia Associated with Use of Ayurvedic Medications

Purchased on the Internet. *Morbidity and Mortality Weekly Report*, 64(32): 883.

Micozzi, M. S. (2015). Traditional medicines of India: Ayurveda and Siddha. In M. S. Micozzi (Ed.), *Fundamentals of Complementary and Alternative Medicine* (5th ed., pp. 545–566). St. Louis, MO: Saunders.

Murray, A. H. (2012). *Ayurveda for Dummies*. Hoboken, NJ: For Dummies, Wiley.

Payyappallimana, U., & Venkatasubramanian, P. (2016). Exploring Ayurvedic knowledge on food and health for providing innovative solutions to contemporary healthcare. *Frontiers in Public Health*. doi: 10.3389/fpubh.2016.00057

Pole, S. (2012). *Ayurvedic Medicine: The Principles of Traditional Practice*. London, UK: Singing Dragon.

Rhyner, H. H. (2017). *Llewellyn's Complete Book of Ayurveda*. Woodbury, MN: Llewellyn Worldwide.

Shukla, S. D., Bhatnagar, M., & Khurana, S. (2012). Critical evaluation of Ayurvedic plants for stimulating intrinsic antioxidant response. *Frontiers in Neuroscience*. doi: 10.3389/fnins.2012.00112

Shunya, A. (2017). *Ayurveda Lifestyle Wisdom.* Louisville, CO: Sounds True.

Tokinobu, A., Yorifuji, T., Tsuda, T., & Doi, H. (2016). Effects of Ayurvedic oil-dripping treatment with sesame oil vs. with warm water on sleep: A randomized single-blinded crossover pilot study. *Journal of Alternative and Complementary Medicine.* doi: 10.1089/acm.2015.0018

Resources

Ayurvedic Herbs—Circle of Health
P.O. Box 719
Ashland, OR 97520
541.944.7243
www.ayurveda-herbs.com

National Ayurvedic Medical Association
620 Cabrillo Avenue
Santa Cruz, CA 95065
800.669.8914
www.ayurveda-nama.org

6

Native American Healing and Curanderismo

Morning Prayer
> *I thank You for another day. I ask that*
> *You give me the strength to walk worthily*
> *this day so that when I lie down at night I*
> *will not be ashamed.*

Evening Prayer
> *At the end of each day, face west and say:*
> *Thank you for all the things that*
> *happened today, the good as well*
> *as the bad.*

Prayers By Bear Heart, Native American Shaman

> *When it comes time to die, be not like*
> *those whose hearts are filled with the fear*
> *of death, so when their time comes they*
> *weep and pray for a little more time to*
> *live their lives over again in a different*
> *way. Sing your death song, and die like a*
> *hero going home.*

Chief Aupumut, Mohican, 1725

There are more than 567 distinct Native American (NA) tribes in the United States, including Alaska Natives (AN), and 44 First Nation tribes in Canada. The term Native Americans in this chapter refers to all of these groups. Although each tribal healing system is unique, the systems share a number of characteristics. This chapter presents the commonalities found among tribes. The population of today's Native American tribes is only a fraction of what it was before Europeans invaded North America, and many customs have been lost forever. Nevertheless, many of the traditions and ceremonies practiced by Native Americans for centuries are still in existence today (Voss, Moerman, & Micozzi, 2015).

BACKGROUND

Non-Indian people can learn a great deal from the Native American approach to life and traditional healing. To learn, people must be open to the ancient wisdom and understand it in the context of the entire Native American experience. It is not something to be trivialized by simply purchasing medicine objects and trying them out at home. As one Sioux leader said, "First they took our land, now they want our pipes . . . all the wannabees, these New Agers, come with their crystals and want to buy a medicine bag to carry them around in. If you want to learn our ways, come walk the red road with us, but be silent and listen" (Johnson, 1994, p. 6).

In their earliest encounters, European–American physicians devalued the skills of Native healers. These encounters have, in a way, come full circle. Western medicine is now advancing toward a holistic point of view that Native Americans have been practicing for thousands of years. Today, medicine women and men practice in a system that parallels conventional medicine. Some of them are traditional, meaning they adhere strictly to the old ways of life and reject any form of biomedicine. Others have acculturated, or adapted to the mainstream culture, and use both Indian medicine and conventional medicine. A third group of Native Americans has become assimilated and has virtually abandoned all traditional ways in favor of the dominant culture and utilizes only biomedicine (Flint, 2015).

Most tribal people have one or more types of health care specialists whose treatments frequently overlap. Some Native healers use herbs, some heal with songs, and some practice spiritual rituals. A midwife or a medicine woman or man might focus on natural medicines such as herbs and hands-on techniques but also use prayer and ceremony. *Shamans*, or holy people, emphasize spiritual healing but are often also knowledgeable about natural medicines. *Kahunas* are people, usually of Hawaiian ancestry, who have developed a level of spirituality that joins them with many of the spirit powers, allowing direct communication about the healing process. Shamans and medicine people are seen as channels the Creator has provided and trained. Some are born into families with medical or ritual skills, while others discover this path through a dream or vision. Selection is based on signs of devotion, wisdom, humility, and honesty. Once called, the individual seeks training, usually by apprenticing to a medicine person for a number of years. All knowledge comes from the Creator, and the elders are charged with the responsibility of keeping knowledge about healing foods, herbs, and medicine and passing it on. Trusted with all secrets, rituals, and legends of their people, Native healers are considered to be inspired individuals with great importance to the tribe. Training is complete when the teacher says it is complete and when the candidate has practiced the skills publicly and with success (Flint, 2015). See Chapter 24 for more information about shamans.

CONCEPTS

Spirituality

Spirituality and medicine are inseparable in Native American tradition. Essentially, no distinction is made between religious and medical practices. "Making medicine" is an important part of traditional life. It is how people give thanks to the Spirit who helps, guides, nourishes, and clothes them. Medicine is the constant pipeline to the Creator. In Indian tradition, making medicine is a process for achieving a variety of positive outcomes: a good hunt, plentiful crops, connecting with someone, healing someone, a successful birthing, and so on. Medicine is the way people keep their balance; it provides them with the opportunity to grow in new and healthier ways (Voss, Moerman, & Micozzi, 2015).

Native Americans believe in a singular living God but also believe that same God may be contacted through many ways, from many cultures. In Native languages, God is given such names as Great Spirit, Creator, Great Being, Great Mystery, Above Being, The One Who Oversees All Things, and He Who Gives Life. Everything is considered a gift from the Creator, and using these gifts is one way to create an atmosphere conducive to addressing the Creator (Bear Heart, 1996).

Gratitude

Gratitude is a central aspect of Native American culture. Every day is a spiritual, sacred day as demonstrated in Bear Heart's prayer at the opening of this chapter. Native Americans give thanks to the Great Power who makes all things possible. They give thanks not only for the good events but also for the bad things that happen throughout the day, because they believe that the more they show their appreciation, the more blessings they will receive.

Native people do not own or possess land but rather see themselves as caretakers of the earth for the Great Spirit. The land is considered the Mother, since all things come from her body. Animals, birds, trees, and grass all come from Mother Earth and are powerful living beings, just like human beings. When Native people take something from the earth, such as herbs or even a stone, they always give an offering, usually tobacco, in return and say a prayer that the item taken will be used in a good manner (Zimmerman, 2016).

Sacred Spaces

Sacred spaces or sites are extremely important to Native Americans. Sacred spaces remain sacred forever. The importance of these spaces includes beliefs about where creation occurred; places where spirits live; sites for ceremonies such as vision quest or sun dance; places where healing occurs; sites of burials, artifacts, and rock art; and resource sites for plants and minerals. Tragically, they are being destroyed by or are under the threat of corporate development such as pipe lines, mining facilities, and power plants.

If we understand the land as sacred, we understand the devastation of past displacement of Native Americans and current development projects. An example of cultural understanding occurred in 2006 when President George W. Bush established the Marine National Monument in Hawaii, and in 2016 when President Obama quadrupled the size of the site. These acts preserved numerous sites sacred to Native Hawaiians.

Healing

Medicine women and men see themselves as channels through which the Great Power helps others achieve well-being in mind, body, and spirit. The only healer is the One who created all things. Medicine people consider that they have certain knowledge to assemble items to help the sick person heal, and that knowledge has to be dispensed in a certain way, often through ritual or ceremony. Healers receive their knowledge through fasting and asking for guidance from above. During the period of fasting, the Great Being might reveal a chant or the location of a particular herb and give instructions on how to use it for different illnesses (Bear Heart, 1996).

Time is often considered an ally in recovery because it allows fears and problems to fade. Love is a key element in the healing process. The healer enters into the healing relationship with love and compassion, and the two individuals experience a joining or merging as this process unfolds. This merger symbolizes the cementing together of people and the Divine Spirit (Zimmerman, 2016).

Circle

The circle represents the cycles of life, which have no beginning, no end, and no time element. The Great Spirit causes everything to be round. The sun, earth, and moon are round. The sky is deep like a bowl. Things that grow from the ground like the stem of a plant or plant roots are round. The circle, symbol of infinity and interconnectedness, is seen in the sweat lodge, the bowl of the Sacred Pipe, the Sacred Hoop, and the Medicine Wheel. In addition, the camp is circular, tepees are circular, and people sit in a circle in all ceremonies. When people come together in a circle, a spirit of oneness and a sense of sacredness come upon them.

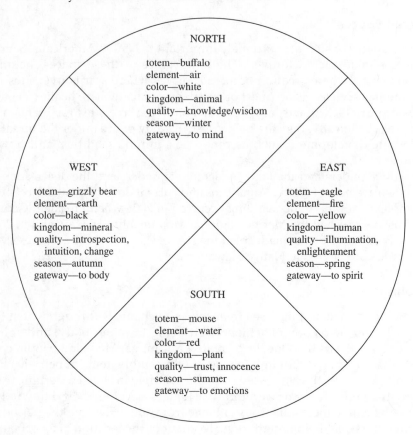

FIGURE 6.1 The Medicine Wheel

Sources: Kapacz (2016); Rutherford (2008).

Medicine Wheel

The Medicine Wheel is both an important conceptual scheme and a major ceremonial observance. The Sacred Hoop makes up the circumference, and the interior of the circle is divided into four quadrants. Each quadrant represents a direction, a totem, an element, a color, a kingdom, a quality, a season, and a gateway to the individual. The four colors—white, black, yellow, and red—represent the races of humanity. See Figure 6.1 for an illustration of the Medicine Wheel.

The Number 4

The number 4 is significant to Native American people and is incorporated into their daily lives through prayers, ceremonies, and activities. It is believed to be the number of completeness. There are four lifespan periods: infancy, childhood, adulthood, and elderhood. Everything that grows from the earth consists of four parts: roots, stems, leaves, and fruit. Earth, air, fire, and water are the four life-giving elements. Four types of things take breath: those that crawl, those that fly, those that walk on four legs, and those that walk on two legs. There are four directions, four seasons, and four races of people—white, black, yellow, and red.

VIEW OF HEALTH AND ILLNESS

Health is viewed as a balance or harmony of spiritual, physical, emotional, mental, and social spheres of life. The goal is to be in harmony with all things, which means first being in harmony with oneself. Harmony is thought to neutralize problems and help one's life become beautiful. Good health makes it easier for all people to do their part in the universe, to serve others, and to fulfill their personal life visions.

Life is considered in all its dualities: winter/summer, cold/hot, day/night, mind/body, spiritual/physical, work/play, and so on. Native people believe that the two sides of everything deserve equal attention and that both should be nourished with love. A healthy person who is walking in balance is energized and alert, and in the presence of disease will still feel alive and fulfilled (Sue & Sue, 2016).

Traditionally, Native American people lived long, happy, healthy, and balanced lives. They did everything to respect and honor Mother Earth and the Great Spirit. They ate wholesome food and considered all food to be blessed as a gift of life from the Creator. They got up with the sun and went to bed with the moon. Exercise was a natural part of their lives, integrated into daily activities. These good health habits, a sense of joy, and a purpose in life are key factors for living into old age (Sun Bear, Mulligan, Nufer, & Wabun, 1989).

Illness occurs when balance is disrupted. It is believed that most illness begins in the head, and people must get rid of ideas that predispose them to illness. If the mind is negative, the body will be drained, making it more vulnerable. Disease is also thought to be caused by "soul loss"—when individuals stop being generous and become selfish and dishonest. When people open up to the universe, learn what is good for them, and find ways to be happier, they can begin to work toward a longer and healthier life. Many ancient people had ways to get rid of this negativity. The Mayan people of Mexico would stand in a stream of flowing water and talk out all their angers, fears, sorrows, or troubles over the water. The moving water would take all the emotions they poured out of themselves into the current and away from them. The Bear Dance was a way the Indian people of Northern California rid themselves of negativity. A man in a bear costume would dance around a circle of people who would use switches to hit him as they spoke about the things in their lives that were bothering them. When the bear had acquired everyone's negativities, he went down into a stream, washing them away. Some Native people of the Southwest had dancers armed with swords who went through the village singing, chanting, and rattling, driving out the negative forces as they went. Behind the dancers came people with brooms to sweep away anything that was left over. Most Indian tribes had some way of letting people get rid of negativity so that they could go on and build new positive patterns (Flint, 2015; Garrett, 2003).

Dreaming is a powerful way for people to learn what is good for them. Dreams are a personal connection to the upper, spiritual realms. Divine guidance is thought to come through dreams and visions. In a period of illness, people may actually dream the healing. Dreaming is important in the healing practices of medicine women and men, because treatment information is often provided through dreams. Dream weavers, dream catchers, or dream nets are special medicine objects that allow the good dreams to reach the person through the hole in the center and catch the bad dreams to keep those away from the person. See Chapter 19 for more detailed information on dreaming.

DIAGNOSTIC METHODS

Healers must diagnose the source of the problem because they want to treat the cause, not just the effect. Much as in Traditional Chinese Medicine and Ayurveda, the diagnostic method takes into account all aspects of one's inner self, lifestyle, emotions, social setting, and natural surroundings. Healers always consider the total person, whether treating someone for physical illness or emotional problems. They look at the overall picture, determine what is out of balance within the whole, and then pinpoint the trouble spots. Some healers diagnose by going into a trance. While in a trance "hand tremblers" pass their shaking hands over the body of the person; when the hands stop trembling, the locale of the illness is found, and the cause is usually identified. "Star gazers" also enter trance states to read cause in the stars. "Listeners" do not go into a trance but listen to the person's story and on that basis identify the cause of the illness (Ingerman, 2014; Struthers, Eschiti, & Patchell, 2004).

TREATMENT

When people fall ill, they often experience anxiety and fear, which may incapacitate them. The healer is not so burdened and is able to supply coherence, calmness, and hope. Power flows through the healer to the patient. Patients' preferences are always respected in determining their own path toward balance and healing. Native healers spend a great deal of time with the ill person and the family. Ceremonies may last a few hours to a few days. Healers use medicine objects to assist them, and treatments consist of ceremony, touch, herbs, singing, drumming, and sometimes peyote.

Items used to help make medicine are called **medicine objects.** Medicine objects can be anything that relates to the Great Spirit in a sacred way. The medicine bag contains healing objects, which vary in size and number but typically are such things as feathers, claws, bird or animal bones, an assortment of herbs or roots, smudges, or paints. The medicine bag may also contain personal items that represent the individual and personal experiences that are sacred to him or to her. Native Americans are protective of their medicine bags because they carry a part of themselves and are among their most prized companions. The Medicine Wheel is a sacred circle usually built from stones. It is entered for the purpose of healing, giving thanks, praying, or meditating. The **Pipe** is one of the most sacred medicine objects and is an instrument of prayer.

The Indian art of healing is *ceremonial* or ritual in nature. Different ceremonies are conducted according to the type of illness or the severity of the person's condition. Healing ceremonies are led by medicine people or holy people. There is a communal aspect of the ceremony—as many people as possible participate to increase the power of the prayers. The primary purpose is to allow connection with the Great Healer, since physical health often fails without the aid of spiritual means. A secondary benefit is a cleansing of the body, mind, and spirit. A healing session is never a casual encounter. It is arranged through a formalized procedure after discussion by the patient, family, advisers, and healer. Acceptance by the healer is followed by instructions on preliminary actions, which may include fasting, abstinences, prayers, or the preparation of offerings or feasts.

Smudging

Smudging is a cleansing and purifying process using smoke from burning sacred herbs, usually sweet grass, sage, cedar, or tobacco. *Sweet grass* is used to bless one's self and one's home to protect from evil spirits. It is also used to purify sacred prayer instruments. *Sage* has a variety of uses. It is used in the blessing of one's home, it is part of the mixture used in the sacred smoking of the Pipe, and it is used in tea to flush out impurities. *Cedar* is considered the "tree of life" because it withstands the four elements no matter how harsh the seasons. Cedar is used in all sacred ceremonies as well as for its medicinal qualities. *Tobacco* is considered a gift from the Creator, and its smoke is a visual representation of people's thoughts and prayers being carried to the Creator. People and all sacred objects are smudged so that all can be centered and focused on the healing process. The smoke clears negativity, purifies the energy field of people and places, and is a prayer to the Creator. In addition to its use in healing ceremonies, smudging is used in the morning or evening as part of daily devotion. Smudging is a practice known to many religions; examples include the use of frankincense in Catholic churches and sticks of incense in Buddhist temples (Ingerman, 2014).

Sweat Lodge

The **sweat lodge** or **purification ceremony** is a ritual to cleanse body, mind, heart, and spirit. It may be held as its own ceremony or in preparation for another ceremony, such as a vision quest. Typically, the sweat lodge is held in a round structure covered with overlapped pieces of tarpaulin or blankets with a small door flap. When the flap is down, the place is nearly dark and almost sealed off from the outer air. Near the lodge is a fire pit, where rocks are heated and then passed into the lodge. Water from a bucket is splashed onto the stones, which creates a dense steam referred to as the Breath of Spirit. Depending on the illness, a variety of herbs are burned on the sweat rocks. Sacred songs and prayers go on for several hours. Everyone in the sweat lodge prays earnestly for the one needing healing, but it is the responsibility of the one being healed to pray that healing energies come to her or to him and to ask the Spirit to give guidance to the medicine person (Sue & Sue, 2016).

The sweat lodge is also a powerful ceremony to keep people healthy, and many view it as the first line of defense in preventing illness. The sweat lodge raises the body's temperature well above normal, killing heat-sensitive viruses and bacteria. The lodge is also a bringing together of the four elements: earth, air, fire, and water. Through sweating and praying, the body is cleansed of toxins, the mind of negativities, the heart of hatred, and the spirit of doubt. The sweat lodge is as sacred a place as a church or a temple (Sue & Sue, 2016).

Drumming and Chanting

Drumming and chanting are powerful ways to bring oneself in balance with self, others, and the world. **Drumming** harmonizes people with the heartbeat of Mother Earth. It is a pulse rather than a tempo. As people dance to the pulse of the drum, they dance in harmony with the Creator and with one another. Symbolically, the drum represents all life. The wood was once a tree, and the skin covering the drum was once life. These objects are related to life that has gone on, yet they are helping present lives (see Figure 6.2). **Chanting** is a form of prayer through music. *Holyway* chants are used to attract good, to cure, and to repair; *ghostway* chants are used to remove evil; and *lifeway* chants are used to treat injuries and accidents (Mackinnon, 2016).

Sing

A **sing** is a healing ceremony that lasts from 2 to 9 days and nights. A highly skilled specialist called a *singer* guides it. Used in healing, sings are attended

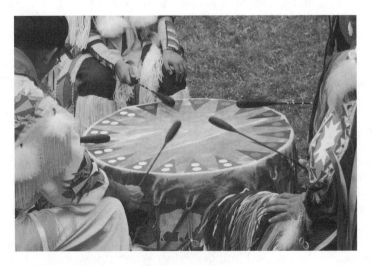

FIGURE 6.2 Peace and Harmony Through Drumming

Source: Bill Perry/Shutterstock.

by as many people in the community as are able to come because just being present is considered healing. Some songs are only for children and call on spirits who take care of little children. Some spiritual songs take care of adults only. Other songs focus on specific problems, such as the song for small burns that will cool them and keep them from blistering. To learn a single chant can take up to several years. It takes some people 40 years of singing before they master the chants and the accompanying herbal preparations (Rutherford, 2008).

Pipe Ceremony

The Pipe ceremony takes many different forms depending on how this sacred knowledge was given to the various tribes. The Pipe is one of the most sacred medicine objects and represents the universe to Native American people. The bowl represents the Mother Earth and the female powers of the universe. The stem represents the plant kingdom and the male powers of the universe. When the bowl and the stem are joined together, the Pipe is sacred. The tobacco smoked in the Pipe is an instrument of prayer and has come to signify the sacredness of the ritual. As the smoke of the Pipe rises, it creates an atmosphere of prayer by symbolizing prayers going up to the Creator (Mackinnon, 2016).

Pipes are used for private and group prayers. Prayers are transmitted in the smoke of the burning tobacco. Participants in the Pipe ceremony are as centered and focused as possible, since everything they think and feel is part of the prayers being offered. As in many other ceremonies, the number 4 has special significance. The Pipe is offered to the four directions and is often passed in four ritual repetitions.

Sun Dance

The **sun dance** includes the sweat lodge, the Pipe ceremony, monthly prayer rituals, and a yearly ceremony. During the monthly ceremony, songs are sung to carry the prayers upward, and people come forth to be healed. The yearly 3- to 4-day sun dance usually takes place in July. It is a very detailed and complex ceremony. The medicine person prays on behalf of the tribe, the world, and all creation. The dancers, who spend all their time praying to the Creator, move to the drumbeat around a center pole. Because the dancers fast for the entire time, many collapse or "take a fall." This fall is often followed by a vision, similar to what happens on a vision quest. The sun dance ends with a purification ceremony so that tribe members can reenter the world refreshed and regenerated (Mackinnon, 2016).

Vision Quest

An extremely powerful ceremony is the **vision quest**. Traditionally, it is a time of fasting, praying, isolation, and exposure to the elements, all of which contribute to a mystic experience with the goal of understanding self and communicating with the Great Spirit. Individuals ask themselves questions such as How can I best serve the people? How can I best serve Mother Earth? How can I best serve future generations? It is hoped that during the vision quest people find out who they are, what they are supposed to do, and what their life's goal should be, as well as discover the purpose and meaning of their lives. The vision quest begins with a sweat lodge for purification, after which the person is taken to an isolated place in nature and begins the period of silence and fasting. During the vision quest, the individual focuses only on prayer and vision and in this way is pushed into the spirit world. After the vision quest, the person returns to the sweat lodge, and a Pipe ceremony is performed (Mackinnon, 2016).

Healing Touch/Acupressure

Native Americans have always considered touch to be therapeutic. The Creator touches patients and transfers power to them through medicine people or shamans who are healing instruments. Touching, an expression of loving care, is essential for the healing process. It cleanses the affected area and relieves pain. The willingness to touch on the part of the healer demonstrates a lack of fear of contamination. Healing touch is a powerful way to remove barriers and create or restore relationships (Ingerman, 2014).

Some tribes have used a form of acupressure since ancient times. Compared with traditional Chinese practitioners, Native Americans use fewer pressure points, but the process is similar. Prior to using acupressure, medicine people warm their hands over a fire so that the Great Being can send healing warmth through them to the patient. It is believed that no harm will be done to a person as long as the pressure is applied slowly and in a relaxed way. Medicine people are taught that acupressure should be performed only with the utmost gentleness and love. Chapter 13 covers acupressure in more detail.

Herbs

Native Americans have long used herbs in maintaining health and treating disease. Botanical remedies are supplemented with ceremony and prayer during the healing process. The beneficial properties of herbs as medicines often depend on the greenness or ripeness of the plant and the part of the plant to be used, such as roots, barks, twigs, bulbs, rhizomes, fruit seed, tubers, leaves, and flowers. Knowing the best time for cutting and digging each type of plant, for peak effectiveness, is part of the knowledge of the Native healer. Whether it be in summer, winter, spring, or autumn, the timing must be appropriate for each plant. An herb gathered with prayers, cut or dug at the correct time, and prepared properly will restore a person from illness to health (Cowan, 2014).

Ancient Native people considered nature to be their pharmacy. They did not have aspirin, but they did have willow bark, which contains salicylic acid. The active ingredient in foxglove is digitalis, which was used in a tea to help people with heart problems. Particular molds, similar to those forming the basis of penicillin, were used to treat infections. Purple coneflower (echinacea) is an immune system booster and antibiotic that is held in high esteem by many people today. Goldenseal, which is a good disinfectant that promotes scab formation, is one of the most important Native American medicinal plants. Currently, it is also used as a gargle for sore throat or as a mouth rinse for canker sores, tonsillitis, and infected gums (Cowan, 2014). For further information on herbs, see Chapter 7.

Peyote

A hallucinogenic herb, peyote has been used by the Indians of North America for a long time. Native people do not use peyote to "get high" but rather to see teaching visions. Using peyote is a sacrament, and it provides a connection to the sacred world. Peyote makes people highly sensitive to sight and sound and more aware of what is around and inside them. It is used to heal all kinds of sickness, for clairvoyance, and in the worship of the Great Being. It is believed that the Creator put peyote on earth as a medicine to help people. Peyote can also be described as an entheogen. Voss and Micozzi (2015, p. 640) state that an entheogen is "a chemical or botanical substance that produces the experience of God within an individual and has been argued to be an essential part of the study of religious experience."

Role of Medicine Women and Men

Although they are the primary care providers in many places, the responsibilities of medicine women and men go beyond healing illness. They also evaluate advice and treatment given by other health care practitioners. Medicine men and women often have a strong influence on the acceptance or rejection of the treatment plans from conventional health care providers. They may also function as tribal social mediators, dispensing traditional wisdom and suggesting action. Medicine people reaffirm and strengthen tribal identity through the recounting of myth and song. They have an extensive knowledge of their communities and of family relationships and interaction. They are the formulators and teachers of the old religion and creators of the new. Medicine people are figures of authority and awe as instruments of the Creator (Mackinnon, 2016).

Navigator Programs

The goal of patient navigator programs is to improve outcomes for indigenous people with cancer. The Native Sisters Program encourages the use of screening programs for breast cancer prevention and identification. The

Walking Forward Program seeks to remove treatment barriers and decrease mortality rates. Both programs are grounded in the traditions and knowledge of Native American populations.

RESEARCH

Formal research into healing ceremonies is almost nonexistent. Native American medicine is a tradition that is subtle and difficult to document and communicate fully outside of its varied traditions and ceremonies. Anecdotally, many ailments and diseases—ranging from skin rashes and asthma to heart disease, diabetes, and cancer—have reportedly been cured by medicine people and shamans. A few studies, such as the following, are beginning to be reported in the scientific literature:

- Native Americans living in rural areas, in contrast to urban/suburban areas, are significantly less likely to have nurses, traditional healers, or shamans on clinic staff. They are also less likely to participate in research or use evidence-based treatments (Rieckmann, Moore, Croy, Novins, & Aarons, 2016).
- A qualitative study was conducted on Native Americans experiencing chronic pain and their use of traditional healing treatments. The findings found that traditional treatments were utilized but there was no recommendation for any specific practice (Greensky et al., 2014).
- Eighteen studies met the criteria for a meta-synthesis of end-of-life experiences of Native Americans. The qualitative theme was "preparing the spirit." A significant finding was that there are barriers within health care systems that interfere with this process (Duggleby et al., 2015).

CURANDERISMO

Curanderismo (pronounced "koo-rahn-dare-EES-mo"), from the Spanish verb *curar*, "to heal," is a cultural healing tradition found in Latin America and among many Hispanic Americans in the United States. In Mexico, many beliefs are shared with Native American cultural traditions. Curanderismo, as described here, is most characteristically practiced by Mexican Americans. Although it is a traditional healing system, curanderismo survives by growing, changing, and incorporating Western biomedical beliefs, treatments, and practices. It is also believed, however, that in certain types of illness and healing, Native healers are more accomplished than practitioners of conventional medicine. Some professional nurses are also Native healers. They combine their knowledge of nursing science with the long tradition of curanderismo (Trotter & Micozzi, 2015).

Natural and Supernatural Illnesses

Illnesses are classified into two types: natural and supernatural. The *natural* source of illness includes genetic disorders, dysfunction of the body, improper self-care, infection, and psychological conditions. *Supernaturally* induced illnesses are said to be caused either by evil spirits or by a person practicing magic and placing a hex on the victim. Supernatural illnesses, which may resemble natural illness, occur when these negative forces damage a person's health. It is believed that conventional medical practitioners are unable to intervene with supernatural illnesses (Trotter & Micozzi, 2015).

Healers

Curanderos (men) and curanderas (women) believe that they work by virtue of *el don*, a gift of healing, often believed to be a gift from God. In some areas, becoming a healer is a matter of inheritance; in other areas, it is a matter of being called. Healers routinely deal with physical ailments as well as with problems of a social, psychological, or spiritual nature. Healers are always one of the people. Their healing awareness comes from living with the people, feeling their pain, knowing their illnesses, and experiencing their suffering (Trotter & Micozzi, 2015).

Three Levels of Healing

Three levels of care are practiced among curanderos and curanderas, namely, the material level, the spiritual level, and the mental level. Healers have the gift for working at only one of these levels because each requires distinct areas of knowledge, methods of diagnosis, and types of healing. The majority of the healers work at the material level, and most combine shamanic healing, herbal medicine, and first-aid techniques (Trotter & Micozzi, 2015).

The *material level* involves the use of physical or supernatural objects to heal or to change the person's environment. Physical healers include midwives, bone setters, herbalists, and people who treat sprains and tense muscles. Objects and rituals are used for their curative powers. Objects include herbs, religious symbols (crucifix, pictures of saints, incense, holy water), and secular items (cards and ribbons). Several types of rituals are used for supernatural cures. One of the most frequently used is a cleansing ritual that includes prayers and invocations designed to remove the negative forces that are causing the illness, and a purification of the environment with incense. At the same time, the patient is given the spiritual strength necessary to achieve recovery.

The *spiritual level* of healing is similar to shamanic healing rituals. It is believed that spiritual beings who exist in another dimension are interested in making contact with the physical world. These spirit entities come from once-living humans. Spiritual-level healers become a direct link or medium with these spirits. They enter a trance state and make contact with the spirit world. Some spirits have left tasks undone in their physical lives; some wish to help or harm others; and some wish to communicate with their friends and relatives. Healers believe that spirits can manipulate a person's health by directing positive or negative forces at them from the spiritual realm.

The *mental level* is the least encountered level of practice. Healers have the ability to transmit, channel, and focus mental vibrations in a way that directly affects a person's mental or physical condition. If healers are working with physical illness, such as cancer, they channel vibrations to the afflicted area to retard the growth of abnormal cells and accelerate the growth of healthy cells. If healers are working with mental conditions, they send vibrations into the person's mind to manipulate energies and modify behavior. Mental healing can be accomplished in person or over long distances (Trotter & Micozzi, 2015). Chapter 24 covers more detailed information on shamans.

Most **research** done on curanderismo is traditional anthropological research such as participant observation and interviewing. Many of the home remedies have been tested for biochemical and therapeutic activities and have demonstrated therapeutic actions that match the healers' uses. Research regarding herbs is presented in Chapter 7.

Related Systems

The **Tarahumara Indians**, who live in the northwest mountains of Mexico, are one of the oldest aboriginal tribes of North America. They believe that disease is due to four possibilities: (1) loss of the soul, (2) as punishment for moral "sins," (3) for breaking cultural "rules," or (4) for disrespecting people, plants, or objects. When people become ill, they first look to themselves, utilizing self-healing skills, including herbs. If that is not effective, they ask their family for help. The next level of healing is asking a wise person of the village (who is not necessarily a healer) for assistance. The wise person may recommend calling a shaman or a conventional medical practitioner.

Shamans are both healers and spiritual leaders who are granted high social status. The owiruame (the one who heals) heals people and animals using dreams to find a lost soul. The waniame sucks on the affected body part withdrawing foreign objects thought to have been inserted by someone else. The Towita limits healing to lifting depressed fontanels in infants. The Jikuri shamans have the highest level of healing skills. They are the only ones who can use the hallucinogenic cactus jikuri (peyote) as part of the healing ceremony (Irigoyen-Rascon, 2015).

Traditional healers in **Africa** have multiple healing traditions. As with other indigenous people, healers are esteemed members of society. Those who would be healers must first suffer a mysterious illness that does not respond to treatment. This is followed by dreams where ancestral spirits call the person to become a healer. The person is then both treated and taken on as an apprentice by an established traditional healer. The apprenticeship is long and strenuous and often lasts a number of years.

In Africa, illness is believed to be caused by emotional or spiritual conflicts or by conflicts with other people, living or dead. Treatment may be herbal, a purification process, and/or appeasing bad spirits. Drumming and dance are used to enhance the treatment process. Spirituality and psychosocial relationships are an important aspect of the healing process (Hewson, 2015).

INTEGRATED NURSING PRACTICE

Just as Native American healers see themselves as channels through which the Great Power helps others achieve a sense of wellness, some nurses see God or the Divine Being at work in their professional practice. Although clients may be unaware of this spiritual impetus, these nurses believe that the spiritual dimension provides the energy and momentum for their practice. Other nurses believe that their desire to care for others is what provides direction for their practice. The *art of nursing*, for many, is in being there, with another person or persons, in a context of caring. As nurses return to their nursing roots in using their hands, heart, and head in creating healing environments, they approach the Native American ideal of healing practices.

Like Native Americans, nurses have traditionally looked at the *total person* in their care. The context of people's lives is critically important to the nursing–healing model. In addition, nurses also believe that feelings or energy or caring flows from nurses to clients. People in distress or who are ill are anxious and fearful. Nurses who are centered and balanced can share their sense of calmness in the face of crisis. Before entering a client's home or room, take a moment to center with a couple of deep, cleansing breaths and focus on what you are about to do with this person who is your client.

When you are with the client, touch may be an appropriate intervention. For some people who are suffering or in crisis, a touch on the arm or holding his or her hand may be the most effective nursing intervention you will provide. It is important to remember that touch must always be appropriate and acceptable to the client.

Just as Native American tribes have rituals for cleansing the mind of negative thoughts and feelings that predispose to disease, nurses can help clients *modify unhealthy thinking* patterns. Negative thinking not only occurs in the brain but also in the body; negative thoughts cause instantaneous chemical changes in every cell. Continuous cellular disruption may contribute to the onset of illness and disease. To counteract negative thinking, some people find it helpful to look at themselves in the mirror and say aloud three good things about themselves. People might say, "I'm a good friend," "I'm an honest person," "I'm a caring person," "My hair looks beautiful today," "I am becoming healthier every day," and so on. The goal is to say different positive qualities about themselves each day. Keeping a journal about feelings immediately after the exercise and feelings throughout the day is helpful in evaluating the impact of positive statements on negative thinking.

Positive affirmations are another way to counteract negative thinking. In this nursing intervention, you encourage people to make a list of positive things in their lives or things they would like to happen. Affirmations are always stated as if they were a fact, even when they are still a dream. For example, an ill client might be thinking, "I'm never going to get better. I'm always going to be miserable." You might suggest that he or she verbalize affirmations such as "I'm feeling better every day. My body is continuing to heal." Encourage clients to write a list of affirmations over several days and repeat them several times a day. Because people tend to live their lives according to their expectations, changing expectations from negative to positive can improve the level of wellness.

Although it might not be reasonable to find a stream of flowing water to take away angers, fears, sorrows, or troubles, you can teach people to *visualize* that process. Direct clients through the relaxation process and have them mentally walk into a stream or actually stand in a shower that is comfortable in temperature and force of the flow. As they stand in the stream, have them visualize the water washing out all their physical, mental, emotional, or relational problems. Similar to the Indian art of healing, this nursing intervention may be beneficial for clients who feel weighted down with their problems or sorrows.

Gratitude is important in Native American culture. As a nurse, you can help others become more grateful for their life experiences. Many people find it extremely beneficial to keep a gratitude journal. At the close of every day, they write at least three things that happened during the day for which they are thankful. They may be thankful for a beautiful sunrise, a smile from a stranger, a hug from a child, an A on an exam, a wonderful dinner, an intimate moment with a partner, and so on. Focusing on gratitude is another way to become more in harmony with oneself and is thought to neutralize problems and negative thinking.

A number of substance abuse programs, both Native American and non-Native American, have added drumming groups to their programs. In addition, drumming is being studied in the treatment of soldiers with post-traumatic stress disorder. *Drumming* enhances hypnotic susceptibility, increases relaxation, improves meditation, and synchronizes brain wave patterns. It facilitates an outlet for rage and a way to regain self-control. Drumming groups may also enhance recovery by encouraging social support and social networks. As a nurse, you can encourage the study and practice of drumming groups in these types of programs (Fancourt et al., 2016).

Most people have *objects* that are significant to them. Although these objects are not medicine objects in the Native American tradition, they may engender a sense of comfort and perhaps protection. Encourage and support clients to have religious symbols or holy books around them if those items are important to them. Secular items can also be of great comfort, such as pictures of family and friends, get-well cards, poems, and beloved books. Most nurses do not have sweat lodges or sings as part of their healing practices, but many clients have a *community* of family or friends who may be sending their love and concern or praying for their healing. Actively support those activities that provide love and hope to counteract the fears and doubts that accompany illness.

Like Native Americans, nurse psychotherapists find the *circle* to be a beneficial design. Group therapy typically occurs with all the participants sitting in a circle, which contributes to the group's sense of oneness and connectedness. Circle arrangements foster cooperation rather than competition. It is often helpful to use a circle arrangement for nursing team conferences or interdisciplinary clinical conferences.

TRY THIS

Positive Thoughts

Often, individuals endure such runs of negative thoughts that they are unaware of the process until they have been "beating themselves up" for 10 to 15 minutes. To become more aware of this habitual process, tap one of your left fingers on a firm surface for every negative thought. When your finger becomes quite sore, you will have another level of awareness of your negativity. Negative thoughts can be countered with positive ones. When you catch yourself thinking and feeling a negative thought, such as how fat your body is or how dumb you are, STOP. Then, look for and substitute a positive thought or feeling in the place of the one you removed, such as how lovely your hair looks or how well you have succeeded at something. Listen to yourself saying the positive phrase out loud. Continue in this way, adding other phrases and wishes for yourself.

References

Bear Heart. (1996). *The Wind Is My Mother.* New York, NY: Berkley Books.

Cowan, E. (2014). *Plant Spirit Medicine.* Boulder, CO: Sounds True.

Duggleby, W., Kuchera, S., MacLeod, R., Holyoke, P., Scott, T., Holtslander, L., . . . Chambers, T. (2015). Indigenous people's experiences at the end of life. *Palliative & Supportive Care.* doi: 10.1017/S147895151500070X

Fancourt, D., Perkins, R., Ascenso, S., Carvalho, L. A., Steptoe, A., & Williamon, A. (2016). Effects of group drumming interventions on anxiety, depression, social resilience and inflammatory immune response among mental health service users. *Public Library of Science.* doi: 10.1371/journal.pone.0151136

Flint, A. (2015). Traditional healing, biomedicine and the treatment of HIV/AIDS. *International Journal of Environmental Research and Public Health.* doi: 10.3390/ijerph120404321

Garrett, J. T. (2003). *The Cherokee Herbal.* Rochester, VT: Bear & Company.

Garrett, M. T., Garrett, J. T., & Melton, J. G. *Native American Faith in America.*

Greensky, C., Stapleton, M. A., Walsh, K., Gibbs, L., Abrahamson, J., Finnie, D. M., . . . Hooten, W. M. (2014). A qualitative study of traditional healing practices among American Indians with chronic pain. *Pain Medicine.* doi: 10.1111/pme.12488

Heart, B. (1998). *The Wind is My Mother: The Life and Teachings of a Native American Shaman.* New York, NY: Berkley Books.

Hewson, M. G. (2015). African healing and becoming a traditional healer. In M. S. Micozzi (Ed.), *Fundamentals of Complementary and Alternative Medicine* (5th ed., pp. 660–666). St. Louis, MO: Elsevier/Saunders.

Ingerman, S. (2014). *Walking in Light.* Boulder, CO: Sounds True.

Irigoyen-Rascon, F. (2015). *Tarahumara Medicine.* Norman, OK: University of Oklahoma Press.

Johnson, S. (1994). *The Book of Elders.* San Francisco, CA: HarperSanFrancisco.

Kapacz, D. (2016). *Walking the Medicine Wheel: Healing PTSD.* Millichap Books. Millichapbooks.com

Mackinnon, C. (2016). *Shamanism*. Carlsbad, CA: Hay House Inc.

Rieckmann, T., Moore, L. A., Croy, C. D., Novins, D. K., & Aarons, G. (2016). A national study of American Indian and Alaska Native substance abuse treatment: Provider and program characteristics. *Journal of Substance Abuse Treatment*. doi: 10.1016/j.jsat.2016.05.007

Rutherford, L. (2008). *The View Through the Medicine Wheel: Shamanic Maps of How the Universe Works*. Ropley, Hants, UK: John Hunt.

Struthers, R., Eschiti, V. S., & Patchell, B. (2004). Traditional indigenous healing: Part 1. *Complementary Therapies in Nursing & Midwifery*, 10(3): 141–149.

Sue, D. W., & Sue, D. (2016). *Counseling the Culturally Diverse: Theory and Practice* (7th ed.). Hoboken, NY: Wiley.

Sun Bear, Mulligan, C., Nufer, P., & Wabun. (1989). *Walk in Balance*. New York, NY: Simon & Schuster.

Trotter, R. T., & Micozzi, M. S. (2015). Latin American curanderismo. In M. S. Micozzi (Ed.), *Fundamentals of Complementary and Alternative Medicine* (5th ed., pp. 643–652). St. Louis, MO: Saunders.

Voss, R. W., & Micozzi, M. S. (2015). Central and South American healing and herbal remedies. In M. S. Micozzi (Ed.), *Fundamentals of Complementary and Alternative Medicine* (5th ed., pp. 639–642). St. Louis, MO: Elsevier/Saunders.

Voss, R. W., Moerman, D. E., & Micozzi, M. S. (2015). Native North American healing and herbal remedies. In M. S. Micozzi (Ed.), *Fundamentals of Complementary and Alternative Medicine* (5th ed., pp. 623–638). St. Louis, MO: Elsevier/Saunders.

Zimmerman, L. J. (2016). *The Sacred Wisdom of the Native Americans*. London: Chartwell Books.

Resources

Association of American Indian Physicians
1225 Sovereign Row, Suite 103
Oklahoma City, OK 73108
405.946.7072
www.aaip.org

Dance of the Deer Foundation, Center for Shamanic Studies
P.O. Box 699
Soquel, CA 95073
888.455.3337
www.shamanism.com

Feathered Pipe Ranch Foundation
P.O. Box 1682
Helena, MT 59624
406.442.8196
www.featheredpipe.com

National Association of Indian Nurses of America
P.O. Box 3002
Northlake, IL 60164
www.nainausa.com

The School of Lost Borders
P.O. Box 796
Big Pine, CA 93513
760.938.3333
www.schooloflostborders.com

Singing with the Wheel (compact disc)
West Winds
P.O. Box 16729
Mobile, AL 36616
www.winddaughterwestwinds.com

UNIT 3

Botanical
Healing

The Lord hath created medicines out of the earth;
and he that is wise will not abhor them.

ECCLESIASTICUS 38:4

Let your food be your medicine and
your medicine your food.

HIPPOCRATES

7

Herbs and Nutritional Supplements

Physicians pour drugs, about which they know little, to cure diseases, about which they know less, into humans, about whom they know nothing.

VOLTAIRE

The Great Spirit is our father, but the earth is our mother. She nourishes us; that which we put into the ground, she returns to us, and healing plants she gives us likewise.

BIG THUNDER

Also known as *botanical medicine* or *phytotherapy* (*phyto* means "plant"), **herbal medicine** is used by 80% of the world's population (Qureshi, Ghazanfar, Obied, Vasileva, & Tariq, 2016). Herbs are also the most popular complementary and alternative (CAM) therapy in the United States, with more than 750 herbs now on the market. According to the National Center for Complementary and Integrative Health (NCCIH), Americans spend more than $14.8 billion a year on herbal remedies and dietary supplements. For many conditions, herbs are the treatment of choice because they are milder and have fewer side effects than prescription drugs. Vitamins, minerals, diet supplements, and specialized diets are beyond the scope of this text. Entire books are devoted to each of those topics, to which the reader is referred.

BACKGROUND

Throughout history, almost all societies have used plants for therapeutic purposes. For example, the oldest surviving garlic prescription, carved into a clay tablet, dates to 3000 B.C. Over thousands of years, a medical pharmacopoeia developed in every culture, from Asia to the Americas, to Europe and Africa. Over an extensive period of time, Chinese herbalists documented the healing properties of more than 7,000 herbs and thousands of herbal combinations. Saint John's wort has a 2,500-year history of safe and effective use and was prescribed as medicine by Hippocrates (460–377 B.C.) himself. Galen (A.D. 129–200) described 130 herbal antidotes and medicines, and Dioscorides (first century A.D.) wrote about the medicinal properties of 500 plants and described how to prepare 1,000 simple remedies. The ancient Egyptians used peppermint and spearmint to relax the digestive tract, while Chinese and Ayurvedic doctors used mint to treat colds, coughs, and fevers (Castleman, 2017).

When Europeans came to the Americas, they found that Native Americans had a vast pharmacopoeia of medicinal plants such as birch, blackberry, coneflower, ginseng, goldenseal, and ginger that had been handed down from generation to generation. Early Jesuit missionaries in Canada discovered American ginseng in the early 1700s and exported it to Asia, where it became a highly revered tonic. The Shakers (Church of the United Society of Believers), who were great friends of Native Americans, were the first to cultivate medicinal plants in mass quantities and became the first reputable pharmaceutical manufacturers in the United States. Until the Civil War disrupted their efforts, the Shakers sold 354 varieties of therapeutic herbs. During the early 20th century, tincture of echinacea was highly valued for its antibiotic properties until synthetic antibiotics became available. Kava, used to calm the nervous system and decrease anxiety, was even sold during the 1920s in the Sears, Roebuck and Company catalog. Many herbs used in ancient times are still in use today throughout the world. Herbal medicine has generally been more widely accepted outside the United States, where health care providers often combine it with conventional therapy (Castleman, 2017).

In the 1960s, the U.S. Food and Drug Administration (FDA) developed the current regulations regarding medications. At that time, herbal medicine was not very popular and thus was virtually ignored by the FDA. Herbs are viewed as dietary supplements and are controlled by the 1994 Dietary Supplement Health and Education Act. Under this act, dietary supplements cannot make specific medical claims, as can prescription and over-the-counter (OTC) drugs. General statements such as "improves memory" or "promotes regularity" can be used as long as a disclaimer notes that the herb is not approved by the FDA and that the product is not intended to diagnose, treat, cure, or prevent any disease.

Researchers are intensifying their efforts to collect and screen more natural products for their medicinal properties. Gordon Cragg, former chief of the Natural Products Branch (NPB) of the National Cancer Institute's (NCI) Division of Cancer Treatment and Diagnosis, stated, "Nature produces chemicals that no chemist would ever dream of at the laboratory bench" (Hallowell, 1997, p. 19). A great variety of some of the most concentrated healing herbs are found in a wide band around the equator. Unfortunately, destruction of these natural plant habitats, especially tropical rain forests, is driving many species to extinction before they can be found and studied.

It is unlikely that most herbal medicines will ever win FDA approval, since the process costs approximately $100 million per drug. Large pharmaceutical companies are willing to invest this fortune in new drugs that can be patented and sold at high profits. In contrast, obtaining exclusive rights or patents to most herbs, such as garlic or ginseng, is nearly impossible, which takes away the financial incentive to get them approved for medicinal use. The lack of profit, rather than the lack of efficacy of herbs, keeps drug companies from advocating for FDA approval of herbs.

Much of what is known about herbs comes from Germany, where an expert panel called Commission E, set up in 1978, has reviewed all available literature on 650 medicinal herbs, issuing recommendations for their use. The National Center for Complementary and Integrative Health is actively involved in researching healing herbs. In addition, NCCIH is screening plants for compounds active against the AIDS virus and nine major types of cancer. Since 1986, NCCIH has received samplings of thousands of plants from ethnobotanists throughout the world. Indigenous people have been testing and using healing plants for thousands of years, but only recently have Western researchers sought their knowledge.

CONCEPTS

Synergism

The active chemicals in herbs work *synergistically*; that is, the combined action of two or more substances produces a greater effect than the sum of the effects of the individual substances acting alone. Most herbal medicines rely on the complex interplay of many chemicals for their therapeutic action, and many lose their activity when purified and isolated. For example, a number of antimicrobial compounds are found in tea tree oil, but studies indicate that no single compound in the oil is responsible for its remarkable germ-fighting ability; rather, the interaction of at least eight distinct chemicals in the oil seems to produce the effects. This complexity makes it nearly impossible for an infectious microbe to build up resistance to tea tree oil. One of the primary problems with conventional antibiotics is the ability of many microbes to develop resistance to them, thus rendering the drugs useless. Antioxidant defenses also operate synergistically. For example, a number of carotenoids working together have higher anticancer properties than does a single carotenoid. Thus, beta-carotene supplements may not provide the same protection as eating fruits and vegetables rich in beta-carotene. Other substances in a plant may help the body utilize its benefits as well as buffer any side effects. Including the whole plant in the final product often ensures that some measure of the natural "checks and balances" will be retained (Castleman, 2017; Chevallier, 2016).

Various herbs and other substances may also work synergistically with one another. A rather dramatic example of this effect was observed during the testing of plant samples from the rain forest in Ecuador for chemicals that could be used to treat diabetes. The leaves from the plant were immersed in an alcohol extract and then a water extract. The researchers debated whether to throw a live crab into the extract, just as native healers did. Some believed it might make a difference, while others believed the crab was simply ritualistic. Amazingly, the only extract that demonstrated therapeutic effect was the one with the crab in it. It turned out that a component in a crab's shell is needed to extract the active chemical compound from the plant (Cray, 1997).

Phytonutrients

Phytonutrients are chemicals present in plants that make the plants biologically active and are responsible for giving plants their color, flavor, and natural disease resistance. Phytonutrients are products of photosynthesis or are substances that serve as defense mechanisms against attacks by insects and other predators. These active components of plants usually occur in groups that complement one another's protective and healing effects. Descriptions of the most important phytonutrients and their uses are found in Table 7.1.

Antioxidants

Antioxidants are a group of vitamins, minerals, enzymes, and herbs that help protect the body against naturally occurring **free radicals,** which are molecular species containing an unpaired electron. In the body, free radicals of both oxygen and nitrogen are produced during normal metabolic processes, as well as being derived from external sources. Free radicals are unstable and highly reactive. They gain stability by either donating or accepting an electron from another molecule, thus creating more free radicals in the process. Because free radicals react so readily with other compounds, they can effect significant changes in the body. Many different factors can lead to the production of free radicals. *Internal sources,* in addition to metabolic processes, include emotional stress and strenuous exercise. *External sources* include air pollution, cigarette smoke, factory and car exhaust, smog, pesticides, herbicides, food contaminants, chemotherapy, and radiation. All cause the overproduction of free radicals. Oxidative damage can be visualized, for example, on the exposed surface of a cut apple, which turns brown as it oxidizes, that is, reacts with the oxygen in air. Humans, however, cannot "see" the damage being done by free radicals in the body. An excess of free radicals is, in part, responsible for the effects of aging and is implicated in cancer and a variety of chronic and degenerative conditions, including arthritis and heart disease (Horne & Easley, 2017; Oschman, 2016).

TABLE 7.1 Phytonutrients

Name	Properties	Use/Effects
Alkaloids	Group of nitrogen-containing compounds; analgesic, local anesthetic, sedating, antispasmodic, hallucinatory; poisonous to varying degrees	Affect both the nervous and circulatory systems. Most familiar are atropine, caffeine, cocaine, morphine, nicotine, and quinine.
Bitter principles	Group of chemicals that have an extremely bitter taste	Through a reflex action via taste buds, stimulate appetite and flow of digestive juices, stimulate liver activity and flow of bile; some act as diuretics. Viewed as overall tonics.
Carbohydrates	Main energy source and structural support of plants	In some herbs, such as coltsfoot and marshmallow, the cellulose combines with other chemicals to form mucilage, a gummy substance that, when ingested by humans, soothes and protects irritated or inflamed internal tissue.
Carotenoids	Yellow, orange, or red pigments in photosynthetic plants; converted to vitamin A in liver	Three most important to humans: Beta-carotene may aid in cancer prevention by neutralizing free radicals; used in conjunction with topical sunscreens for better prevention of sunburn and skin damage. Lycopene may prevent prostate cancer and decrease risk of heart attacks. Lutein may be useful in prevention of macular degeneration, a leading cause of blindness in the elderly.
Essential oils	Vaporize when heated; combinations give plants their particular smell	Garlic is an antiseptic, thyme is an expectorant; chamomile relieves gaseous distention and painful intestinal spasms.
Fatty oils	Mixture of triglycerides, glycerol, fatty acids	Omega-3 fatty acids are used against cardiovascular disease and depression; improve cognition.

(continued)

TABLE 7.1 Phytonutrients (*Continued*)

Name	Properties	Use/Effects
Glycosides	Complex organic substances; some of the most potent herbal remedies and among the most toxic substances known	Cardiac glycosides include foxglove and lily of the valley, which affect cardiac contractions; used to correct arrhythmias.
		Mustard glycosides are used externally and have antiseptic and analgesic effects.
		Cyanogenic glycosides release hydrogen cyanide when chewed or digested, resulting in antispasmodic, purgative, and sedative effects. Found in some nuts, vegetables, and the seeds of some fruits. Hydrogen cyanide, sometimes called prussic acid, is highly poisonous.
		Phenolic glycosides include salicylic derivatives found in willow and other plants; salicylic acid derivative is main ingredient in aspirin; antiseptic, analgesic, and anti-inflammatory effects.
		Coumarin glycosides strengthen capillary walls and act as an anticoagulant.
		Anthraquinone glycosides are used as laxatives.
		Flavonoid glycosides, known as bioflavonoids or flavonoids, improve circulation, stimulate bile production, lower cholesterol levels, and strengthen the liver.
Isoflavones	Compounds similar to human estrogen; found primarily in soy products	May prevent hormone-related cancers; lower cholesterol, relieve menopausal symptoms, prevent osteoporosis by increasing bone density.
Tannins	Chemical substances with astringent and antiseptic properties	Form a protective layer on the skin and mucous membranes and are useful in treatment of burns and local inflammation; used for eye and mouth infections.

Free radicals are normally kept under control by antioxidant enzymes, which act as scavengers to search out and neutralize dangerous free radicals. As people age, they produce fewer of these enzymes, and they may benefit from dietary antioxidants such as vitamin C, vitamin E, carotenoids, the mineral selenium, and the hormone melatonin. Herbs with antioxidant properties include bilberry, ginkgo, grape seed extract, green tea, and flavonoids. Fruits and vegetables are the primary sources of antioxidants.

Plant-Derived Products

Herbal medicines were in use even before pharmaceutical companies came into existence. In many parts of the world, treating illness with herbs is still the only medicine available. Even though only a tiny fraction of plants have been studied for medicinal benefits, conventional physicians use plant-derived products regularly. Fifty percent of all prescription and over-the-counter (OTC) drugs sold in the United States are derived from plants. Examples of herbal remedies that have been synthesized into modern drugs are reserpine from Indian snakeroot, digoxin from foxglove, quinine from Peruvian bark, aspirin from willow tree bark, morphine from opium poppy, cocaine from coca leaves, and atropine from deadly nightshade. Paclitaxel (Taxol, Abraxane) is found in Pacific yew bark and is currently being used in the treatment of early and advanced breast cancer and ovarian tumors. The drug vincristine (Oncovin) has been isolated from the Madagascar periwinkle and has been found to arrest cell division so dramatically that it is being used to treat acute leukemia and Hodgkin's disease (Chevallier, 2016; Standish, Alschuler, Weaver, & Nezami, 2014).

Safety

Not all plant life is beneficial. Most plant-related poisonings are due to accidental consumption of toxic ornamental plants such as jade, holly, poinsettia, schefflera, philodendron, and dieffenbachia rather than herbs. Data compiled by the American Association of Poison Control Centers indicate that medications such as analgesics, sedatives, antipsychotics, antidepressants, cold/cough preparations, and cardiovascular drugs are much more likely to cause adverse reactions and fatalities than are herbs.

Although the safety of herbs has not been completely established through an evidence-based approach, it is thought that the vast majority of herbal medicines present no danger if taken appropriately. Some can, however, cause serious side effects if taken in excess or, for some individuals, if taken over a prolonged period. For example, *comfrey* (a digestive remedy), *coltsfoot* (used to treat cough), and *kava* (used for anxiety) can cause liver damage if taken in large doses. *Beta-carotene* increases the risk of lung cancer among smokers. *Vitamin E* supplements increase the incidence of prostate cancer among healthy men. *Yohimbe* may lower blood pressure and contribute to a heart conduction disorder that may result in death. *Willow bark* may result in Reye's syndrome in children. *Ephedra* can increase blood pressure and contribute to seizures, myocardial infarctions, or strokes. *Bitter orange* contains synephrine that is similar to ephedra. *Kava* has been linked to severe liver damage (Horne & Easley, 2017).

Herbs can also interact with drugs, and caution should be used when combining herbs with prescription and OTC medications (see Table 7.2). The majority of people who use herbs do not inform their medical providers of this fact. Such lack of communication can lead to herb–drug interactions that might otherwise have been avoided. Any herbs that act as anticoagulants or those that potentiate anesthesia must be discontinued before surgery if at all possible.

TABLE 7.2 Herb Interactions

Herb/Supplement	May Interact with	Potential Effects
Black cohosh	Hormone replacement medications	May potentiate one another
Capsicum	Anticoagulants, aspirin	May prolong bleeding time
	Theophylline	Increases absorption, may cause toxicity
Echinacea	Immunosuppressants	Reduces effectiveness of immunosuppressants
	Antifungals; drugs known to elevate liver enzymes	May cause liver damage
Evening primrose oil	Phenothiazine medications, Wellbutrin	May increase risk of seizures
Feverfew	Anticoagulants, aspirin	May increase anticoagulant effects
Garlic	Anticoagulants, aspirin	May increase anticoagulant effects
	Hypoglycemics	May cause hypoglycemia
	Antihypertensives	May require decreased dose of antihypertensive
	HIV medications	May increase or decrease effectiveness of medications
Ginger	Anticoagulants, aspirin	May increase anticoagulant effects
Ginkgo	Anticoagulants, aspirin	May increase anticoagulant effects
	Anticonvulsants	May decrease effectiveness of anticonvulsants
Ginseng	Oral contraceptives	Increases the potency of estrogen in oral contraceptives causing side effects such as weight gain, breast pain, and vaginal bleeding
	MAO inhibitors	May result in mania
	Caffeine	May cause irritability
	Glaucoma medications	May decrease effectiveness of glaucoma medications

TABLE 7.2 *(Continued)*

Herb/Supplement	May Interact with	Potential Effects
Goldenseal	Anticoagulants, aspirin	Decreases effectiveness of anticoagulants
	Diuretics	Increases diuretic effect
	General anesthetics	May increase hypotensive effect of anesthetic
Licorice	Hypoglycemics	May interfere with regulation of blood sugar levels
	Lanoxin, Lasix, Hygroton, Lozol, Bumex	Licorice depletes potassium; may cause hypokalemia
	Thyroid replacement medication	May require higher doses of thyroid replacement drugs
	Oral contraceptives	May cause high blood pressure, fluid retention, hypokalemia
	Antihypertensives	Decreases effectiveness of antihypertensives
Ma huang	Most antihypertensives	May increase blood pressure and risk of cardiac arrhythmia
	Antidepressants	May increase blood pressure and risk of cardiac arrhythmia
	Decongestants	May increase blood pressure and risk of cardiac arrhythmia
	Lanoxin	Increases risk of cardiac arrhythmia
	Hypoglycemics	May interfere with regulation of blood sugar levels
Milk thistle	Oral contraceptives	Reduces effectiveness of oral contraceptives
Psyllium	Laxatives	May increase effects
Saint John's wort	Oral contraceptives	Reduces effectiveness of oral contraceptives
	Tetracyclines, sulfa drugs, Feldane, Prilosec, Prevacid	Extreme photosensitivity may occur; increasing risk for severe sunburn
	Antidepressants	May potentiate one another, causing severe agitation, nausea, confusion, and possible cardiac problems
	Anticonvulsants	May decrease effectiveness of anticonvulsants
	Anticoagulants	May increase anticoagulant effect

(continued)

TABLE 7.2 Herb Interactions (*Continued*)

Herb/Supplement	May Interact with	Potential Effects
	Dioxin, immunosuppressants, protease inhibitors	May reduce effectiveness of these medications
	Theophylline	May decrease serum theophylline levels
	General anesthetics	May prolong effect of anesthesia
Saw palmetto	Proscar	May potentiate each other, resulting in overdose
Valerian	Anti-anxiety medication, Benadryl, Vistaril, anticonvulsants	May increase sedative effects
	General anesthetics	Prolongs anesthesia
Vitamin A	Accutane for acne	Toxicity may occur, resulting in severe headaches, dry eyes and skin, hair loss, and possible liver damage
Vitamin B_6	Carbidopa, levodopa	May decrease effectiveness, resulting in breakthrough symptoms such as tremors

The processing and manufacturing of herbal products varies from country to country, with varying degrees of quality assurance. Contamination with heavy metals, pesticides, herbicides, insects, animals, and/or animal excreta can result in unsafe herbal products. In the United States, herbs are sold as dietary supplements and have significantly fewer requirements compared with prescription and OTC drugs. The requirements apply only to how the final product is manufactured, not to suppliers of the herbal ingredients.

TREATMENT

Medicinal herbs are available at health food stores, herb shops, supermarkets, and pharmacies. They can be used as a preventive, a tonic, or a treatment. Herbs can be prepared and used in a number of ways. **Extracts** or **tinctures** are made by pressing herbs with a heavy press and soaking them in alcohol or water, which after evaporation yields a concentrated extract. Extracts are generally measured in drops and diluted in a small amount of water for ingestion. A preparation of the delicate parts of plants—that is, leaves, flowers, and seeds—is called an **infusion**, a process similar to making tea. Hot water is poured over the herb, steeped for 3 to 5 minutes, and strained before drinking. Honey or lemon may be added to taste. **Decoction** is the preparation of the more resilient parts of plants, such as the bark, roots, and berries. These parts of the herb are usually boiled for 10 to 20 minutes and strained before drinking. A *compress* is a cloth soaked in a warm or cool herbal solution and applied directly to an injured area. An herbal *poultice* is made by mixing powered herbs with enough hot water to make a thick paste that is then applied directly to the skin. Poultices are used to reduce swelling, relieve pain, decrease muscle spasms, draw out toxins from the body, increase circulation, and speed healing. Table 7.3 lists some of the more common herbs as well as their action, dosage, and side effects.

TABLE 7.3 Common Herbs		
Name	**Properties/Use**	**Side Effects/Contraindications**
Asian ginseng	Improve mental and physical performance; lower blood glucose; improve immune function	Headaches, sleep problems, GI problems People taking medicine to lower blood sugar should use extra caution NOT for people with hypoglycemia
Bilberry	Diarrhea; menstrual cramps; varicose veins; venous insufficiency	High doses or extended use of the leaf or extract may lead to possible toxic effects
Black cohosh	Menopause; dysmenorrhea	Minimal side effects May increase bleeding NOT for people with a liver disorder NOT to be used with hormone replacement therapy NOT to be used with hormone-sensitive breast cancer
Blessed thistle	Prepared as a tea for anorexia, indigestion, diarrhea, colds, cough	May decrease the effectiveness of antacids NOT for pregnant or lactating women NOT for inflammatory intestinal problems NOT for people who have allergies to ragweed and related plants
Butterbur	Antihistamine for allergy symptoms; migraines	Belching, GI issues, asthma, fatigue. Raw, unprocessed butterbur can cause liver damage NOT for children
Calendula	1.5% ointment for diaper rash, skin inflammation due to radiation therapy; 7.5% ointment for leg ulcers caused by poor circulation	Increase the sedative effect of medications NOT for pregnant or lactating women NOT for people who have allergies to ragweed and related plants

(continued)

TABLE 7.3 Common Herbs (Continued)

Name	Properties/Use	Side Effects/Contraindications
Chamomile	Anxiety, sleeplessness, GI upset, infant colic, mouth ulcers from cancer treatment; drug withdrawal	NOT for those with extreme allergy to ragweed. NOT for pregnant or lactating women
Cranberry	Prevent urinary tract infections or *H. pylori* infections that can lead to stomach ulcers; antioxidant	Use with caution for people taking anticoagulants or medications that affect the liver
Dong quai	Premenstrual syndrome Menopause symptoms	Photosensitivity Increased bleeding
Echinacea	Prevent colds, flu; stimulate immune system	Few side effects
Evening primrose oil	Eczema; rheumatoid arthritis; breast pain; diabetic neuropathy	Well tolerated by most people NOT for pregnant or lactating women NOT for people taking anticoagulants
Fenugreek	Diabetes; loss of appetite; stimulate milk production in breastfeeding women; skin inflammation	Gas, bloating, diarrhea NOT for pregnant women NOT for women with hormone-sensitive cancers
Feverfew	Migraines; rheumatoid arthritis; psoriasis, allergies; tinnitus; dizziness	No serious side effects NOT for pregnant women
Garlic	High cholesterol; slow development of atherosclerosis; hypertension; immunomodulating	Nausea, garlicky scent NOT for people with clotting disorders NOT prior to surgery
Ginger	Nausea and vomiting of various causes; arthritis. Ginger tea and crystallized ginger calm coughs; settle digestive distress	Safe during pregnancy
Ginkgo	Memory impairment; intermittent claudication; tinnitus	Headache, nausea, GI upset NOT for people with clotting disorders NOT prior to surgery
Goldenseal	Respiratory tract infections; eye infections; vaginitis; canker sores	Few side effects
Grape seed extract	Hypertension; high cholesterol; poor circulation; vascular fragility; edema; antioxidant	Few side effects NOT prior to surgery

TABLE 7.3 *(Continued)*

Name	Properties/Use	Side Effects/Contraindications
Green tea	Cancer; mental alertness; weight loss; high cholesterol; immunomodulating	Contains caffeine
Horse chestnut	Venous insufficiency	Do NOT use raw or unprocessed plant parts, as they are poisonous
Licorice root	Stomach ulcers; bronchitis; sore throat; hepatitis C	Use with caution with diuretics, as potassium levels could drop dangerously low; use with caution for people with hypertension
Milk thistle	Liver disorders; high cholesterol; immunomodulating	NOT for pregnant or lactating women Use with caution for people with diabetes or hypoglycemia
Noni	Antioxidant; immunity stimulating; tumor fighting properties	High in potassium; use with caution for people with renal disease
Red clover	Menopause; high cholesterol; osteoporosis; prostate enlargement	Few side effects Unclear if it is safe for pregnant or lactating women or hormone-sensitive cancers
Saint John's wort	Minor depression	Photosensitivity, anxiety, dry mouth, sexual problems NOT for use with other antidepressants NOT for children NOT for pregnant or lactating women
Saw palmetto	Urinary antiseptic; benign prostatic hyperplasia	Few side effects Increase bleeding NOT for pregnant or lactating women
Tea tree oil	Antifungal, antiseptic; acne; minor wounds and cuts; athlete's foot; nail infections; herpes; douche for yeast infections	ONLY for topical use
Turmeric	Anti-inflammatory, antimicrobial, antioxidant; osteoarthritic pain; control blood sugar	Increased bleeding Uterine contractions in pregnant women
Valerian	Insomnia; menopause; menstrual and intestinal cramps	Excitability, uneasiness, fatigue, headache; increase sedative effects

RESEARCH

Most herbal medicines have not been tested as thoroughly as have prescription drugs in the United States, although the National Center for Complementary and Integrative Health, the National Cancer Institute, and the Society for Integrative Oncology fund many herbal research trials. South Africa has more than 20,000 plant species, several thousand of which are used by traditional healers. Research teams from the United States are teaming up with the South African Herbal Science and Medicine Institute to study the medicinal properties, safety, and effectiveness of several of these African plants. In contrast, many scientific studies have been conducted outside the United States on a variety of herbal remedies, such as those by Commission E in Germany, mentioned previously. In the coming years, the pharmacopoeia of useful herbs is likely to expand, since research in the field of herbal medicine is on the rise worldwide.

In 1995, the American Herbal Pharmacopoeia (AHP) was organized as an educational foundation to disseminate information regarding the pharmacology, actions, indications, dosages, side effects, contraindications, drug interactions, and toxicology of herbs. To date, their information covers 140 medicinal plant species, representing 90% of the herb sales in the United States. The goal of AHP is for health care providers in the United States to integrate herbal medicines into treatment plans, as their contemporaries have done in other countries.

The quality of herbal products can affect study outcomes and the degree to which herbs can be integrated into evidence-based medicine. Quality can be affected by environmental conditions; herb collection practices; handling, storage, and manufacturing conditions; and contamination.

The following is a small sample of the research:

- A systematic review was conducted to determine the effects of herbs on hot flushes and at least one other symptom of menopause. Black cohosh mixed with other herbs, *Rheum rhaponticum*, and French maritime pine bark had significant effects on hot flushes and at least one or more symptoms such as sleep, mood, cognition, or pain (Ismail et al., 2015).
- Many women use black cohosh as a treatment for menopausal symptoms. Since it has estrogenic activity, there is a question of its use in women with or at risk for breast cancer. A systematic review found that there was no significant association between black cohosh and increased risk of breast cancer (Fritz et al., 2014).
- A systematic review of preoperative melatonin, compared to a placebo, significantly reduced preoperative anxiety, and may reduce postoperative anxiety (Hansen, Halladin, Rosenberg, Gogenur, & Moller, 2015).
- A systematic review examined the evidence of both topical and ingested turmeric to treat skin diseases. There was significant improvement in disease severity in both topical and ingested turmeric groups compared with control groups (Vaughn, Branum, & Sivamani, 2016).

- A randomized, parallel-group, double-blind, placebo-controlled trial considered the effect of topical saffron for men with diabetes and erectile dysfunction. Compared to the placebo, the saffron gel significantly improved erectile dysfunction (Mohammadzadeh-Moghadam et al., 2015).
- A randomized, double-blind, placebo-controlled trial was conducted to see if cocoa flavanol improved vascular function in patients on hemodialysis. There was significant vascular improvement in high-risk population (Rassaf et al., 2016).

INTEGRATED NURSING PRACTICE

Because herbs are marketed as "natural" or promoted as foods, consumers may assume incorrectly that herbs are safe and without side effects. It is important to remember that natural remedies must be approached with respect. They work because they have strong pharmacological activity. It is important to teach clients that although herbs are generally safer than prescription drugs, if herbs are abused or overused, they can cause harm.

Although herbs can be quite effective, it is important to caution people about becoming overzealous about their use. If they have a life-threatening illness such as asthma or if they experience chest pain or if they notice more benign symptoms that persist for longer than a few days, they should seek medical attention. While it may be helpful to take echinacea for an incipient cold, any serious ailment should first be diagnosed by a health care practitioner. Self-diagnosis and self-care are by nature subject to limits. Conventional medicine is best used in crisis situations, and herbs are best used in noncrisis situations. Professionals can save consumers from treating something that does not exist or failing to treat something that does. Further, health practitioners can help individuals evaluate the extent of their progress on the herbal regimen. Consultation is especially important if people are taking other medications; although some herbs can work with prescription drugs, others may not. Some herbs potentiate the effects of drugs, so individuals may need a lower dose of their regular medication. Suddenly stopping a prescription can be hazardous to one's health. Pregnant and lactating women should always consult their primary care practitioner before taking any herbal medicines.

Herbs should be used with caution with children. Children are not "small adults" and may experience side effects that are different from those experienced by adults. Parents or caregivers should consult with the child's primary care professional before using any herbs with children.

Nurses must be open to exploring and discussing their clients' use of and questions about herbal medicine. This clinical screening allows evaluation of herbal intake against known and potential adverse interactions with prescription and over-the-counter (OTC) medications. Prior to surgery, clients must tell health care providers what herbs and supplements they are taking. Some may affect the response to anesthetics or to other medication and some may increase the risk of bleeding.

As a nurse, you need to educate consumers about potential actions and interactions of herbal remedies. People cannot expect to take an herb for a few days to undo 10 years of poor health habits nor to replace a healthy diet with herbal supplements. If people eat a healthful, varied diet that is high in fresh foods, especially fruits, vegetables, and whole grains, they do not need to take supplements unless they have special needs (Weil, 1998).

Sometimes, walking into a health food store or pharmacy is highly confusing. Many people are overwhelmed by the wide assortment of products and brands. As a nurse, you can teach consumers the following basic guidelines in selecting herbal medicines:

- Store clerks are not experts. They do not have an adequate scientific background to counsel people.
- Go with a name brand. Since the industry is unregulated, it is best to choose products made by large, reputable companies that have been in business for a long time. Many excellent products are produced in Germany and France, where they must meet strict production standards.
- Check the label. Look for the word *standardized*, which tells you that the product consistently contains a certain percentage of a specific chemical.
- Check to see whether the claims are reasonable. Be wary of promises of instant cures for complicated disorders. If something sounds too good to be true, it probably is.
- Consider the product's form. A liquid, powder, or solid extract is generally best. Bulk herbs can lose their potency quickly. Many herbal tinctures are 50% grain alcohol, which may be a problem for people with a history of alcohol abuse or for those who take drugs that can interact with alcohol.
- Be wary of ultracombination products. If the product has more than six ingredients, it probably contains a small amount of each. A combination of herbs does not necessarily make the product better. If you need ginkgo to boost your memory, it is better to get it full strength than to get a product diluted with ginseng, garlic, and other herbs.
- Take the right dose. Do not take higher doses than the label recommends. Exceeding the recommended dose can lead to toxicity. Most herbal remedies are not to be given to children under the age of 1 unless directed by an experienced practitioner. Children ages 1 to 6 are typically given one-third the adult dose, while children ages 6 to 12 receive half the adult dose. People over the age of 65 may need a reduced dosage.
- Watch for side effects. If you have any unusual symptoms, such as allergies, rashes, heart palpitations, or headaches, stop taking the herb immediately and see a health care practitioner.
- Give the product time to work. Evaluate how it makes you feel. After 30 days, ask yourself whether the product has made a difference in your health. If you are not sure, stop taking the herb to gauge the difference.

- Inform your primary health care practitioner about the herbal remedies you are taking.
- If you plan on regularly using herbal remedies, invest in a good herbal reference guide to ensure your access to proper information, or consult with the one of the organizations in the resource list. The U.S. Department of Agriculture provides free access to 80,000 records, developed by Dr. James A. Duke, on herb taxonomy and use of herbs worldwide.

As a nurse, it is also important that you warn consumers about remedies that can be risky. Chaparral, sold as teas and pills to fight cancer and "purify blood," has been linked to serious liver damage. Dieter's teas, containing such ingredients as senna, aloe, rhubarb root, buckthorn, cascara, and castor oil, act as laxatives that when consumed in excessive amounts can disrupt potassium levels and contribute to cardiac arrhythmias. Ephedra is a cardiac and nervous system stimulant that can cause anxiety, psychotic episodes, hypertension, stroke, tachycardia, arrhythmias, and cardiac arrest. The Food and Drug Administration has banned the sale in the United States of supplements containing ephedra. The ban does not apply to traditional Chinese herbal remedies that are regulated as conventional foods.

TRY THIS
Herbal Remedies

Peppermint Tea

Used to soothe an upset stomach, aid digestion, relieve menstrual cramps, soothe sore throats, improve alertness.

How to

Combine 1 to 2 teaspoons of dried peppermint leaf with 8 ounces of water. Steep for 3 to 5 minutes. Strain and drink the tea.

Chamomile

An excellent home remedy for indigestion, heartburn, and infant colic. It also soothes skin and has mild relaxant and sedative properties.

How to

For an infusion, use 2–3 heaping teaspoons of dried or 1/3 cup of fresh flowers per cup of boiling water. Steep for 10–20 minutes. Strain and drink up to 3 cups a day. Diluted infusions may be given to infants for colic.

For a relaxing herbal bath, fill a cloth bag with a few handfuls of dried or fresh flowers and let the water run over it.

For allergic skin rashes, tightly pack a jar of flower heads, and cover them with olive oil. Cover and set in a sunny place for 3 weeks. Strain and apply to rashes.

(continued)

Comfrey

External use only. Promotes the growth of new cells and has a mild anti-inflammatory action. Used in wound and burn treatment.

How to

Mix the powdered root with water to make a paste. Apply to the injured area and cover with a clean bandage. Change daily.

Ginger

Decreases nausea, boosts the immune system, lowers blood pressure.

How to

Use 2 teaspoons of powdered or grated root per cup of boiling water. Steep for 20 minutes, strain, and add juice from half a lemon and honey to taste. Drink hot up to 3 cups a day. Dilute ginger infusion to treat infant colic. If you buy whole root, refrigerate it.

Mint

Relaxes the digestive tract; used to treat colds, coughs, and fevers.

How to

For an infusion, use 1 teaspoon of fresh herb or 2 teaspoons of dried leaves per cup of boiling water. Steep for 10 minutes, strain, and drink up to 3 cups a day. Peppermint has a sharper taste than spearmint and feels cooler in the mouth.

For a relaxing herbal bath, fill a cloth bag with a few handfuls of dried or fresh leaves and let the water run over it.

Rosemary

Stimulates circulation and relaxes tired and sore muscles.

How to

For tired, sore feet, make a footbath by adding 10 drops of essential oil to a basin of hot water large enough to hold both feet. Stir the oil into the water with your hand.

The U.S. public is demanding more information about herbal remedies. In the best of all worlds, consumers would have an educated professional—a nurse, a pharmacist, or a doctor—to help guide them through the process of using herbal remedies. That is the situation in Germany, where health care practitioners and pharmacists must be knowledgeable about natural remedies, their approved uses, their potential side effects, and how they should be prescribed. This is not the case in the United States, but it surely will change in the near future. Schools of nursing and schools of medicine are including courses on complementary and alternative medicine in their curriculum. Pharmacy schools now require their students to take a course in herbal therapy.

As nurse–author Carolyn Kresse Murray (1996) said, "Part of patient advocacy is making sure you help your patient with all his [her] therapies. Equipping yourself with knowledge about herbal therapies is another way to keep him [her] from harm" (p. 59).

References

Burlin, N. C. (1907). *The Indians' Book: An Offering by the American Indians of Indian Lore, Musical and Narrative, to Form a Record of the Songs and Legends of Their Race*. Harper and Brothers.

Castleman, M. (2017). *The New Healing Herbs*. Emmaus, PA: Rodale Books.

Chevallier, A. (2016). *Encyclopedia of Herbal Medicine* (3rd ed.). New York, NY: Penguin Random House.

Cray, D. (1997). Money that grows on trees. *Time*, Fall special issue, 150(19): 21.

Fritz, H., Seely, D., McGowan, J., Skidmore, B., Fernandes, R., Kennedy, D. A., . . . Fergusson, D. (2014). Black cohosh and breast cancer: A systematic review. *Integrative Cancer Therapies*. doi: 10.1177/1534735413477191

Hallowell, C. (1997). The plant hunter. *Time*, Fall special issue, 150(19): 17–22.

Hansen, M. V., Halladin, N. L., Rosenberg, J., Gogenur, I., & Moller, A. M. (2015). Melatonin for pre- and postoperative anxiety in adults. *Cochrane Database of Systematic Reviews*. doi: 10.1002/14651858.CD009861.pub2

Hippocrates. (1983). *Hippocratic Writings Classic Series*, Vol. 451 of Penguin Classics.

Horne, S., & Easley, T. (2017). *The Modern Herbal Medicine Reference Guide*. Berkeley, CA: North Atlantic Books.

Ismail, R., Taylor-Swanson, L., Thomas, A., Schnall, J. G., Cray, L., Mitchell, E. S., & Woods, N. F. (2015). Effects of herbal preparations on symptom clusters during the menopausal transition. *Climacteric*. doi: 10.3109/13697137.2014.900746

Mohammadzadeh-Moghadam, H., Nazari, S. M., Shamsa, A., Kamalinejad, M. Esmaeeli, H., Asadpour, A. A., & Khajavi, A. (2015). Effects of a topical saffron (*Crocus sativus* L) gel on erectile dysfunction in diabetics. *Evidence-Based Complementary and Alternative Medicine*. doi: 10.1177/2156587215583756

Murray, C. K. (1996). Cultivating your knowledge about herbal remedies. *Nursing*, 26(12): 58–59.

Murray, C. K. (1996). *Walking the Spiritual Walk*. Virginia Beach, VA: A.R. E. Press.

Oschman, J. L. (2016). *Energy Medicine: The Scientific Basis* (2nd ed.). St. Louis: Elsevier.

Qureshi, R., Ghazanfar, S. A., Obied, H., Vasileva, V., & Tariq, M. A. (2016). Ethobotany: A living science for alleviating human suffering. *Evidence-Based Complementary and Alternative Medicine*. doi: 10.1155/2016/9641692

Rassaf, T., Rammos, C., Hendgen-Cotta, U. B., Heiss, C., Kleophas, W., Dellanna, F., . . . Kelm, M. (2016). Vasculoprotective effects of dietary cocoa flavanols in patients on hemodialysis: A double-blind, randomized, placebo-controlled trial. *Clinical Journal of the American Society of Nephrology*. doi: 10.2215/CJN.05560515

Standish, L. J., Alschuler, I. N., Weaver, M., & Nezami, M. (2014). Botanical and mycological medicine in integrative oncology. In D. I. Abrams & A. T. Weil (Eds.), *Integrative Oncology* (2nd ed., pp. 160–245). New York, NY: Oxford University Press.

Sutton, J. (1991). *Words of Wellness: A treasury of Quotations for Well-Being.* Carson, CA: Hay House.

Vaughn, A. R., Branum, A., & Sivamani, R. K. (2016). Effects of turmeric (*Curcuma longa*) on skin health: A systematic review. *Phytotherapy Research.* doi: 10.1002/ptr.5640

Vintage Archives Staff. (1999). Ecclesiasticus 38:4. *King James Bible* 1611.

Weil, A. (1998). Ask the experts. *Natural Health,* (January–February): 24–28.

Resources

American Botanical Council
P.O. Box 144345
Austin, TX 78714-4345
512.926.4900
www.abc.herbalgram.org

American Herbalists Guild
P.O. Box 3076
Ashville, NC 28802-3076
617.520.4372
www.americanherbalistsguild.com

American Herbal Pharmacopoeia
P.O. Box 66809
Scotts Valley, CA 95067
831.461.6318
www.herbal-ahp.org

British Herbal Medicine Association
P.O. Box 583
Exeter EX1 9GX
44(0)845.680.1134
www.bhma.info

Herb Research Foundation
4140 15th St.
Boulder, CO 80304
800.748.2617
www.herbs.org

NAPRALERT (NAtural PRoducts ALERT)
The Program for Collaborative Research in the Pharmaceutical Sciences

College of Pharmacy
University of Illinois at Chicago
833 South Wood St.
Chicago, IL 60612
312.996.9035
www.napralert.org

National Naturopaths and Herbalists Association of Australia
P.O. Box 696
Ashfield, NSW 2131, Australia
61.2.9797. 2244
www.nhaa.org.au

Ontario Herbalists Association
P.O. Box 123, Station D
Etobicoke, ON M9A 4X2
877.642.4372
www.herbalists.on.ca

U.S. Food and Drug Administration
10903 New Hampshire Ave
Silver Spring, MD 20993-0002
888.463.6332
www.fda.gov

Wise Woman Apprentice Program
P.O. Box 64
Woodstock, NY 12498
845.246.8081
www.susunweed.com

8

Aromatherapy

Earth laughs in flowers.

RALPH WALDO EMERSON

Aromatherapy is the therapeutic use of essential oils of plants to heal the body, mind, and spirit. It is an offshoot of herbal medicine, and its basis of action is the same as that of modern pharmacology. The chemicals found in the essential oils are absorbed into the body, resulting in physiological or psychological benefit. Aromatherapy is used to treat symptoms, so it has neither a theory of health and illness nor a system of diagnosis, in contrast with biomedicine, Traditional Chinese Medicine, and the like.

Scientists have long known that certain scents have the power to evoke strong physical and emotional reactions, but rarely has that knowledge been used in conventional medicine. Healthy humans can smell as many as 10,000 different odors, ranging from the deep fragrance of jasmine to the putrid stench of sewage. Most people, however, do not realize how much the sense of smell affects their daily lives.

Aromatherapy has been forgotten and ignored for many years but is now one of the fastest growing alternative therapies in Europe and the United States. The term *aromatherapy* has become more than a buzzword since the mid-1980s. In the United States, it is now a generic term in the public domain and, as such, cannot be trademarked by an individual or business.

Aromachology is a term coined by the Sense of Smell Institute to describe the scientific study of fragrances, both natural and synthetic, as applied to psychology and human behavior. A systematic review of 18 studies found that odors can affect mood and behavior in humans (Herz, 2009).

Essential oils come from all over the world—lavender from France, sandalwood and jasmine from India, rose from Turkey and Bulgaria, geranium from the island of Réunion, eucalyptus and tea tree from Australia, and mint from the United States, to name a few examples. Today, only 3% of essential oils are used in therapy; the remaining 97% are used in the perfume and cosmetic industry. Owing to increased popularity, aromatherapy has become a $1 billion industry.

BACKGROUND

Almost all ancient cultures recognized the value of aromatic plants in maintaining health. Ancient Egyptians used scented oils daily to soften and protect their skin from the harsh, dry climate. They created various fragrances for personal benefit as well as for use in rituals and ceremonies. Fragrances were considered a part of the personal purification necessary to reach a realm of higher spirituality. Oils were dispersed into the air to purify the environment and to protect against evil spirits. Egyptians were the first to perfect embalming with the use of aromatic plants and oils.

Priests and physicians used oils thousands of years before the time of Christ. The Ebers Papyrus, discovered in 1817, dates to 1500 B.C. and mentions more than 800 different formulas of herbal prescriptions and remedies. The Romans diffused oils in their temples and political buildings and bathed in hot tubs scented with oils. Ancient Arabian people studied the chemistry of plants and developed the process of distillation for extraction of essential oils. Throughout Asia, perfumes were prized for both medicinal and cosmetic properties. Hundreds of references are made to oils in the Bible such as frankincense, myrrh, and cinnamon. Many were used as protection against disease and for anointing and healing the sick (Butje, 2017). Hippocrates, the father of Western medicine, reportedly said, "The way to health is to have an aromatic bath and scented massage every day" (Thomas, 2002, p. 10).

In the 12th century, trade routes from the Middle East introduced spices, herbs, and exotic scents to Europe, leading to the compilation of many books on therapeutic plant remedies. In the Americas, shamans also used herbs and aromatics in bathing patients to transform their energy field. Smoke from plants was often blown over patients as part of healing ceremonies (Stiles, 2017).

Although oils were used with great effectiveness in ancient times, they were largely forgotten by the Western world until resurrected in the 20th century by a French cosmetic chemist, Maurice-Rene Gattefosse. While working in his laboratory in 1920, he had an accident that resulted in a third-degree burn of his hand and forearm. He plunged his arm into a vat of lavender oil, thinking that it was water. To his surprise, the burning stopped within a few moments. With the continual application of lavender oil over the next few weeks, the burn healed completely without a trace of a scar. This incident was the beginning of Gattefosse's fascination with the therapeutic properties of essential oils. He carried out experiments using oils to cure burns, to treat wounds, and to prevent gangrene and in 1937 coined the term *aromatherapie* (Lewis, 2015).

PREPARATION

Since the 1980s, numerous schools of massage and aromatherapy have opened in the United Kingdom, France, and Japan. Training in aromatherapy has grown, and courses in it are part of the nursing degree program in some nursing colleges and universities. Aromatherapists practice in a number of settings, including private practices, general medical clinics, and hospitals.

Some people in the United States, after a weekend course, call themselves "aromatherapists." They may know little about plant chemistry and the specific ways in which the oils need to be formulated. Their self-proclaimed title is fine if they use oils only for fragrance and perfume. However, it is inappropriate for individuals with this limited knowledge to use oil formulas for a specific therapeutic action. Jane Buckle, PhD, RN (www.rjbuckle.com) offers a 45-hour CEU program that is available only to registered nurses (RNs) and licensed massage therapists (LMTs). Those who successfully complete the program become certified Clinical Aromatherapy Practitioners (Buckle, 2015). Valerie Cooksley, RN, OCN, FAAIM, and Laraine Kyle Pounds, RN, MSN, who founded the Integrative Institute of Aromatherapy, offer an Integrative Aromatherapy® Certification Program, which consists of 310 contact hours for RNs (Valerie@aroma-rn.com).

Both these programs have been developed in conjunction with and approved by the American Holistic Nurses Association. In addition, the National Association for Holistic Aromatherapy has established certification guidelines and Standards of Training Levels.

CONCEPTS

Essential Oils

Essential oils are volatile liquids that are distilled or cold pressed from plants. Although chemically they are oils and as such do not mix with water, the term *oil* is somewhat misleading, since essential oils feel like water rather than oil. Varying amounts of essential oil can be extracted from a particular plant, which influences the price of the oil. For example, 1 ounce of jasmine may cost $150, while the same amount of tea tree oil may cost only a few dollars. The orange tree is a good example of a plant from which oils are extracted from various parts. Neroli oil comes from the orange tree blossoms, orange oil from the fruit itself, and petitgrain oil from the leaves of the tree. The following are other examples of plant parts from which oils are derived:

Leaves: eucalyptus, peppermint, petitgrain
Flowers: lavender, rose
Blossoms: neroli
Fruits: lemon, mandarin, orange
Grasses: lemongrass
Wood: camphor, sandalwood
Barks: cinnamon

Gum: frankincense
Bulbs: garlic, onion
Dried flower buds: clove

Essential oils are stored in tiny pockets between plant cell walls. As the oil is released, it circulates through the plant and sends messages that help the plant function efficiently. Oils activate and regulate such activities as cellular metabolism, photosynthesis, and cellular respiration. They may also trigger immune responses to assist in coping with stressful changes in the environment and climate. Some oils protect the plant from predators, especially microorganisms, and in so doing are essentially antibacterial, antiviral, and antifungal. Some oils protect the plant by repelling harmful insects, while others attract insects or animals that are useful for propagation (Lara et al., 2016).

Plant oils are highly concentrated, and it is important to respect their power. One drop of oil is the medical equivalent of 1 ounce of the parent plant material used in herbal medicine. Essential oils are chemically diverse and may contain a mixture of more than 100 organic compounds, including esters, alcohols, aldehydes, ketones, phenols, and acids. Each oil may contain more of some compounds than others, which impart to the oil its particular therapeutic properties. Table 8.1 lists some of the major chemical components and their therapeutic effects.

Hydrosols

Hydrosols, sometimes called *plant waters,* are extracted from plants during the process of steam distillation. In addition to the essential oil, a condensate water is produced that contains all the components of the plant. In essence, a hydrosol is equivalent to a homeopathic version of the essential oil and is diluted in the same manner (see Chapter 9 for information on dilution). The use of hydrosols in aromatherapy is quite new but growing, since they are gentle, safe, and highly effective in extremely low dilutions (Kennedy, 2016b).

How Essential Oils Work

The sense of smell is an important part of aromatherapy. Inside the human nose is a small cavity called the *vomeronasal organ* (VNO), which is lined with a cell type that is unlike any other in the human body. The VNO is far less prominent in people than in animals, which depend more heavily on smell for guidance. Pheromones are chemical substances produced by an animal that cause a specific reaction in another, usually of the same species, through smell. The VNO appears to specialize in detecting pheromones without people's conscious awareness. In other words, people do not "smell" pheromones in the same way they smell freshly baked apple pies or essential oils. The scent, however, is registered at some brain level, and people respond to it emotionally and/or physically (Salazar, Barrios, & SaNchez-Quinteiro, 2016).

TABLE 8.1 Chemical Compounds of Essential Oils and Their Therapeutic Actions

Chemical Compound	Therapeutic Action	Examples of Oils
Aldehydes	Anti-inflammatory, vasodilators, calm central nervous system	Citronella, melissa, cinnamon bark, lemongrass, lemon, lime, verbena
Esters	Similar to alcohols; antifungal, anti-inflammatory, antispasmodic; generally safe; low toxicity	Ylang-ylang, neroli, bergamot, lavender, clary sage, petitgrain, geranium, citronella
Hydrocarbons Terpenes	Antiseptic, bactericidal, antiviral; may be expectorant, decongestant, stimulant	Bay, verbena, pine, juniper, tea tree
Ketones	Calming, sedative, analgesic, promote wound healing; not for long-term use; never used in pregnancy	Caraway, dill, spearmint, peppermint, jasmine, rosemary, sage, fennel
Lactones	Calming; potentially photocarcinogenic; triggered by action of light; never use before sun exposure	Bergamot, orange, mandarin, lemon
Oxygenated hydrocarbons Alcohols	Antiviral, bactericidal, stimulate immune system; non-skin irritating; generally safe for children and the elderly	Rose, geranium, citronella, rosewood, coriander, eucalyptus
Phenols	Antiseptic, bactericidal, stimulate immune system, stimulate central nervous system; very potent; handle with great care, since these can irritate the skin and mucous membranes	Thyme, sage, oregano, clove, cinnamon leaf, ylang-ylang

Sources: Butje (2017); Kennedy (2016a); Tisserand and Young (2014); Young (2017).

In addition to the VNO, the nose contains 5 million smell-sensing cells that allow people to consciously register smells. Each cell has 6 to 12 hairlike receptors (cilia) that hang down into the stream of air rushing into the nose. These olfactory receptors are the only sensory pathways that open directly to the brain. The cilia detect scents, and the nerve cells relay this information directly to the limbic system, triggering memories and influencing behavior. The amygdala of the limbic system, which stores and releases emotional memories, is most sensitive to odor or fragrance. Thus, the sense of smell can evoke powerful memories in a split second and change people's perceptions and behaviors. Odors are powerful memory stimulants even when they are not actually present. Just thinking or talking about a particular odor can unleash many memories. Olfactory stimulation can trigger negative responses such as intense fear or panic, or can trigger positive feelings with increased release of endorphins and neurotransmitters. Odors stimulate the pituitary gland and hypothalamus and thus affect the production of hormones that control appetite, insulin production, body temperature, metabolism, stress levels, and sex drive. Unlike vision and hearing, the sense of smell is fully functional at birth. Newborns can recognize their mothers by smell, and this sensory response is an important part of bonding. In adult relationships, the sense of smell has a significant role in sensual and sexual attraction (Parma, Ferraro, Miller, Ahs, & Lundstrom, 2015).

Perception of odors falls along a continuum from one person to another. The ability to normally detect odors is referred to as *normosmia*. A decreased sense of smell is *hyposmia* and an inability to detect odors is *anosmia*. The sense of smell is an important aspect of food enjoyment. As people age, the ability to detect and identify odors decreases, which may lead to a lowered or even inadequate food intake (Seow, Ong, & Huang, 2016).

In addition to activating the central nervous system, inhaled oil molecules enter the respiratory system. There, the molecules attach to oxygen molecules and circulate throughout the body, bringing with them the potential for activating self-healing processes. The equivalent in conventional medicine is the use of inhalers in the treatment of asthma. Essential oils can be inhaled directly or mixed with a carrier oil. Electrical and fan-assisted equipment or an aromatherapy lightbulb ring may be used to scent a room for therapeutic purposes or to simply make the environment more pleasant. Steam inhalers can be used in the treatment of respiratory infections.

Applied externally, essential oils can calm inflamed or irritated skin, soothe sore muscles, decrease muscular tension, and release muscle spasms. Molecules of essential oils are so tiny that they are quickly absorbed through the skin and enter the intercellular fluid and the circulatory system, bringing healing nutrients to the cells. Some oils such as basil, tea tree, and thyme encourage the production of white blood cells, while others such as lavender and eucalyptus fight harmful bacteria, viruses, and fungi. Oils may be applied just about anywhere: neck, face, wrists, over the heart, back, arms, legs, and feet. Massage therapists and acupuncturists often use essential oils in their treatments. Benefits are gained not only from the penetration of the oil through the skin but also from inhalation of the vapor and from direct massage of the skin and muscles. Essential oils do not remain in the body but are excreted in urine, feces, perspiration, and exhalation, usually in 3 to 6 hours (Benjamin, 2016).

A diffuser is a special air pump designed to disburse the oil as an extremely fine vapor into the atmosphere, where it stays suspended for several hours. Diffusing releases antiviral, antibacterial, and antiseptic properties. Unlike commercial air fresheners, which mask odors, essential oils clean the air by altering the structure of the molecules that create an unpleasant smell. Essential oils help remove dust particles from the air and, when diffused in the room, can be an effective air filtration system. Diffusers should be used with caution by people with respiratory problems and/or allergies, by children, and by pregnant women.

It is also believed that there is a psychological component to the effect of essential oils. Odors associated with either positive or negative emotional feelings and experiences trigger the same feelings when smelled at a later date. For example, a person may smell bus fumes and instantly recall a bus trip taken as a young child. The olfactory nerve is only two synapses away from the amygdala (involved in emotions) and three synapses away from the hippocampus (involved in memory). Thus, both feeling and memories are an almost instantaneous response to certain odors (Parma et al., 2015).

TREATMENT

Essential oils influence health on physical, mental, and emotional levels. They have the ability to penetrate cell membranes and transport oxygen and nutrients to the cell, and many have antiviral, antibacterial, antifungal, and antiseptic properties. This property of oils may be significant in the future as microbes continue to mutate and develop resistance to known medications. Aromatherapy can be used to

- prompt the body and mind to function more efficiently,
- decrease and manage stress,
- refresh or recharge oneself,
- regulate moods, by either energizing or sedating,
- aid restful sleep,
- act as a first-aid measure,
- reduce weight,
- boost the immune system,
- minimize the discomforts of illness and speed recovery, and
- refresh a room environment.

The purity and authenticity of essential oils is critical to their effectiveness. Oils that are diluted, adulterated, or synthetic should not be used for aromatherapy. Those identified as commercial-grade essential oils are likely to be diluted or adulterated in some way. Some are diluted with chemical carriers and passed on to the consumer as "pure essential oils." These are often found in bath and cosmetic shops. Those labeled as "infused oils" are also adulterated. "Nature identical" oils are synthetic petrochemical-based products. They have been developed to closely mimic the smell and composition of essential oils. They are not identical, however, and lack many of the healing components of essential oils. Other names for synthetic oils are *aroma-chemicals, perfume oils,* and *fragrance oils.* Manufacturers are not restricted in labeling essential oils. In general, those described with terms such as *genuine, authentic,* or *premium* are more likely to be pure essential oils. Informed consumers read labels carefully and buy from reputable dealers.

Essential oils are quite potent and can irritate the skin, so they should be diluted with a carrier oil before being used on the skin. Carrier oils contain vitamins, proteins, and minerals that provide the body with added nutrients. Some carrier oils can be purchased at supermarkets, while others may be available only at health food stores. Carrier oils include apricot kernel oil, sunflower oil, soy oil, sweet almond oil, grapeseed oil, sesame oil, avocado oil,

---

BOX 8.1

Blending Oils According to Effects

Soothing oils: Chamomile
Uplifting oils: Black pepper, coriander, jasmine, juniper, eucalyptus, peppermint, tea tree
Balancing oils: Cypress, lavender
Uplifting and soothing oils: Basil, bergamot, frankincense, ginger, neroli, orange, patchouli, sandalwood
Uplifting and stimulating oils: Cedarwood, lemon, lemongrass, myrrh, pine, rose, rosemary, ylang-ylang
Uplifting and balancing oils: Clary sage, geranium

Examples of Blends

Basil, lavender
Bergamot, cypress, jasmine
Chamomile, lavender
Clary sage, lavender, sandalwood
Eucalyptus, chamomile, lavender, bergamot
Geranium, bergamot, lemon, lavender
Ginger, lavender, orange, neroli
Jasmine, rose, lemon, black pepper
Juniper, bergamot, geranium, frankincense
Lemon, tea tree, ylang-ylang
Pine, eucalyptus, lavender
Patchouli, bergamot, geranium
Peppermint, lavender
Sandalwood, ylang-ylang, black pepper, neroli

jojoba, and wheat-germ oil. The fragrance does not have to be intense to be effective. In fact, the more intense the odor, the less pleasant it becomes.

Blending together two or more pure essential oils can create a synergistic effect; that is, the blend can be more powerful than the sum of its parts. The interaction of the oils also adds vibrancy to the blend. Essential oils that complement each other are combined. For example, the calming effects of lavender and bergamot or rosemary work well together. Oils that produce opposite effects, such as a soothing oil and a stimulating oil, should not be blended. It is also important that the blend have a pleasing scent. See Box 8.1 for categories of oils to consider when formulating blends. See books on essential oils for amounts of oils to use.

RESEARCH

The research basis for aromatherapy is in its infancy. Much of the research has been performed on animals and isolated tissue cultures. Few trials have been conducted on humans under clinical conditions. Many of the studies are practice-based and anecdotal, and little is known at this time about possible interactions with conventional medications or treatments. Nurses are conducting much of the aromatherapy research in conventional health-care settings. A number of studies are being done in intensive care settings and in the fields of midwifery, palliative care, and geriatric care. Difficulties with research include chemical inconsistencies across laboratories, the impact of culture on odor perception, individual experiences with odors, and gender differences in sensitivity to odors.

The following is a small sample of findings of aromatherapy studies:

- A systematic review was conducted regarding olfaction and depression. Subjects who presented with primary depression were found to have hyposmia and subjects who presented with olfactory dysfunction were found to have depressive symptoms that worsened with the severity of hyposmia (Kohli, Soler, Nguyen, Muus, & Schlosser, 2016).
- A systematic review was conducted investigating the relationship between chronic rhinosinusitis and olfactory loss. It was found that a significant percentage of subjects experienced olfactory problems with scores in the hyposmia range (Kohli et al., 2016).
- Some previous studies found that people with visual impairment have increased olfactory abilities. A study found that the olfactory abilities of early-blind and late-blind people were no different than sighted people (Sorokowska, 2016).
- A randomized controlled trial was designed to determine the effects of massage with lavender oil on restless leg syndrome (RLS) in patients on hemodialysis. It was found that lavender oil massage effectively reduced the severity of RLS in the intervention group through a combination of muscle relaxant and sedative effects of lavender oil (Hashemi, Hajbagheri, & Aghajani, 2015).

INTEGRATED NURSING PRACTICE

Worldwide, nurses are increasingly providing aromatherapy in a variety of health care settings. Essential oils can be combined with carrier oils and used for back rubs and foot rubs to help clients relax and decrease their levels of anxiety. Other essential oils can be used as an adjunct to conventional approaches to boost the production of white blood cells and to utilize their antibacterial or antiviral action. Acute-care and long-term care settings often have unpleasant smells in rooms and hallways. Essential oils such as rosemary, lemon, tangerine, mandarin, and lemongrass can be diffused into the air to alter the structure of the molecules creating the odor, thus refreshing the environment. Diffusion of essential oils can also help boost the client's immune system, decrease anxiety and stress, aid restful sleep, and speed recovery. Essential oils can be used to enhance sedation, thereby decreasing the need for nighttime medication.

Nurses can teach people a number of things about the **safe** use of essential oils. As a general rule, people should purchase essential oils in natural and health food stores rather than stores selling beauty products and perfumes. Oils should be stored in tightly closed dark vials away from heat, light, or dampness. Essential oils should not be ingested, because even modest amounts can be fatal. They must be kept away from children and pets. Pregnant or lactating women, children, and persons with pulmonary disorders, allergies, or epilepsy should consult a knowledgeable health care practitioner or a qualified aromatherapist before using essential oils. Some oils can trigger bronchial spasms, so persons with asthma should consult their primary health-care provider before using oils. Oils other than lavender or tea tree oil must always be diluted before being applied to the skin. Individuals who have sensitive skin or allergies should take extra care in massaging the oils into the skin or inhaling the essential oil aromas. People should not rub their eyes if they have any essential oil on their hands. Several oils are photosensitive or phototoxic and can cause severe sunburn if the skin is exposed to the sun within 6–48 hours after application. These oils include clove, bergamot, angelica, verbena, bitter and sweet orange, lemon, lime, and mandarin. People with hypertension should avoid the use of hyssop oil. Those who have a seizure disorder should not use camphor, fennel, hyssop, rosemary, sage, and lavender. Certain oils can be highly toxic, so their use should be limited to qualified aromatherapists. These oils include boldo leaf, calamus, yellow camphor, horseradish, rue, sassafras, savin, tansy, wintergreen, wormseed, and wormwood (Keniston-Pond, 2015).

Professional aromatherapists use up to 50 oils. Most people can meet their home needs with just 10: chamomile, clove, eucalyptus, geranium, lavender, lemon, peppermint, rosemary, tea tree, and thyme. Box 8.2 describes helpful oils you can encourage people to have available at home.

BOX 8.2

Helpful Oils to Have at Home

Oil	Use
Basil	Decrease sinus congestion; soothe GI tract, aid digestion; decrease headache; decrease anxiety; decrease menstrual cramps
Bergamot	Decrease anxiety, decrease depression; urinary antiseptic; acne, disinfectant for wounds, abscesses, boils
Cedarwood	Decrease respiratory congestion and coughs, expectorant; for pain swelling of arthritis; antifungal for skin rashes
Chamomile	Soothe muscle aches, sprains, swollen joints; GI antispasmodic; rub on abdomen for colic, indigestion, gas; decrease anxiety, stress-related headaches; decrease insomnia; can be used with children
Clary sage	Induce sleep; increase sense of well-being; massage or warm compress for menstrual cramps; do not use in pregnancy until onset of labor
Coriander	Improve digestion, decrease colic, decrease diarrhea; decrease muscle aches and stiffness in joints; decrease mental fatigue, and increase memory and mental function
Cypress	Massage or cold compress for rheumatic aches; bruising or varicose veins; respiratory antispasmodic (put couple of drops on handkerchief or tissue and inhale deeply), decrease coughs, asthma, bronchitis
Elemi	Boost immune system; cystitis; speed bone healing (massage in prior to casting); speed healing of cuts, sores, wounds; cool inflamed skin; sedative
Eucalyptus	Feels cool to skin and warm to muscles; decrease fever; relieve pain; anti-inflammatory; antiseptic, antiviral, and expectorant for respiratory system in steam inhalation; boost immune system
Frankincense	Bronchodilatory, acts on mucus, enabling sputum to be expelled; infected sores; deepen breathing to induce calmness; incense creates a state conducive to prayer or meditation
Geranium	Antibacterial; insecticidal; antidepressant; improve yeast infections; first aid on minor cuts and burns
Ginger	Help ward off colds; calm upset stomach, decrease nausea; soothe sprains, muscle spasms
Green apple	Reduce headache severity; decrease anxiety; aid in weight reduction program; reduce symptoms of claustrophobia
Jasmine	Uplifting and stimulating, antidepressant; massage abdomen and lower back for menstrual cramps
Juniper	Calming, decrease stress; diuretic; muscle aches and pains

(continued)

Lavender	Calming, sedative, for insomnia; massage around temples for headache; inhale to speed recovery from colds, flu; massage chest to decrease congestion; heal burns
Lemongrass	Sedative; skin antiseptic for acne
Marjoram	Insomnia, decrease tension; muscle and joint pain; inhale to clear sinuses and clear congestion; massage abdomen for menstrual cramps
Neroli	Gentle sedative for insomnia, panic attacks; massage abdomen for irritable bowel syndrome
Orange	General tonic; decrease anxiety; GI antispasmodic for colic and indigestion; massage abdomen for constipation; can be used with children
Peppermint	Increase alertness and mental clarity; GI antispasmodic for colic and indigestion; massage on temples for headache; decongestant for colds, flu
Petitgrain	Useful for acne and oily skin; decrease muscle spasms; gentle sedative
Rose	Antidepressant; increase alertness; compress for eyestrain, headaches; use in massage for PMS
Rosemary	Stimulating; increase circulation to skin; compress on swollen joints; decrease respiratory congestion; antifungal, antibacterial; deodorize the air
Sandalwood	Calm and cool body; decrease inflammation; drops on handkerchief for sore throat, congestion; in bath water for cystitis; improve chapped dry skin; increase sense of peace in meditation or prayer
Tea tree	First-aid kit in a bottle; antifungal, good for athlete's foot; soothe insect bites, stings, cuts, wounds; in bath for yeast infection; drops on handkerchief for coughs, congestion
Vetiver	Stimulate production of red blood cells; increase circulation; induce restful sleep; decrease tension
Ylang-ylang	Soothe CNS, decrease depression, increase euphoric mood; decrease blood pressure; regulate respiration; calm heart palpitations

Sources: Alexander (2015); Buckle (2016); Rhind (2016).

TRY THIS
Soothing Potions

Rosewater

Instead of using soap, try splashing your face with rosewater, a simple infusion from rose petals containing some of the flowers' essential oils. Rose oil has mild antiseptic and anti-inflammatory action, and it can reduce redness in the skin by constricting the tiny blood vessels. It is also used in aromatherapy to calm the nerves and elevate mood. You can buy rosewater in any natural food store, but you can also make your own. Put a handful of fresh rose petals into a small saucepan, add enough water to cover the petals completely, simmer for 15 minutes, and then remove the pan from the heat. When the mixture is completely cooled, strain away the petals and transfer your rosewater to a clean glass bottle.

Adult Cold Care

> 2 drops eucalyptus
> 5 drops geranium
> 3 drops peppermint
> 5 drops rosemary

Mix oils together. Use in any of the following ways:

- Put several drops in a diffuser.
- Put 2 drops on a tissue and breathe in the aroma.
- Put 4 drops in a bath.
- Add 8 drops to 2 tablespoons of carrier oil and massage the chest, back, neck, forehead, nose, and cheekbones.

Leg Cramps

- Add 10 drops of rosemary, 10 drops of sweet marjoram, 5 drops of geranium, and 5 drops of lavender and blend together. Add 5 drops of the blended mixture to 1 teaspoon of carrier oil. Before bed, massage entire leg up from the ankle. Massage feet.

Natural Sleep Aid

- Put 2 drops of lavender on your pillowcase.
- Combine 3 drops chamomile, 4 drops lavender, 3 drops orange, and 5 ounces of water. Using a spray bottle, spray linens and room air before sleeping.

Body Scrub

- 2 parts small-grain salt or sugar
- 1 part oil (olive, coconut, almond, safflower, vegetable, baby)
- 5 drops of preferred essential oil
- Use on dry skin to exfoliate. Rinse well.

Sources: Hoffman and Fox (2006); Kennedy (2016b); Young (2017).

Considering the Evidence

Watson, K., Chang, E., & Johnson, A. (2012). The efficacy of complementary therapies for agitation among older people in residential care facilities: A systematic review. *Joanna Briggs Institute Library of Systematic Reviews*, 10(53): 3414–3486.

(continued)

What Was the Approach of the Research?

Systematic review of randomized clinical trials (RCTs).

What Was the Aim/Purpose/Objective(s) of the Research as Related to Complementary and Integrative Therapies?

The review objective was to determine types of complementary therapies implemented in residential care facilities focusing on agitation management and identify specific therapies that are effective in reducing agitation.

How Was the Study Done?

A comprehensive search strategy using the Joanna Briggs Institute protocol for systematic reviews incorporated 11 electronic databases to identify randomized controlled trials (RCTs) focused on specific complementary therapies. The review included both published and non-published studies, as well as reference lists from selected papers. Ten randomized controlled trials that met inclusion criteria were reviewed with a total of 584 participants. Participants in 9 out of 10 studies were living with dementia. The selected RCTs focused on aromatherapy, exercise, music therapy, and therapeutic touch relative to the frequency and severity of verbal, nonphysical aggressive, and physical aggressive agitation in older persons.

What Were the Significant Findings of the Research?

All 10 of the included studies in the final review reported all interventions (aromatherapy, exercise, music therapy, and therapeutic touch) effective in decreasing nonphysical and verbal agitation in older persons. However, aromatherapy (lavender) and music therapy purported to have a significant effect in reducing physical aggressive agitation in this population.

What Additional Questions Might I Have?

Can these findings be applied to persons not residing in a residential care facility? Are there any adverse effects of the proposed therapies? Is the type of music relevant to decreasing agitation in these individuals? While the review mainly focused on persons living with dementia, would these complementary therapies be effective in others living with other mental health/brain injury diagnosis who frequently experience outbursts of agitation and aggression? Do educational programs exist that would allow for nurses to become proficient in initiating these therapies? Can these therapies be integrated within the "normal routine" for the person living with dementia and experiencing agitation? What outcomes might be expected if other combinations of therapies are implemented? What is the comfort level of nurses in initiating these therapies?

What Is the Clinical Significance of This Study?

The findings of this systematic review have considerable value to nurses working with a growing population of older persons experiencing agitation. While the focus of the review was on participants living in residential care facilities, perhaps, the findings can be shared with the many families caring for these individuals in their homes. These therapies are not complicated to initiate and may be more cost effective than traditional pharmacological interventions. Perhaps, the decrease in the incidence of agitation behaviors may also lower workplace stress for nurses, the patients, and their families.

Source: Contributed by Dolores M. Huffman, RN, PhD.

References

Alexander, J. (2015). *Wellbeing & Mindfulness*. London: Carlton Books.

Benjamin, P. J. (2016). *Tappan's Handbook of Massage Therapy* (6th ed.). Boston: Pearson.

Buckle, J. (2016). Aromatherapy. In B. M. Dossey & L. Keegan (Eds.), *Holistic Nursing: A Handbook for Practice* (7th ed., pp. 345–364). Burlington, MA: Jones & Bartlett Learning.

Buckle, J. (2015). *Clinical Aromatherapy* (3rd ed.). St. Louis, MO: Elsevier/ Churchill Livingstone.

Butje, A. (2017). *The Heart of Aromatherapy.* Carlsbad, CA: Hayhouse Publishing.

Emerson, R. W. (1847). *Poems.* J. Munroe & Company.

Hashemi, S. H., Hajbagheri, A., & Aghajani, M. (2015). The effect of massage with lavender oil on restless leg syndrome in hemodialysis patients: A randomized controlled trial. *Nursing and Midwifery Studies.* doi: 10.17795/nmsjournal29617

Herz, R. S. (2009). Aromatherapy facts and fictions: A scientific analysis of olfactory effects on mood, physiology and behavior. *International Journal of Neuroscience.* doi: 10.1080/00207450802333953

Hoffman, R., & Fox, B. (2006). *Alternative Cures That Really Work.* New York, NY: Rodale.

Keniston-Pond, K. (2015). *Essential Oils for Health.* Avon, MA: Adams Press.

Kennedy, A. (2016a). *The Portable Essential Oils.* Berkeley, CA: Althea Press.

Kennedy, A. (2016b). *Aromatherapy for Natural Living.* Berkeley, CA: Althea Press.

Kohli, P., Naik, A. N., Harruff, E. E., Nguyen, S. A., Schlosser, R. J., & Soler, Z. M. (2016). The prevalence of olfactory dysfunction in chronic rhinosinusitis. *Laryngoscope.* doi: 10.1002/lary.26316

Kohli, P., Soler, Z. M., Nguyen, S. A., Muus, J. S., & Schlosser, R. J. (2016). The association between olfaction and depression: A systematic review. *Chemical Senses.* doi: 10.1093/chemse/bjw061

Lara, V. M., Carregaro, A. B., Santurio, D. F., Facco de Sa, M., Santurio, J. M., & Alves, S. H. (2016). Antimicrobial susceptibility of *Escherichia coli* strains isolated from *Alouatta* spp. Feces to essential oils. *Evidence-Based Complementary and Alternative Medicine.* doi: 10.1155/2016/1643762/

Lewis, R. (2015). Aromatherapy and plant essential oils. In M. S. Micozzi (ed.), *Fundamentals of Complementary and Alternative Medicine.* (5th ed., pp. 411–426). St. Louis, MO: Saunders.

Parma, V., Ferraro, S., Miller, S. S., Ahs, F., & Lundstrom, J. N. (2015). Enhancement of odor sensitivity following repeated odor and visual fear conditioning. *Chemical Senses.* doi: https://doi.org/10.1093/chemse/bjv033

Rhind, J. P. (2016). *Aromatherapeutic Blending.* London, UK: Singing Dragon.

Salazar, I., Barrios, A. W., & SaNchez-Quinteiro, P. (2016). Revisiting the vomeronasal system from an integrated perspective. *Anatomical Record (Hoboken).* doi: 10.1002/ar.23470

Seow, Y. X., Ong, P. K., & Huang, D. (2016). Odor-specific loss of smell sensitivity with age as revealed by the Specific Sensitivity Test. *Chemical Senses.* doi: 10.1093/chemse/bjw051

Sorokowska, A. (2016). Olfactory performance in a large sample of early-blind and late-blind individuals. *Chemical Senses.* doi: 10.1093/chemse/bjw081

Stiles, K. G. (2017). *The Essential Oils Complete Reference Guide.* Salem, MA: Page Street Publishing Co.

Thomas, D. V. (2002). Aromatherapy: Mythical, magical, or medicinal? *Holistic Nursing Practice*, 17(1): 8–16.

Tisserand, R., & Young, R. (2014). *Essential Oil Safety* (2nd ed.). London: Elsevier/ Churchill Livingstone.

Young, K. Y. (2017). *The Healing Art of Essential Oils.* Woodbury, MN: Llewellyn Worldwide.

Resources

Aromatherapy Registration Council
    5940 SW Hood Ave.
    Portland, OR 97039
    503.244.0726
    www.aromatherapycouncil.org

Institute of Integrative Aromatherapy
    P.O. Box 19241
    Boulder, CO 80308
    303.545.2002
    www.aroma-rn.com

International Federation of
    Aromatherapists
    20A The Mall
    Ealing, London W5 2PJ
    44(0).567.2243
    www.ifaroma.org

National Association for Holistic
    Aromatherapy (NAHA)
    P.O. Box 1868
    Banner Elk, NC 28604
    828.898.6161
    www.naha.org

Smell & Taste Treatment and Research
    Foundation
    233 E. Erie St., Suite 712
    Chicago, IL 60611
    847.274.2267
    www.smellandtaste.org

9

Homeopathy

*Miracles do not happen in contradiction
of nature, but in contradiction to what we
know about nature.*

SAINT AUGUSTINE

The term **homeopathy** is derived from the Greek words *omoios*, meaning "similar," and *pathos*, meaning "feeling." It is a self-healing system, assisted by small doses of remedies or medicines, that is useful in a variety of acute and chronic disorders. The practice of homeopathy in the United States has increased tremendously since the 1980s, corresponding to the increase in other forms of alternative medicine. Homeopathic medicine is practiced worldwide, especially in Europe, Latin America, and Asia.

In the United States, the homeopathic drug market has grown into a multimillion-dollar industry. Most of these remedies are not regulated by the U.S. Food and Drug Administration (FDA) and are available as over-the-counter medications.

BACKGROUND

As a therapeutic system, homeopathy is approximately 200 years old. It was developed by Samuel Hahnemann (1755–1843), a German physician and chemist. Homeopathy spread through most of Europe and to the United States, Russia, and Latin America in the 1830s. During epidemics of cholera, typhus, and scarlet fever, homeopathy was significantly more effective than the conventional medical approaches of the times. In 1869, the American Institute of Homeopathy opened free dispensaries for the poor and voted to admit female physicians, unheard of in conventional medicine. By the 1890s, 15% of U.S. physicians were using some homeopathic remedies in their practice, were being educated in the 22 homeopathic medical schools, and were practicing in more than 100 homeopathic hospitals (Chambers, 2016).

During and after the Civil War, the practice of medicine began to change with technical achievements such as anesthesia, antisepsis, surgery, microbiology, vaccines, and antibiotics. State legislatures began to license physicians and to accredit medical schools. The American Medical Association (AMA) invited homeopaths to become members in exchange for licensing, seeking to create a monopoly against lay healers, midwives, and herbalists. When homeopaths chose not to join forces, the AMA began to persecute homeopathy and, in 1914, proposed uniform standards of medical education. The AMA also assumed the power of accreditation, using it to phase out homeopathic colleges. Between the 1920s and 1970s, homeopathic education in the United States was almost nonexistent (Chambers, 2016).

PREPARATION

About half the homeopaths in the United States are physicians. The others are licensed health-care practitioners such as nurse practitioners, dentists, naturopathic physicians, chiropractors, acupuncturists, and veterinarians. Nonlicensed homeopathic practitioners can "counsel" people, but they cannot state or imply that they can diagnose or treat illnesses. The Council for Homeopathic Certification administers the certification process, which involves 500 hours in the theory and foundations of homeopathy in an accredited program, 250 hours of clinical training, and written and oral examinations. Certification gives one the right to place the designation *DHt* after one's name.

CONCEPTS

Law of Similars

Hahnemann proposed the use of the **law of similars,** which claims that a natural substance that produces a given symptom in a healthy person cures it in a sick person. The substance whose symptom-picture most closely resembles the illness being treated is the one most likely to initiate a curative response for that person—hence the name *homeopathy*—"similar feeling."

If taken in large amounts, these natural compounds will produce symptoms of disease. In the doses used by homeopaths, however, these remedies stimulate a person's self-healing capacity. As Andrew Weil stated, "The difference between a poison and a medicine is the dose" (Frye, 1997, p. 846). An example is the use of ipecac, which in large doses causes severe nausea and vomiting. People who are experiencing nausea and vomiting, however, can use a remedy made with ipecac to cure those same symptoms (Rost, 2017).

Law of Infinitesimals

Natural healing compounds are specially prepared for homeopathic use through a process of serial dilution. The compound is first dissolved in either water or a water/alcohol mixture and is called the "mother tincture." One drop of the tincture is then mixed with 9 drops of water/alcohol to form a 1:10 dilution, and this dilution process is repeated many times depending on the potency being prepared. At each step of the dilution, the vial is vigorously shaken, a process called **succussion,** which is an essential step. Thus, the notation 6X on a remedy means that the procedure (diluting and succussing) has been repeated sequentially six times. The concentration of the active substance is then one part in 10 raised to the sixth power (10^6), or one part per million. Dilutions of 30X and 200X are common. The homeopathic belief is that the more the substance is diluted, the more potent it becomes as a remedy.

The remedies are diluted beyond the point at which any molecules of the substance can theoretically still be found in the solution. This paradox, that the remedy becomes more potent through dilution, is the reason many biomedical scientists reject homeopathic medicine. Just as the mechanisms of many conventional drugs are not fully understood, it is not presently known how homeopathic remedies work, but a number of theories have been proposed.

A remedy may be like a hologram. No matter how many times a substance is diluted, a smaller but complete essence of the substance remains. Modern chaos theory supports the observation that major changes occur in living organisms when bodily substances are activated only slightly. The basic assumption of the chaos theory is that minute changes can have huge effects. Advances in quantum physics have led some scientists to suggest that the imprinting of electromagnetic energy in the remedies interacts with the body on some level. Gas discharge visualization technology may provide an electromagnetic probe into the properties of homeopathic remedies in the future. Researchers in physical chemistry have proposed the memory-of-water theory in which the structure of the water/alcohol solution is altered during the process of dilution and retains its new structure even after the substance is no longer present. It seems likely that remedies work through a bioenergetic or subatomic mechanism that is not yet capable of being understood. The situation may be likened to any number of advances in the understanding of energy such as radio, television, microwave ovens, and cordless telephones that previously were virtually unimaginable (Ives & Jones, 2015; Ostermann, Reinhold, & Witt, 2015).

In the 1920s and 1930s, Dr. Bach, a bacteriologist, a pathologist, a homeopathic physician, and an intuitive healer, discovered **flower essences.** He believed that emotions such as anger, hate, or fear negatively affect the immune system, leading to stress, pain, and illness. He experimented with a number of flowers, eventually creating a treatment system involving 38 different types of wildflowers. Flowers are placed in a clear glass bowl filled with purified water and placed in direct sunlight, which transfers the energy of the blossom into the water—a process called **infusion.** Bach's flower essences are diluted but not as much as homeopathic remedies. The remedies are placed under the tongue or in a glass of liquid four times a day. They are usually safe for even infants and the elderly and are thought to contribute to physical, emotional, mental, and spiritual healing. The best known remedy is the Bach Rescue Remedy, which is used to calm people (and pets) in any stressful situation (Stengler, Balch, & Balch, 2016).

VIEW OF HEALTH AND ILLNESS

Homeopathy is a method for treating the sick rather than a set of hypotheses about the nature of health and illness. However, the underlying assumption is that a vital force—known as qi or prana in other traditions—exists. It is necessary to have adequate nutrition, exercise, rest, good hygiene, and a healthy environment to establish and to maintain homeostasis. In other words, health is the ability of people to adapt their equilibrium in response to internal and external changes. Illness is primarily a disturbance of the vital force manifesting as symptoms of distress. Vital force or life energy is the ultimate origin of health and illness alike, ending only with the death of the person (Bellavite, 2015).

Symptoms of illness represent a body's attempts to heal itself. Thus, homeopathy views symptoms as an *adaptive reaction* that is the best possible response that can be made in the present circumstances. For example, a cough is the body's attempt to clear the bronchi; inflammation is the body's effort to wall off and burn out invading foreign bodies; and fever is the body's way of creating an internal environment that is less conducive to bacterial or viral growth. Given this perspective, the therapeutic approach is to aid the body's efforts to adapt to stress or infection. Thus, for someone with a high fever, homeopaths may recommend belladonna, which increases the natural healing response of body heat. The law of similars is a stimulation of immune and defense responses leading to spontaneous resolution of symptoms as the illness is conquered. In like manner, two of the few conventional therapies that seek to stimulate the body's own healing reaction, immunization and allergy treatment, have the homeopathic law of similars as their basis. Other applications in conventional medicine include the use of radiation in the treatment of cancer and Ritalin in the treatment of children with hyperactivity disorders. The majority of interventions in biomedicine, however, attempt to oppose symptoms by exerting a greater and opposite force. Medicines are designed to "cure" by suppressing symptoms, such as when aspirin is used in an effort to control or limit fevers. The danger is that, over time, suppressive treatments may actually strengthen disease processes instead of resolving them (Chambers, 2016).

DIAGNOSTIC METHODS

Homeopathic diagnosis is holistic and detailed; the initial assessment may last several hours. Practitioners assess the whole person, examining every aspect of physical, emotional, and mental life. A multitude of factors are considered, such as nutritional status, emotional imbalance, and environmental stress. It is believed that no part can be isolated from the whole person. The homeopathic interview itself is a powerful healing experience because clients are encouraged to tell their story in its entirety. They are encouraged to speak for as long a time as possible. This process of sharing pain and suffering begins the healing process. During the interview, the practitioner observes everything about the person, including posture, dress, facial expression, tone of voice, rate of speech, and so forth. The physical exam is a head-to-toe assessment with the inclusion of laboratory work as needed to establish a diagnosis. Answers to questions are elicited in an attempt to fully understand the significance of symptoms:

- Subjective symptoms such as pain, vertigo, fatigue, or anger
- Localization of symptoms such as one sided, wandering, radiating, or diffuse
- Factors that modify the symptoms, making them better or worse, such as time of day, hot or cold, weather, diet, or emotional state
- Quality of symptoms such as burning, aching, or throbbing
- Rate of onset or resolution of the symptoms, such as sudden or gradual
- Symptoms that appear simultaneously or in sequence

Symptoms are classified into three categories—the general physical symptoms, the local symptoms, and the mental and emotional symptoms. *General physical symptoms* include such factors as sleep, appetite, energy, temperature, or generalized body pain. *Local symptoms* occur in particular parts of the body, such as swelling in the right elbow or pain in the left leg. Included in local symptoms are those related to a specific organ function, such as shortness of breath or palpitations. *Mental and emotional symptoms* include anxiety, irritability, anger, tearfulness, isolation, or suspiciousness. This composite picture of the person is far more important than any isolated laboratory findings or abstract disease category in formulating the diagnosis. Homeopathic practitioners do not hesitate to refer to biomedical specialists for conventional drugs or surgery.

TREATMENT

Homeopathy is not a complete system of medicine in itself and should be used in conjunction with biomedicine. As in other complementary and alternative practices, the initial question is always, who is the person? rather than, what is the disease? This focus ensures an individualized approach to treatment. Each person with the same presenting complaint may be treated with different remedies depending on the totality of physical, mental, and emotional symptoms. A person with a sore throat may be prescribed one of six or seven common remedies for sore throats, depending on whether the pain is worse on the right or left side, what time of day it is worse, how thirst and appetite are affected, and the individual's emotional state (Bellavite, 2015).

Homeopathic practitioners see the purpose of treatment as stimulating the individual's self-healing powers. The science and the art of homeopathy is to find the remedy with the ability to mimic most closely the sick person's pattern of symptoms. Practitioners use only one remedy at a time, since administering different remedies for different symptoms makes it difficult to know which remedy was effective. Not only are the smallest possible doses used but typically only one dose is given, which allows time for the remedy to complete its action without further interference. If necessary, a dose may be repeated or another remedy may be tried. A temporary worsening of the symptoms may occur after receiving the remedy, which is usually mild and short-lived and may be an indication that the correct remedy was chosen (Rost, 2017).

Homeopathy is used to treat both acute and chronic health problems as well as for health promotion. It cannot cure conditions resulting from structural, long-term organic changes such as cirrhosis, diabetes, chronic obstructive lung disease, advanced neurological diseases, or cancer. In some of these cases, homeopathy can palliate the symptoms and increase the client's comfort level. Traumatic injuries affect nearly everyone in similar ways, and thus the remedies are fairly standard. Epidemic infectious diseases also tend to affect most victims in the same way, and individuals are usually treated with the same remedy. Common infectious illnesses such as urinary tract infections, respiratory infections, and ear infections demonstrate more individual symptoms and require more individualization in selecting the remedy. Chronic illnesses such as ulcerative colitis, rheumatoid arthritis, asthma, and skin disorders are considered to be constitutional. Thus, these disorders require the most skillful assessment, individualized prescription, and follow-up (National Center for Complementary and Integrative Health, 2016).

The Homeopathic Pharmacopoeia of the United States (Borneman & Foxman, 1989), listing more than 2,000 remedies, is the official standard for preparation and prescription. Most remedies come from plants used in traditional herbal medicine. A few remedies come from animal sources, and others from naturally occurring chemical compounds. Box 9.1 lists examples of remedies. Some, such as mercury and belladonna, would be poisonous in large doses but are safe in the superdilute homeopathic doses. These remedies rank among the safest medicines available (Stengler et al., 2016). Homeopathic medicines found in most health food stores are called *combination medicines* or *formulas* because they contain between three and eight different homeopathic medicines mixed together. The various manufacturers choose the medicines most commonly prescribed for specific symptoms and assume that one of them will help cure the ailment of each consumer. Professional homeopaths believe that the remedy individually chosen for the person tends to work more often and more effectively than these combinations.

RESEARCH

As in other areas of medical research, the two questions to be answered are, how does it work? and how well does it work? Many researchers are studying the physics of how homeopathic remedies work. It currently seems likely that remedies work through a bioenergetic or subatomic mechanism that is not yet understood or measurable. Research in the areas of quantum physics, physical chemistry, and biochemistry may someday be able to explain how the remedies work.

BOX 9.1

Examples of Homeopathic Remedies

Plant	Mineral	Animal
Herbs: comfrey, eyebright, mullein, yellow dock	**Metals:** copper, gold, lead, tin, zinc	**Venoms:** jellyfish, insects, spiders, mollusks, crustaceans, fish, snakes, amphibians
Foods and spices: cayenne, garlic, mustard, onion	**Salts:** calcium sulfate, sodium chloride, potassium carbonate	**Secretions:** ambergris, musk, cuttlefish ink
Fragrances, resins, residues: amber, petroleum, charcoal, creosote	**Acids:** hydrochloric, nitric, phosphoric, sulfuric	**Milks**
Mushrooms, lichens, mosses	**Elemental substances:** carbon, hydrogen, iodine, phosphorus, sulfur	**Hormones**
	Constituents of earth's crust: silica, aluminum oxide, ores, rocks, lavas, mineral waters	**Glandular and tissue extracts**
		Disease products: vaccines, abscesses, tuberculosis, gonorrhea, syphilis

One of the difficulties in using the standard randomized, placebo-controlled paradigm for homeopathic remedies is that the treatments are individualized. Unlike with biomedicine, each person with the illness is likely to be prescribed a different remedy based on holistic assessment. In addition, there is no uniform prescribing standard for homeopaths.

A small sampling of studies included the following findings:

- A systematic review of options for otitis media found that homeopathy should be integrated into the treatment strategy for these children (Marom et al., 2016).
- A systematic review and meta-analysis found a small, statistically significant treatment effect of individualized homeopathic treatment. The overall quality of the studies was low requiring improved studies in the future (Mathie et al., 2014).

- A blind, randomized, placebo-controlled trial was designed to study the prevention of flu and acute respiratory infection in children aged 1–5 years. Homeopathic medicines significantly minimized the number of these illnesses compared to the placebo group (Siqueira et al., 2016).
- A randomized, double-dummy, double-blind, placebo-controlled trial studied the impact of homeopathic treatment versus placebo versus placebo and fluoxetine in menopausal women with moderate to severe depression. There was a significant difference between the homeopathic group compared to the placebo group but not compared to the placebo and fluoxetine group. The homeopathic group was significantly better than the other two groups in treatment of other menopausal symptoms (Macias-Cortes, Llanes-Gonzalez, Aguilar-Faisal, & Asbun-Bojalil, 2015).

INTEGRATED NURSING PRACTICE

Nurses, like homeopathic practitioners, emphasize listening to clients' stories of their lives. It is within the context of people's lives that nurses identify patterns of response to illnesses and disorders and formulate nursing diagnoses. Nursing diagnoses and outcome criteria focus attention on adaptations that may help people live healthier lifestyles. The study of mental health nursing in the basic educational program teaches the value of listening and attending to people's pain as an intervention to help them begin the process of healing. These principles are common to both nursing and homeopathy, illustrating, once again, the broad base of nursing practice. Some nurse practitioners, valuing the contributions of homeopathy to well-being, continue their education and achieve licensure to practice homeopathic medicine. Nurses educated in Western approaches are more likely to suppress symptoms in an attempt to "cure" the disease. In many situations, it may be more beneficial to follow the homeopathic approach and view symptoms as the body's attempt to heal itself. Clients may improve more quickly when non-life-threatening symptoms are supported rather than suppressed, such as low- to moderate-grade fevers or productive coughs.

People who are interested in homeopathic remedies can find low-potency remedies in health food stores. Higher potency remedies are obtained from homeopathic pharmaceutical companies under the direction of experienced homeopathic prescribers. Because remedies are inactivated by direct sunlight and heat, nurses should teach people to store the preparations in a dark, dry place, away from other strong-smelling substances. When taking a remedy, patients should have nothing by mouth for at least 30 minutes before and after the dose. Many homeopaths discourage the use of coffee, mint, camphor, and other strongly aromatic substances while undergoing treatment, since such substances may reverse the effects of the remedy. Camphor is a component in chest rubs as well as in many cosmetics, skin creams, and lip balms. If the remedy is in the form of a pellet, it should be held under the tongue and allowed to dissolve slowly. If the remedy is a liquid, it should be held in the mouth for 1 to 2 minutes before swallowing.

Prescription medications, especially those given for potentially life-threatening disorders such as asthma, should not be stopped abruptly when homeopathic care is begun. As the person improves, however, a downward titration of the biomedical prescription may be needed. Acupuncture and chiropractic medicine should not be started at the same time as homeopathic remedies, but if already instituted, may be continued (Stengler et al., 2016).

A number of homeopathic remedies can be used to speed recovery and prevent recurrences of acute conditions such as colds, stomachaches, coughs, and headaches. Although many remedies are used for conditions that subside on their own, remedies can dramatically speed recovery and often prevent recurrences. Because homeopathic medicines are considerably safer than conventional drugs, it often makes sense to use them first and then consider using conventional drugs if the homeopathic remedies work too slowly or not at all. Individuals should read all the information on the label to select the right remedy. If the label states, for example, that the remedy is best used when the symptoms appear suddenly, then that remedy is not likely to be effective for a condition that emerged almost unnoticed over several days. Nurses can teach clients the following three guidelines for the use of homeopathic remedies:

1. *The more the better.* The more the symptoms match that of the remedy, the more likely it will work.
2. *The less the better.* The more dilute the remedy, the more powerful it is.
3. *It's working if you feel better within 24 hours.* If not, you may have the wrong remedy and may need a different remedy or may need to see a health-care practitioner.

Many people keep homeopathic remedies on hand and ready to use. See "Try This: Top 10 Remedies and Bach Flower Essences" for the most popular remedies that help with the majority of common physical problems and emotional difficulties.

TRY THIS

Top 10 Remedies and Bach Flower Essences

1. *Bryonia (wild hops):* Used for coughs that are worsened by simple breathing; headaches that are increased by bending over, walking, or even moving the eyes; constipation with dry, hard stools.
2. *Allium cepa (onion):* Used for colds or respiratory allergies in which symptoms resemble the reaction of a person exposed to the mist produced when an onion is cut: watery eyes, clear nasal discharge, and sneezes, all of which are aggravated by exposure to heat.

(continued)

3. *Pulsatilla (windflower):* Need is based on the type of person, rather than a specific ailment. Helpful for people who are highly emotional, weepy, impressionable, easily influenced, fearful of abandonment, and worried about what others think of them. May also be used for digestive disorders, allergies, earaches, headaches, insomnia, and premenstrual syndrome.
4. *Ignatia (St. Ignatius bean):* Used by persons experiencing anxiety or grief.
5. *Arsenicum album (arsenic):* Used for many conditions, especially when symptoms are worse after midnight, when burning symptoms are predominant, when great thirst occurs, or when the person is high strung and restless.
6. *Belladonna (deadly nightshade):* Used for fever or inflammation that begins rapidly, with a red or flushed appearance; the person is hypersensitive to touch or light.
7. *Gelsemium (yellow jessamine):* Used for classic flu symptoms accompanied by lack of thirst. Helpful for headaches in the back part of the head.
8. *Nux vomica (poison nut):* Useful after overdosing with food or drink, indigestion, constipation, and headaches that are worse at night and on waking.
9. *Aconitum (monkshood):* Used for colds, flu, coughs, and sore throats with rapid onset.
10. *Rhus toxicodendron (poison ivy):* Helpful for arthritis syndromes, flu, sprains and strains, and sore throats; used by people who feel pain on initial motion that eases with continued motion and who have symptoms that worsen in cold or wet weather.

Bach Flower Essences

1. *Fear:* rockrose, centaury, willow
2. *Worry:* crab apple, chicory, willow, red chestnut, heather
3. *Anger:* holly, elm
4. *Anxiety:* Rescue Remedy

Sources: Chambers (2016); Noriega (2016); Rost (2017); Stengler et al. (2016).

TRY THIS

Pet Remedies

Mercurius solubilis: Inflamed gums; swollen nasal bones and a greenish thick discharge

Podophyllum: Diarrhea with gushy feces containing mucus

Baryta carb: Diarrhea in puppies and young dogs

Arsenicum album or allium cepa: Respiratory symptoms with thin, watery nasal and ocular discharge

Sulfur: Red, itchy skin

Lycopodium or thallium acetas: Hair loss secondary to skin disorders

Sources: Kachnic (2012); Macleod (2012); Madrewar and Glencross (2011).

References

Bellavite, P. (2015). Homeopathy and integrative medicine: Keeping an open mind. *Journal of Medicine and the Person.* doi: 10.1007/s12682-014-0198-x

Borneman, J. P., & Foxman, E. L. (1989). *Homeopathic Pharmacopoeia of the United States.* Southeastern, PA: Homeopathic Pharmacopoeia.

Bryson, A. (2000). *Healing Mind, Body, and Soul.* Sterling Publishers Pvt. Ltd.

Chambers, B. (2016). *Homeopathy Plus Whole Body Vibration.* London: Quartet Books.

Frye, J. (1997). Homeopathy in office practice. *Primary Care,* 24(4): 845–864.

Ives, J. A., & Jones, W. D. (2015). Energy medicine. In M. S. Micozzi (Ed.), *Fundamentals of Complementary and Alternative Medicine* (5th ed., pp. 197–212). St. Louis, MO: Elsevier/Saunders.

Kachnic, J. (2012). *Your Dog's Golden Years.* Denver, CO: Wallingford Vale.

Macias-Cortes, E. d. C., Llanes-Gonzalez, L., Aguilar-Faisal, L., & Asbun-Bojalil, J. (2015). Individualized homeopathic treatment and fluoxetine for moderate to severe depression in peri- and postmenopausal women. *Public Library of Science.* doi: 10.1371/journal.pone. 0118440

Macleod, G. (2012). *Dogs: Homoeopathic Remedies.* London, UK: Rider.

Madrewar, B. P., & Glencross, M. (2011). *Therapeutics of Veterinary Homeopathy & Repertory.* New Delhi, India: B. Jain.

Marom, T., Marchisio, P., Tamir, S. O., Torreta, S., Gavriel, H., & Esposito, S. (2016). Complementary and alternative medicine treatment options for otitis media: A systematic review. *Medicine.* doi: 10.1097/ MD0000000000002695

Mathie, R. T., Lloyd, S., Legg, L. A., Clausen, J., Moss, S., Davidson, J. R. T., & Ford, I. (2014). Randomised placebo-controlled trials of individualised homeopathic treatment: Systematic review and meta-analysis. *Systematic Reviews.* doi: 10.1186/2046-4053-3-142

National Center for Complementary and Integrative Health. (2016). Accessed October 25, 2016 at www.nccih.nih. gov/health/homeopathy

Noriega, P. (2016). *Bach Flower Essences and Chinese Medicine.* Rochester, VT: Healing Arts Press.

Ostermann, J. K., Reinhold, T., & Witt, C. M. (2015). Can additional homeopathic treatment save costs? A retrospective cost-analysis based on 44500 insured persons. *Public Library of Science.* doi: 10.1371/journal.pone.0134657

Rost, A. (2017). *Natural Healing Wisdom & Know How.* New York, NY: Black Dog & Leventhal.

Siqueira, C. M., Homsani, F., da Veiga, V. F., Lyrio, C., Mattos, H., Passos, S. R., . . . Quaresma, C. H. (2016). Homeopathic medicines for prevention of influenza and acute respiratory tract infections in children. *Homeopathy.* doi: 10.1016/j.homp.2015.02.006

Stengler et al. (2016). *Prescriptions for Natural Cures* (revised 3rd ed.). Nashville, TN: Turner Publishing Co.

Resources

American Institute of Homeopathy
c/o Sandra M. Chase
10418 Whitehead St.
Fairfax, VA 22030
888.445.9988
www.homeopathyusa.org

Australian Homoeopathic
Association
P.O. Box 7108
Toowoomba South, QLD 4350
07.4636.5081
www.homeopathyoz.org

European Council for Classical
   Homeopathy
School House
Market Place
Kenninghall, Norfolk NR16 2AH
44.1953.888163
www.homeopathy-ecch.org

Hahnemann Center for Heilkunst
9-4338 Innes Rd.
Ottawa, ON K4A 3W3
613.692.1700
www.homeopathy.com

Homeopathic Educational Services
www.homeopathic.com

The Academy of Veterinary
   Homeopathy
www.theavh.org

10
Naturopathy

It is more important to know what sort of person has a disease than to know what sort of disease a person has.

Naturopathic medicine is not only a system of medicine but also a way of life with emphasis on client responsibility, client education, health maintenance, and disease prevention. It may be the model health system of the future with the movement toward healthy lifestyles, healthy diets, and preventive health care.

BACKGROUND

The basic precepts of naturopathy are similar to those of ancient medical systems throughout the world. Naturopathy can trace its philosophical roots to the Hippocratic school of medicine around 400 B.C. Hippocrates had a holistic approach to clients and instructed his students to prescribe only wholesome treatments and to avoid causing harm or hurt. Furthermore, Hippocrates thought that the entire universe followed natural laws, and the role of the physician was to understand and support nature's own cures (Pizzorno, Snider, & Micozzi, 2015).

Naturopathic medicine grew out of the 19th-century medical systems of the United States and Europe. Dr. John Scheel of New York City coined the term **naturopathy** in 1895, although it was Benedict Lust who formalized it in 1902 as both a system of medicine and a way of life. By the early 1900s, more than 20 naturopathic schools of medicine were operating in the United States. In the 1920s and 1930s, naturopathic journals encouraged a diet high in fiber and low in red meat, the same type of diet promoted by the National Institutes of Health and the National

161

Cancer Institute in the 1990s. With the development of antibiotics and vaccines in the 1940s and 1950s, the popularity of naturopathy began to decline as people began to rely on these medical breakthroughs. The 1970s saw a renewal in the importance of nutrition, healthy lifestyles, and environmental cleanup programs. This interest continued to grow into what is now the U.S. interest in complementary and integrative medicine (Pizzorno & Murray, 2012).

PREPARATION

For naturopathic medicine to become recognized as a legitimate health-care system required that accredited schools be established and credible research be conducted. Currently, there are seven schools in the United States and Canada: Bastyr University in Kenmore, Washington; National University of Natural Medicine in Portland, Oregon; the Southwest College of Naturopathic Medicine and Health Science in Tempe, Arizona; University of Bridgeport College of Naturopathic Medicine in Bridgeport, Connecticut; National University of Health Sciences in Lombard, Illinois; Canadian College of Naturopathic Medicine in North York, Ontario; and Boucher Institute of Naturopathic Medicine in New Westminster, British Columbia. There is an additional candidate program: Universidad del Turabo, School of Health Sciences, in Gurabo, Puerto Rico.

The Council on Naturopathic Medical Education is the accrediting agency for programs in the United States and Canada. Schools in Australia include Southern Cross University, the University of Western Sydney, and Victoria University.

In the United States, state law determines the scope of naturopathic practice, since there is no national licensure for naturopathy. The laws typically allow standard diagnostic procedures, a range of therapies, vaccinations, and limited prescriptive rights. Some states allow the practice of natural childbirth. In states that do not license naturopathic doctors, anyone can call herself or himself a naturopathic doctor after completing some correspondence courses. These individuals may give seminars and advise people on healthy lifestyles, but they are not permitted to diagnose illness or to prescribe treatment. When seeking a naturopathic doctor as a primary care physician, people must ask for verification of graduation from an accredited naturopathic medical school.

The education of naturopathic physicians is extensive and similar to conventional medical education. Four years of medical school follow a college degree in a biological science. The first two years of medical school include courses in anatomy, cell biology, nutrition, physiology, pathology, neurosciences, histology, pharmacology, biostatistics, epidemiology, and public health as well as alternative therapies. Some differences are significant. For example, conventional medical students may have only 4 course hours in nutritional education, while naturopathic medical students have 138 course hours in nutrition. The third and fourth years of medical school are oriented toward clinical experience in diagnosis and treatment. The profession has redefined itself in terms of current advances in health care and the evolution of scientific knowledge. Today's naturopathic doctor is an extensively educated primary care physician able to utilize a broad range of conventional and alternative therapies.

CONCEPTS

Naturopathic medicine holds the same view of human physiology, bodily functions, and disease processes as does conventional medicine. Although many alternative health-care professions are defined by the therapies used, naturopathy is defined by basic concepts.

Healing Power of Nature

It is believed that the body innately knows how to maintain health and heal itself. Natural laws of life operate inside and outside the body, and the physician's job is to support and restore them by using techniques and medicines that are in harmony with the natural processes. These natural methods are geared to strengthen the body's own healing ability. Faith, hope, and beliefs may be the most significant aspects of any treatment. Many studies have documented the ability of the mind to affect the process of disease, either positively or negatively. Physicians consider issues such as What does it mean, for this person, to be in balance? and What healing powers are available for this person?

First Do No Harm

Iatrogenic illness, an inadvertent complication as a result of medical treatment—either traditional or alternative—is a major health problem in the United States. Adverse drug reactions send thousands of people to hospital emergency departments, and hospital-acquired (*nosocomial*) infections have become a major problem in the United States.

As Hippocrates said, "Above all else, do no harm." Naturopathic physicians prefer noninvasive treatments that minimize the risk of harmful side effects. Questions considered are, will a delay in treatment be of benefit? and what is the potential for harm with this particular treatment plan?

Find the Cause

Naturopathic physicians look for the underlying causes of disease and try to help patients eliminate them. These causes are often found in people's lifestyles, habits, and/or diets. Physical, mental, emotional, and spiritual factors are important in determining cause. Issues considered are, what are the causative factors contributing to "disease" in this person? Of these causative factors, which are avoidable or preventable? and what are the limiting factors in this person's life?

Treat the Whole Person

Naturopathic medicine has a holistic approach in caring for clients. Practitioners consider the physical, genetic, dietary, mental, emotional, spiritual, and environmental factors influencing clients' health or illness status. In other words, they treat the person rather than the disease.

Preventive Medicine

Conventional medicine is reductionistic with a focus on body parts and symptoms of disease independent of mind and spirit. Naturopathic physicians focus on healthy living as a way to prevent major diseases and chronic illness. The goal is to support people's inherent healing abilities. They do not believe that disability is inevitable as people age.

Wellness and Health Promotion

More than prevention, wellness promotion is a proactive state of being healthy. People are encouraged to make decisions and change negative lifestyle patterns that interfere with a state of wellness. Interventions include removing obstacles to healing in the process of restoring normal function.

Physician as Teacher

The word *doctor* comes from the Latin *docere*, meaning "to teach." Unlike many conventional medical physicians who have little time to teach, naturopathic physicians focus on teaching people how to achieve health and avoid disease by assuming responsibility for themselves and their well-being. Consumers are becoming increasingly aware that good health is dependent to a great extent on treating the body properly. They are seeking health-care practitioners who can teach them how to conduct all aspects of their life in a healthy manner. Thus, naturopathic physicians are an appropriate choice for many. These consumers need to ask such questions as What type of patient education does the physician provide? and In what ways does the physician encourage and support patient's responsibility?

VIEW OF HEALTH AND ILLNESS

Naturopathy views health as more than the absence of disease. Health is a dynamic process that allows people to thrive despite various internal and external stresses. Health arises from a complex interaction of physical, mental, emotional, spiritual, dietary, genetic, environmental, lifestyle, and other components. Health is characterized by positive emotions, thoughts, and actions. Healthy people are energetic and creative as they live goal-directed lives. Health does not come from doctors, pills, or surgery but rather from people's own efforts to take appropriate care of themselves.

Naturopathic physicians recognize the role of bacteria and viruses in illness but view these as secondary factors. They believe that most diseases are the direct result of ignoring natural laws. These violations include eating processed foods, not getting enough exercise and rest, living a fast-paced lifestyle, focusing on negative thoughts and emotions, and being exposed to environmental toxins. Disease-promoting habits lead people away from optimal function toward progressively greater dysfunction in body, mind, and spirit. Naturopathy recognizes that death is inevitable but believes progressive disability is often avoidable.

DIAGNOSTIC METHODS

Naturopathic physicians practice as primary care providers. They see people of all ages suffering from all types of disorders and diseases. They make conventional medical diagnoses using standard diagnostic procedures such as physical examinations, laboratory tests, and radiology. They also perform a detailed assessment of lifestyle, looking for physical, emotional, dietary, genetic, environmental, and family dynamics contributing to a disorder. Since health or disease is a complex interaction of factors, naturopathic physicians treat the whole person, taking all these elements into account. Careful attention to each person's individuality and susceptibility to disease is critical to accurate diagnosis. When necessary, naturopathic physicians, like family practice physicians, refer patients to other health-care professionals for hospitalization, surgery, or other specialized care.

TREATMENT

Naturopathic physicians do not provide emergency care, nor do they perform major surgery. They rarely prescribe drugs, and they treat clients in private practice and outpatient clinics, not in hospitals. Some physicians practice natural childbirth at home or in a clinic.

The therapeutic approach of the naturopathic doctor is to help people heal themselves and to use opportunities to guide and educate people in developing healthier lifestyles. The goal of treatment is the restoration of health and normal body function, rather than the application of a particular therapy. Virtually every natural medical therapy is utilized, most of which are described in this text. Physicians mix and match different approaches, customizing treatment for each person. The least invasive intervention to support the body's natural healing processes is a primary consideration. A primary focus is on the return to nature—that is, diet, exercise, and rest. Cleansing and detoxification consists of decreasing the amount and number of toxins entering the body by eating organic whenever possible and avoiding processed foods, sugar, caffeine, and alcohol. A goal is also to increase the elimination of toxins from the body by increasing intake of fluids, fruits, and vegetables, and increasing sweat through exercise or the use of saunas. The colon is cleansed with high-fiber foods, herbs such as aloe vera juice, liquid fasting for short periods of time, and, sometimes, colonic irrigation.

Chemical remedies used by naturopathic physicians include botanicals and homeopathy. Mechanical remedies include physical therapy, spinal manipulation, acupuncture, yoga, and massage. Mental and spiritual remedies include prayer, positive thinking, and stress management.

Counseling is an important intervention because mental, emotional, and spiritual factors are part of the holistic approach. Lifestyle modification is crucial to the success of naturopathy. While it is relatively easy to tell a person to stop smoking, get more exercise, and reduce stress, such lifestyle changes are often difficult for people to make. The naturopathic physician is educated to assist people in making the needed changes. This process involves helping people acknowledge the need to change habits; identifying reinforcers for unhealthy habits; setting realistic and progressive goals; establishing a support group of family, friends, and others with similar difficulties; and giving people positive recognition for their gains (Hechtman, 2014; Pizzorno & Snider, 2015).

RESEARCH

The American Association of Naturopathic Physicians publishes the *Journal of Naturopathic Medicine*, which includes articles on original research, research reviews, and news and review articles relating to naturopathic medicine. Naturopathic schools of medicine have active research departments investigating a number of healing therapies. Because treatment programs are individually designed, it is nearly impossible to compare naturopathic medicine with conventional medicine; too many variables are involved. Scientific research in particular therapies has been conducted in China, India, Germany, France, and England. In the United States, substantial scientific information is readily available on the effectiveness of diet and lifestyle in modifying the risk of severe illnesses such as heart disease and cancer. Hundreds of scientific papers address diet, nutritional supplements, herbs, exercise, and acupuncture. Some of the other natural healing therapies have not been fully investigated from the Western scientific perspective. Currently, there is no adequate scientific basis for naturopathic evidence-based medicine. It may be many years before science is sophisticated enough to understand some of these therapies.

INTEGRATED NURSING PRACTICE

Interestingly, the bond between nursing and naturopathy is demonstrated by the enrollment in U.S. naturopathic colleges of medicine: one-third of the students are nurses who have chosen this path to continue their post-baccalaureate education. The profession of nursing, like naturopathy, has traditionally embraced the concept of the healing power of nature and the belief that the locus of restoring health is within each person and cannot be "given" to a client by health-care practitioners. Drugs, herbs, procedures, surgeries, or mind–body techniques may be helpful or necessary but by themselves do not cure disease. People must, and do, rebalance and repair themselves. The profession of nursing was founded on this philosophy and view of life as noted by Florence Nightingale (1860) in her basic premise that healing is a function of nature that comes from within the individual. She saw the role of the nurse as putting the "patient in the best condition for nature to act on him."

Nursing has always focused on education of those who have been entrusted to our care. We believe that through education we empower others by providing the knowledge, skills, and support to tap into their inner wisdom and make healthy decisions for themselves. This concept is basic to the practice of nursing and is evidenced in the American Nurses Association's Standard of Nursing Practice, which includes health teaching as one of the standards. The goal of nursing, as in naturopathy, is one of healing and, if possible, the restoration of health.

Because we nurses spend so much more time with clients than do physicians, we are often in a position to prevent or respond quickly to iatrogenic illnesses. To this end, it is critically important that we monitor closely the impact of medications on the recipients. We must know the physiological action, expected effects, side effects, and adverse effects of every medication we administer. We must assess and reassess clients who are receiving medications. Likewise, we must understand procedures and their potential problems for all clients in our care. It is up to each one of us to maintain clinical skills through self-study and continuing education.

TRY THIS

Visualization

Visualization is one of the many interventions used by nurses. This visualization is called "Winched up the Hill." Whenever you are faced with a hill to ascend, imagine a winch at the top and a cord from it to your solar plexus. Invite the winch to draw you upward, easily and effortlessly. At first it may make little difference, but keep practicing the visualization at every opportunity until you train yourself to tune into this extra source of energy.

Source: Rutherford, L. (1996).

References

Amenta, M. O'R. , & Bohnet, N. L. (1986). Nursing Care of the Terminally Ill. Boston, MA: Little Brown.

Hechtman, L. (2014). *Clinical Naturopathic Medicine* (revised ed.). Philadelphia, PA: Churchill Livingstone.

Hippocrates. (1983). *Hippocratic Writings Classic Series*, Vol. 451 of Penguin Classics.

National Conference of Jewish Communal Service. (1948). *The Jewish Social Service*, Quarterly, Vol. 25.

Nightingale, F. (1860). *Notes on Nursing.* New York, NY: D. Appleton.

Pizzorno, J. E., & Murray, M. T. (2012). *Textbook of Natural Medicine* (4th ed.). St. Louis, MO: Elsevier.

Pizzorno, J. E., & Snider, P. (2015). Contemporary naturopathic medicine. In M. S. Micozzi (Ed.), *Fundamentals of Complementary and Alternative Medicine* (5th ed., pp. 366–386). St. Louis, MO: Elsevier/Saunders.

Pizzorno, J. E., Snider, P., & Micozzi, M. S. (2015). Nature cure, naturopathy, and natural medicine. In M. S. Micozzi (Ed.), *Fundamentals of Complementary and Alternative Medicine* (5th ed., pp. 347–365). St. Louis, MO: Elsevier/Saunders.

Rutherford, L. (1996). *Principles of Shamanism.* San Francisco, CA: Thorsons.

Resources

American Association of Naturopathic Physicians
4435 Wisconsin Ave., NW, Suite 403
Washington, DC 20016
866.538.2267
www.naturopathic.org

Australian Naturopathic Practitioners Association
Suite 36/123 Camberwell Rd.
East Hawthorn, VIC 3123
613.9811.9990
www.anpa.asn.au

British Naturopathic and Osteopathic Association
2 Clifton Road
Southbourne, Dorset BH6 3PA
United Kingdom
bnoa.org.uk

Canadian Association of Naturopathic Doctors
20 Holly St., Suite 200
Toronto, ON M4S 3B1
416.496.8633
www.cand.ca

Manual Healing Methods

All things are connected.
Whatever befalls the earth
befalls the sons of the earth.
Man did not weave the
web of life.
He is merely a strand in it.
Whatever he does to the web
he does to himself.

CHIEF SEATTLE, UPON SURRENDERING HIS TRIBAL LANDS IN 1856

11

Chiropractic

*It is most necessary to know the nature of
the spine. One or more vertebrae may or
may not go out of place very much and if
they do, they are likely to produce serious
complications and even death, if not
properly adjusted. Many diseases are
related to the spine.*

HIPPOCRATES

The word **chiropractic** comes from two Greek words, *cheir* (hand) and *praktikos* (practical), which were combined to mean "done by hand." Chiropractic, by numbers of practitioners, is the third largest independent health profession in the United States, following conventional medicine and dentistry. It is also the most frequently used form of complementary medicine. Chiropractors are primary health-care providers, licensed for both diagnosis and treatment. The practice is limited by procedure (manipulation of the spine) and excludes surgery and prescription medications.

BACKGROUND

Manipulation, as a healing technique, was practiced long before chiropractic. Chinese artifacts dating to as early as 2700 B.C. describe manipulation of the spine. In 1500 B.C., the Greeks gave written instructions on how to manipulate the lumbar spine for back care. Hippocrates (born c. 460 B.C.), considered the father of Western medicine, used spinal manipulation to reposition vertebrae and cure a variety of dysfunctions. Galen (born c. A.D. 130), a Greek physician, anatomist, and physiologist, also used manipulation and reported the cure of a patient's hand weakness and numbness through manipulation of the seventh cervical vertebra. Hippocrates and Galen helped form the foundation of Renaissance medicine, during which manipulative healers were known as "bone-setters." Regarded by some as the father of surgery, Ambroise Paré (born c. A.D. 1517) incorporated manipulation into his treatment of patients. In the centuries that followed, manipulative techniques were passed down from generation to generation, often within families (Redwood, 2015).

Daniel David Palmer, a self-educated American healer, founded chiropractic in 1895. Palmer administered the first chiropractic adjustment to Harvey Lillard, a janitor who had gone deaf 17 years earlier while stooping in a mine. Palmer found what he called a misaligned vertebra, which he manipulated, allowing Lillard to stand up straight, free of back pain, and with his hearing restored. Within 2 years of this discovery, Palmer founded his Chiropractic School and Cure while at the same time developing the underlying concepts. In 1906, a split in the profession occurred that still exists today. Several faculty members, including John Howard, left Palmer College because of significant differences with Palmer's son, B. J. Palmer. B. J. Palmer believed that spinal subluxation or misalignment of the spinal vertebrae was the cause of all disease, whereas Howard believed that additional causes were generally present. Howard opened his National School of Chiropractic around a broad-based and scientific educational curriculum. To this day, those who follow Palmer's path are called "straight" chiropractors, while those who follow the Howard model are called "mixer" chiropractors (Redwood, 2015).

PREPARATION

Chiropractors are licensed in all states of the United States as well as in many other countries. The 21 U.S. chiropractic colleges graduate more than 3,000 chiropractors each year. There are also colleges in Canada, Australia, England, Europe, South Africa, and Japan. Chiropractic education requires at least 90 undergraduate credit hours, including many in the basic sciences. Chiropractic college is a 4-year program that includes courses in anatomy, physiology, pathology, and diagnosis, as well as spinal adjusting, nutrition, physical therapy, and rehabilitation. Course work also includes public health and research methods. Educational standards in the United States are supervised by a government-recognized accrediting agency, the Council of Chiropractic Education (Redwood, 2015).

Chiropractors practice in more than 60 countries and function almost entirely in freestanding private practices. Some continue their education with postdoctoral training in specialty areas such as radiology, orthopedics, neurology, behavioral medicine, family practice, occupational health, and sports medicine. The majority of states have mandated health insurance coverage for chiropractic treatment.

CONCEPTS

Anatomy

The **craniosacral system** is composed of the brain and spinal cord, the cerebrospinal fluid, the meninges, and the bones of the spine and skull. The adult vertebral column is composed of 7 cervical, 12 thoracic, 5 lumbar, 1 sacral, and 1 coccygeal vertebrae. The vertebrae provide attachment for various muscles and protection for the spinal cord and are separated by intervertebral disks. Several curves in the vertebral column increase its strength. The spinal cord, housed in the vertebral canal, conducts sensory and motor impulses to and from the brain and controls many reflexes. Thirty-one pairs of spinal nerves originate from the cord: 8 cervical, 12 thoracic, 5 lumbar, 5 sacral, and 1 coccygeal.

The vertebrae, with the exception of the first and the second cervical, are much alike and are composed of a body, an arch, and seven projections called *processes* (see Figure 11.1). The two processes at the top are the superior articular processes, and the two at the bottom are the inferior articular processes; these four processes are of particular interest to the chiropractic physician. At the end of each of these processes is a facet, which, like the facet of a diamond, is smooth and capped with cartilage to allow for friction-free movement. The two superior articular processes from each vertebra join with the two inferior articular processes of the vertebra above. The resulting structure is called a *facet joint*, which is encased in a strong, fibrous joint capsule that prevents the joint from coming apart. The other anatomical feature that is of concern to chiropractic is the sacroiliac joint, which is formed where the sacrum attaches to the ilia.

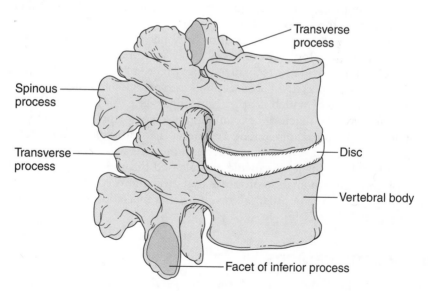

FIGURE 11.1   The Vertebrae

Assumptions

Chiropractic practitioners believe that the body possesses a unique internal wisdom that continually strives to maintain a state of health within the body. This body wisdom means that every person has an innate healing potential. Accessing this internal healing system is the goal of the healing arts. In addition, it is believed that a balanced, natural diet and regular exercise are essential to proper bodily function and good health.

VIEW OF HEALTH AND ILLNESS

Chiropractic practitioners believe that health is a state of balance, especially of the nervous and musculoskeletal systems. When the spine is fully aligned, nerve energy flows freely to every cell and organ in the body. This free flow of energy nurtures the innate ability of the body to work effectively and coordinate normal body functions.

Traditionally, chiropractic viewed illness and disease as caused by misalignment of the spinal vertebrae, referred to as **vertebral subluxation**, leading to irritation and dysfunction of nerves and blood vessels. The disrupted flow of impulses was thought to interfere with normal muscle function, respiration, heartbeat, arterial tone, digestion, and resistance to disease. A more recent theory is that of **intervertebral motion dysfunction.** This motion theory contends that loss of mobility in the facet joints (see Figure 11.2), rather than misalignment, is the key factor in the concept of subluxation. Subluxation can be caused by just about anything—falls, injuries, genetic spinal weaknesses, improper sleeping habits, poor posture, obesity, stress, and occupational hazards (Redwood, 2015).

Although this "one cause" philosophy has been a central concept in chiropractic history, few chiropractors today would endorse this simplistic formulation of illness. They recognize the existence of bacteria and viruses in creating disease, especially in a susceptible person. Susceptibility depends on many factors, one of which is spinal misalignment. Although chiropractic now embraces a multifactorial explanation of disease, the chiropractic treatment of choice is spinal adjustment. The biomechanical explanation states that range of motion is improved when fibrous adhesions within joints are broken or small tags from the joint capsule are released through manipulation. The neurophysiologic explanation proposes that mechanoreceptors in the joint are stimulated through manipulation, resulting in a relaxation of the paraspinal muscles (VanDehey, 2015).

DIAGNOSTIC METHODS

Ninety percent of those seeking chiropractic services have neuromusculoskeletal symptoms or disorders, primarily back pain, neck pain, and headaches. The central focus of chiropractic diagnosis is the determination of when and where **spinal manual therapy** (SMT) is appropriate. The diagnostic process

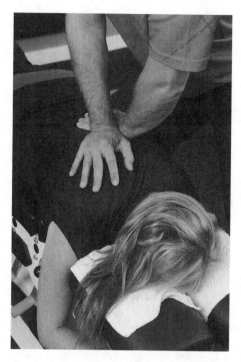

FIGURE 11.2   A practitioner uses her hands to discover which spinal joints are moving freely and which joints are stiff.

Source: Rainer Plendl/123RF.

also determines what type of adjustment would be most appropriate. Unlike practitioners of conventional medicine, who typically assume that the site of a pain is the site of its cause, chiropractors evaluate the site of pain in a regional and whole-body context. Joint pain in the upper extremities, for example, not only can be caused by injury or pathology in the joint but may also originate from cervical spine dysfunction. Similarly, the source of joint pain in the lower extremities can be in the lumbar spine. The chiropractic assumption is that the source of the pain should be sought along the path of the nerves leading to and from the site of the symptoms. This whole-body approach is a hallmark of chiropractic (Redwood, 2015).

The process for assessing a client is much the same as that followed by any other physician or nurse practitioner. The chiropractor may spend as much as 60 to 90 minutes with a new client, examining and explaining the results of the examination, the diagnosis, and the proposed treatment plan. The quality of the relationship is primary to chiropractic.

A detailed history is the first step in chiropractic diagnosis. The chiropractor asks about the pattern and quality of the pain and its chronology. Is the pain constant or intermittent? Is the pain a dull ache, a nagging sensation, or a burning sensation? What causes the pain to get worse? What causes the pain to get better? The answers to these types of questions are key to the diagnostic process. The physical examination includes postural assessment, range-of-motion studies, inspection and palpation of affected areas, muscle strength testing, and neurologic screening.

A number of back pain risk factors are critical to diagnosis and are consistently assessed by the physician. *Individual factors* contributing to back pain include older age, tallness, obesity, smoking, decreased muscle strength, decreased flexibility, lack of physical conditioning, and multiple pregnancies. Other health conditions are considered, such as osteoporosis, multiple myeloma, osteoarthritis, scoliosis, and ruptured disk. *Psychological factors* include the person's levels of anxiety, stress, and pain tolerance. *Occupational risk factors* for back pain include heavy physical work; frequent bending, twisting, lifting, pushing, and pulling; repetitive strain; and injury or accidents. *Recreational risk factors* include hockey, football, gymnastics, golf, racquetball, bowling, squash, handball, tennis, backpacking, wrestling, skiing, and other high-impact sports. All applicable risk factors are noted during the history.

The chiropractic physician relies heavily on hands-on procedures using palpation to determine both structural and functional problems. These hands-on procedures are complemented by a neurologic physical examination, which is the same as performed by a physician practicing conventional medicine. In the motion palpation exam, the chiropractor physically examines the spine, noting how it feels as well as how the client says it feels. The client is gently moved into and out of various postures during this part of the exam. Some postures are done standing, while others are done lying down. This process often informs the chiropractor what movements or positions reproduce or aggravate the pain. X-rays to confirm diagnostic findings may or may not be done.

Hypermobility of spinal joints is diagnosed by the sound of a repeated click when a joint is moved through its normal range of motion. This unstable type of subluxation is related to flaccid ligaments and is more problematic than the fixated type of subluxation. Hypermobile joints should not be forcibly manipulated, since manipulation can move the joint beyond the safe range of motion and increase the degree of hypermobility. Rather, nearby joints that have become fixated to compensate for the unstable joint can be manipulated, and muscle strength and tone can be increased with exercise (Redwood, 2015).

The chiropractor rules out pathologies that contraindicate SMT. For example, advanced, degenerative joint disease would rule out all forms of SMT that use significant force on the joint. Chiropractic treatment is not appropriate in the case of spinal infections, fractures, or tumors, which fortunately are fairly rare. In addition, SMT is not done on a woman in late pregnancy or on people whose pain is increased with manipulation. Diagnosis determines appropriate chiropractic treatment, referral for appropriate conventional medical care, or concurrent care. In the past, there has been some concern that spinal manipulation may be related to cervical artery dissection and stroke. However, multiple studies have found the rate to be 1 to 3 incidents per 1 million treatments (Biller et al., 2014; Redwood, 2015).

TREATMENT

Three primary clinical goals guide chiropractic intervention. The *first clinical goal* is to reduce or eliminate people's pain. Typically, this goal is the client's primary—and often only—goal. The *second clinical goal* is to correct the subluxation, thereby restoring biomechanical balance to reestablish shock absorption, leverage, and range of motion. In addition, spinal rehabilitative exercises are encouraged to strengthen muscles and ligaments to increase resistance to further injury. The *third clinical goal* is to perform preventive maintenance to ensure that the problem does not recur. This goal is comparable to the practice of having teeth cleaned periodically to prevent decay. Maintenance intervals vary from person to person depending on lifestyle.

Back pain is a leading cause of disability and the second most common reason (after the common cold) people visit a doctor. Chiropractors have twice the number of visits for back pain as do biomedical physicians. Most chiropractors also treat peripheral joints—elbows, knees, and shoulders. In 1994, a panel from the Agency for Healthcare Research and Quality (AHRQ) of the U.S. Department of Health and Human Services concluded that spinal manual therapy speeds recovery from acute low back pain and recommended it either in combination with or as a replacement for the use of nonsteroidal anti-inflammatory drugs. At the same time, the panel rejected many methods used for years by conventional medicine, such as bed rest, traction, and various other physical therapy modalities, and cautioned against spinal surgery except in the most severe cases (Theberge, 2008). **Spinal manipulation** is an assisted (chiropractor) passive (client) motion applied to the spinal facet joints or the sacroiliac joints. Chiropractors use their hands to apply pressure in a specific location and direction. The skill lies in the ability to be specific about which joint is being manipulated, which is especially important in the presence of any unstable joints. A chiropractor has 10 to 20 different ways of manipulating every movable joint in the body. Chiropractors also practice soft-tissue manipulation to stretch contracted muscles and decrease muscle spasms.

High-velocity, low-amplitude (HVLA) thrust adjustment is the most common form of manipulation. It is performed by manually moving a joint to the end point of its normal range of motion, isolating it by local pressure on bony prominences, and then giving a swift, specific, low-amplitude thrust. Often, a series of these thrusts are applied to the back and neck. When the facet joints are forced apart, a small vacuum is created and then released, which creates a popping sound much like that produced when people crack their knuckles. This manipulation does not cause pain, though people may feel a little discomfort the next day owing to rebalancing of the contracted muscles. This sensation can be compared to muscular soreness at the beginning of a weight training program. Other adjusting methods include low-velocity thrust adjustment with mechanically assisted drop-piece tables, various light-touch techniques, ultrasound, and electrical muscle stimulation. Some chiropractors use an activator adjusting instrument (AAI) instead of their hands to do the adjustment. This is a low-force, high-speed adjustment that is especially good for children and the elderly (Souza, 2014).

Safety is always a concern in any form of health-care treatment. HVLA is *absolutely contraindicated* in malignancies, bone and joint infections, acute myelopathy, acute fractures and dislocations, acute rheumatoid or rheumatoid-like joint pathology, and unstable joints. Adverse effects with cervical adjustment may be more serious, such as disk injury, vertebrobasilar infarction, or vertebral fracture (Souza, 2014).

Network chiropractic spinal analysis blends chiropractic and energy field principles. This approach assesses two types of subluxations: structural, involving the joint facets; and soft tissue, involving tension in the muscles and other soft tissue connected to the spine. Network chiropractors treat the soft-tissue subluxations with energy techniques before correcting the structural subluxations with manipulation. Similar to network chiropractic is **Bio-Energetic Synchronization Technique** (BEST). Chiropractors using BEST look at the part of the body responsible for misalignment of the spine and use energy balancing to treat the malfunction (Souza, 2014).

Craniosacral therapy involves manipulation of the sutures in the skull, resulting in decreased cerebrospinal fluid pressure and increased mobility of the cranial bones. Stimulating nerve endings in the scalp triggers the nervous system to turn off stress signals. The goal of craniosacral therapy is to reestablish structural stability and improve neurologic function. It is used to treat problems of the brain and spinal cord, such as chronic pain, headache, temporomandibular joint (TMJ) syndrome, stroke, epilepsy, cerebral palsy, dizziness, and tinnitus. Craniosacral therapy is rapidly gaining acceptance in Western medicine. In addition to chiropractors, nurses, physicians, dentists, and physical therapists are incorporating craniosacral techniques into their practice (Oschman, 2016).

As holistic practitioners, chiropractors work with many facets of clients' lifestyles. Chiropractors provide nutrition education, design exercise programs, plan rehabilitation measures, explain correct posture and lifting techniques, and assess and improve activities of daily living. Conditions commonly seen by a chiropractor include the following:

- Lower back syndromes
- Midback conditions
- Neck syndromes
- Headaches
- Carpal tunnel syndrome
- Sciatica
- Muscle spasms
- Sports-related injuries
- Whiplash and accident-related injuries
- Arthritic conditions
- Shoulder conditions
- Torticollis
- Extremity trauma

RESEARCH

Procedures have been researched since the early days of chiropractic, though researchers frequently had difficulty in finding a source for publication. The most significant research in the 1980s and 1990s was done outside the United States. The quality and quantity of chiropractic research in the United States has increased, however, as chiropractors have become more accepted by bio-medical physicians. Professional groups such as the American Back Society, the North American Spine Society, the International Society for the Study of the Lumbar Spine, and the American Public Health Association all accept chiropractic physicians as full members.

The National Center for Complementary and Integrative Health has established a Developmental Center at the Palmer College of Chiropractic. The purpose of this center is to enhance research and build relationships with institutions of conventional medicine. The following is a small sampling of studies:

- A systematic review and meta-analysis found that there was moderate level evidence to support the immediate effectiveness of cervical spine manipulation in people with cervical radiculopathy (Zhu, Wei, & Wang, 2016).
- A systematic review found that chiropractic intervention was not effective for sleep difficulties in postmenopausal women (Goto et al., 2014).
- A review of systematic reviews found that chiropractic interventions demonstrated improvement in conditions such as shoulder and neck trigger points, neck pain, and sport injuries. In the case of asthma, infant colic, fibromyalgia, and autism spectrum disorder, the recommendation is for larger sample sizes and high-quality research methodology (Salehi, Hashemi, Imanieh, & Saber, 2015).
- A systematic review found that chiropractic was as effective as physical therapy in persons with low back pain (Blanchette et al., 2016).

Chiropractic researchers are examining the effectiveness of chiropractic in organic or somatovisceral disorders. With growing medical–chiropractic cooperation and new federal funding of studies, more widely disseminated research findings are anticipated.

INTEGRATED NURSING PRACTICE

Observing a client's posture and gait is a key component of basic nursing assessment. Normally, a person's posture should be erect and at ease with the shoulders level and straight. Movements should be smooth and relaxed. A normal walk is rhythmic, in a straight, upright position with the arms swinging naturally at each side. General nursing assessment data provided by the client includes the following:

- Description of current mobility, mobility 2 months ago, and mobility 2 years ago

- Description of changes in the ability to walk, sit, or stand
- History of injuries and treatments
- Description of daily exercise routine
- List of sport activities
- Description of repetitive movements related to work or other activities

During a nursing assessment, clients are asked to walk across the room and back as the nurse looks for any difficulties with gait or posture that require further evaluation. An older client's gait may include short, shuffling, uncertain, and sometimes unsteady steps with a decreased arm swing. As people age, they often develop slumped shoulders and a more stooped body posture. Pregnant women often experience changes in body posture and gait as their pregnancy advances. The pelvis tips forward, increasing the lumbosacral curve, creating a gradual lordosis—an exaggerated lumbar curve in the spine. The enlarging breasts may pull the shoulders forward, contributing to a stooped body posture. As the pelvic joints relax and the weight and size of the fetus increase, the woman's center of gravity, stance, and gait are altered, contributing to the common complaint of backaches.

As a nurse, you can intervene to help with minor difficulties of gait and posture. Teach people to warm up and stretch before exercising, and cool down and stretch afterward. Many people can participate in low-impact aerobic activity that does not stress muscles and joints, such as walking, swimming, dancing, weight training, and bicycling. Other activities you can encourage are yoga, t'ai chi, and qigong, which are presented in other chapters in this text. Help people become aware of problems they are experiencing in posture, and encourage them to walk and sit "straight, tall, and relaxed." Good standing posture is with one's feet facing forward, knees slightly flexed, chest up, shoulders back, and chin parallel to the floor. Good sitting posture includes feet flat on the floor, with knees, ankles, and hips at right angles, and chin parallel to the floor.

Nursing practice and chiropractic medicine support the belief that prevention of injuries is preferred over treatment of injuries. Many nursing activities such as lifting, transferring, or positioning clients require muscle exertion by the nurse. To reduce the risk of injury to your clients and yourself, practice proper body mechanics. The coordinated motion of the body depends on the integrated functioning of bones, joints, muscles, and the nervous system. You achieve better body balance from a wide base of support created by separating your feet to a comfortable distance. Bending your knees and flexing your hips, thus bringing the center of gravity closer to your support base, will also improve your balance. When you are lifting an object or person, use your legs to lift and your arms to support. Facing the direction of movement and pivoting with your feet prevents abnormal twisting of the spine. Balancing activity between arms and legs protects the back from strain.

A referral to chiropractic evaluation and treatment is appropriate for the conditions listed earlier in the chapter. Chiropractors view themselves as contributing members of the health-care team and refer to conventional physicians for problems outside their scope of practice. Although chiropractors have clear guidelines for referring to conventional practitioners, biomedical professionals have not developed formal guidelines for referring to chiropractors. It is time for communication and cooperation to be broadened between conventional practitioners and chiropractors in an effort to create the most effective health-care system for the greatest number of people.

TRY THIS

Energy Boosters

Poor posture robs your body of energy. You may spend many hours of your day walking incorrectly or slumped in a chair, which interrupts the flow of energy and oxygen through your body and spinal cord. Take a moment to sit up or stand straight. Imagine that a cord is attached to the top of your head, pulling it gently toward the sky. This image helps readjust your posture. Feel your head, neck, shoulders, and spine relax as they realign from a constricting position. This imagery, practiced either sitting or standing, will revive you.

Take your shoes off; sit on the floor with your legs stretched out in front of you and your palms facing down at your sides. Point your toes as hard as you can and hold for 5 seconds, then flex your feet as hard as you can and hold for 5 seconds. Repeat 10 times.

References

Biller, J., Sacco, R. L., Albuquerque, F. C., Demaerschalk, B. M., Fayad, P., Long, P. H., . . . Tirschwell, D. L. (2014). Cervical arterial dissections and association with cervical manipulative therapy. *Stroke.* doi: 10.1161/STR.0000000000000016

Blanchette, M. A., Stochkendahl, M. J., Borges, D. S., Boruff, J., Harrison, P., & Bussieres, A. (2016). Effectiveness and economic evaluation of chiropractic care for the treatment of low back pain: A systematic review of pragmatic studies. *Public Library of Science.* doi: 10.1371/journal.pone.0160037

Goto, V., Frange, C., Andersen, M. L., Junior, J. M., Tufik, S., & Hachul, H. (2014). Chiropractic intervention in the treatment of postmenopausal climacteric symptoms and insomnia. *Maturitas.* doi: 10.1016/j.maturitas.2014.02.004

Hippocrates. (1983). *Hippocratic Writings* Vol. 451). Edited by G. E. R. Lloyd, J. Chadwick, & W. N. Mann. Penguin Books Limited.

Oschman, J. L. (2016). *Energy Medicine: The Scientific Basis* (2nd ed.). St. Louis, MO: Elsevier/Saunders.

Redwood, D. (2015). Chiropractic. In M. S. Micozzi (Ed.), *Fundamentals of Complementary and Alternative Medicine* (5th ed., pp. 300–325). St. Louis, MO: Elsevier/ Saunders.

Salehi, A., Hashemi, N., Imanieh, M. H., & Saber, M. (2015). Chiropractic: Is it efficient in treatment of diseases? Review of systematic reviews. *International Journal of Community Based Nursing and Midwifery.* Retrieved from www.ncbi.nim.nih.gov/pmc/articles/ PMC4591574

Smith, H. A., (1887). Chief Seattle's Speech. *Seattle Sunday Star*, October 29, 1887.

Souza, T. A. (2014). *Differential Diagnosis and Management for the Chiropractor.* Burlington, MA: Jones & Bartlett Learning.

Theberge, N. (2008). The integration of chiropractors into health care teams. *Sociology of Health and Illness*, 30(1): 19–34.

VanDehey, D. (2015). Innate intelligence—Chiropractic and your onboard healing mechanisms. In D. Friedman & R. V. Ittersum (Eds.), *A Cup of Coffee with 10 Leading Chiropractors in the United States* (pp. 34–54). Ramseur, NC: Rutherford Publishing House.

Zhu, L., Wei, X., & Wang, S. (2016). Does cervical spine manipulation reduce pain in people with degenerative cervical radiculopathy? A systematic review of the evidence, and a meta-analysis. *Clinical Rehabilitation.* doi: 10.1177/0269215515570382

Resources

American Chiropractic Association
1701 Clarendon Blvd.
Arlington, VA 22209
703.276.8800
www.acatoday.org

British Chiropractic Association
0118.950.5950
enquiries@chiropractic-uk.co.uk
www.chiropractic-uk.co.uk

Canadian Chiropractic Association
186 Spadina Ave, Suite 6
Toronto, ON M5T 3B2
877.222.9303
www.chiropracticcanada.ca/

The Chiropractors' Association of Australia
Level 1, 75 George St.
P.O. Box 255, Parramatta, NSW 2124
1800.075.003
www.chiropractors.asn.au

Federation of Chiropractic Licensing Boards
5401 West 10th St., Suite 101
Greeley, CO 80634-4400
970.356.3500
www.fclb.org

World Chiropractic Alliance
800.347.1011
www.worldchiropracticalliance.org

12
Massage

If you want to go faster, go alone
If you want to go farther, go together.

AFRICAN PROVERB

Massage therapy, the scientific manipulation of the soft tissues of the body, is a healing art, an act of physical caring, and a way of communicating without words. Massage, a hands-on touch therapy, is experiencing an ever-widening U.S. audience. Massage is the most prevalent complementary therapy offered in hospitals in the United States. The goal of massage therapy is to achieve or increase health and well-being and to help the body heal itself. Although massage therapists may hold general views of health and well-being, massage therapy has no specific theoretical framework or diagnostic system of disease.

Touch, from the moment of our birth, is critical for our physical, mental, and spiritual well-being. In some cultures, social touch is considered to be warm and friendly while in other cultures it is considered intrusive or even inappropriate. Cultural values surround what body parts may/may not be touched, who is allowed/forbidden to touch, and who is allowed to receive social touch. Compared with members of other cultures, people in the United States are generally touch phobic and touch deprived.

Concerns have escalated about "inappropriate" touch, sexual abuse, and sexual harassment in schools and workplaces in the United States. Touch, unfortunately, has become associated with sex. Some schools have instituted "teach, but don't touch" policies. It is rare to see teachers put their hands on the shoulder of a child who is crying. Sadly, to protect themselves from being accused of inappropriate touch, many people are not touching at all. While concern for protecting children from those who would touch inappropriately is valid, the implications of a "hands-off" barrier have significant negative effects on growth, development, and emotional well-being.

BACKGROUND

The idea that touch can heal is an old one. Cave paintings in the Pyrenees show that 15,000 years ago people treated injuries with what looks like massage, and references to massage are found in 4,000-year-old Chinese medical texts. In the fourth century B.C., Hippocrates wrote, "The physician must be acquainted with many things and assuredly with rubbing" (the ancient Greek and Roman term for massage). Some of the greatest physicians in history advocated massage, including Celsus (25 B.C.–A.D. 50), Galen (130–200), and Avicenna (980–1037). Ambroise Paré (1517–1590), called by some the father of surgery, William Harvey (1578–1657), who demonstrated the circulation of blood, and Herman Boerhaave (1668–1738), who introduced the clinical method of teaching medicine, all utilized massage as a healing technique. Roman gladiators were massaged before entering the arenas, and 18th-century Swedish cavalrymen were rubbed down between battles. In the Middle Ages, Christians viewed massage as the work of the devil, and many therapists were burned at the stake as witches. Remnants of this attitude have continued into the 20th century, as massage is sometimes assumed to be a front for prostitution (Rose, 2012).

The 13th-century German Emperor Frederick II was curious to know what language children would speak if they were raised without hearing any words at all. Having stolen a number of newborns from their parents, he gave them to nurses who physically cared for the infants but were forbidden to cuddle or talk to them. All the children died before they could talk, which revealed a critical fact: tactile stimulation can be a matter of life and death. Most recently, a similar situation occurred in the early 1990s in Romania when thousands of infants were stockpiled in orphanages. Some were virtually left alone in their cribs for 2 years and were discovered to be severely impaired as a result of this isolation (Colt, 1997).

Two New York physicians who were trained in Sweden introduced massage into the United States in the mid-19th century. The first massage therapy clinics were opened by Swedish physicians after the Civil War and had among their clients members of Congress and Presidents Harrison and Grant. At first, physicians performed massage, but they eventually delegated the technique to nurses and physical therapists. By the mid-20th century, massage therapy had virtually been abandoned by most health-care professionals except nurses. For many years, during the time of relatively little technology, it was standard nursing practice to give back rubs after bathing clients, and back rubs were also a routine part of hour-of-sleep care. Advanced medical technology, sophisticated equipment, and the assumption by nurses of more management roles left little time for hands-on nursing care. There was an upsurge of interest in the field in the 1970s when

Drs. Dolores Kreiger and Martha Rogers, two nurse pioneers, advocated the art and caring form of touch in nursing practice. Nurses are now returning to their tradition in providing comfort and care through the use of touch and massage. Most communities of Catholic sisters have at least one sister trained in massage therapy, and massage is routinely offered at spiritual retreats. These sisters have come to recognize the power of spiritual renewal from physical contact in their healing ministries. If clients choose, they also pray with them. Going beyond what most massage therapists do, sisters often set aside time after the massage if the client wants to talk about a problem or issue.

In the United States, some insurance companies will pay for massage that has been ordered by a primary health-care provider, but most do not. In many areas of the world, massage is an integral part of health systems. In Russia, much of Europe, China, and Japan, massage therapists work along with physicians in the hospital setting as important members of the health-care team. Some U.S. hospitals have a massage therapist available for outpatient and inpatient clients.

PREPARATION

Therapists who have 600 or more hours of education from a recognized school are eligible to take the National Certification Examination offered by the National Certification Board for Therapeutic Massage and Bodywork. The International Association of Infant Massage also certifies instructors who take 4 days of training, read course material, and pass a take-home exam. There is also a certification process for those therapists who wish to practice prenatal massage therapy. The Federation of State Massage Therapy Boards facilitates communication among board members, which includes 47 state boards and the boards in the U.S. Virgin Islands and Puerto Rico. The goal of the organization is to improve standards of massage therapy education, licensure, and practice.

CONCEPTS

Skin

In many ways, human beings are wired for touch. The skin is the body's largest organ, covering almost 20 square feet and accounting for nearly one-quarter of the body's total weight. As many as 5 million touch receptors in the skin—3,000 in a fingertip—send messages via the spinal cord to the brain. The skin has four main functions: it protects against mechanical and radiation injuries and from invasion by foreign substances; it is a sense organ; it regulates temperature; and it is a metabolic organ. Of all the sensory organs, the skin is the most important. People can survive without the senses of sight, sound, smell, and taste but would find it difficult to survive without the functions performed by the skin.

Touch

Touch is a primal need, as necessary for growth and development as food, clothing, or shelter. The sense of touch is the earliest to develop in the human embryo, and at less than 6 weeks of gestation, a light stroking of the face will cause the neck and trunk to bend away from the source of stimulation. Touch continues to function even after seeing and hearing begin to fade with age. Touch can be thought of as a nutrient transmitted through the skin in many different ways: holding, cuddling, nuzzling, caressing, and massage. From the bonding of parent and newborn to holding the hand of a dying loved one, touch is the most intimate and powerful form of communication between people. It can be aggressive, as the spanking of a child or a punch in the face. It can be tender, as the hug that comforts a crying friend or the touch of a lover.

The importance of the sense of touch is evident in many English expressions. Some people have to be "handled" carefully because they are "thin-skinned," while others are "thick-skinned." "Touchy" people are overly sensitive or easily angered. Some people are "soft touches," and others have "the human touch." Some people "rub" others the wrong way. "Feeling" for another person is a description of empathy. A "touching" experience is something that is deeply felt. As biomedicine continues to make incredible advances in technology, it leaves behind one of the most valuable senses of a human being—that of touch. This sense of isolation may explain, in part, the increasing interest in healing practices, most of which include the experience of touch.

Trigger Points

When a person is injured or bodily systems are malfunctioning, trigger points or pain reflexes appear throughout the body. A trigger point is a "knot" of tensed muscles that when stimulated triggers a referred pain response in other parts of the body. Some of the trigger points are in the area of the injury or problem, while others are at a distance. Rubbing and exerting pressure on these points have been found to have a positive effect on the healing process (Benjamin, 2016).

Fascia and Fascial Restrictions

The fascia is the tough connective tissue in the body that is almost like a three-dimensional web from head to foot. If somehow every structure of the body were removed except the fascia, the body would retain its shape. Every muscle, bone, organ, nerve, and blood vessel of the body is covered with fascia like a continuous plastic wrapping. Fascia varies in thickness and density and in the amount of collagenous fiber, elastic fiber, and tissue fluid it contains. The function of the fascia is to support cells, muscles, groups of muscles, and organs and act as a shock absorber. At the cellular level, fascia creates the interstitial spaces and is important in cellular respiration, elimination, metabolism, fluid, and lymphatic flow.

Each time a person experiences a trauma, undergoes an inflammatory process, or suffers from poor posture over time, the fascial system becomes restricted, and the individual loses flexibility and spontaneity of motion. As the fascia continues to slowly tighten, an abnormal pressure develops on the nerves, muscles, bones, or organs, resulting in poor cellular efficiency, necrosis, pain, and dysfunction throughout the body (Delany, 2015).

VIEW OF HEALTH AND ILLNESS

It is believed that massage aids the ability of the body to heal itself, so the aim of massage is to achieve or increase health and well-being. Only now are scientists coming to appreciate the importance—and the power—of touch. The Touch Research Institute (TRI) at the University of Miami School of Medicine brings together researchers from Duke, Harvard, the University of Maryland, and other universities to study touch and how it might be used to promote health and treat disease.

A stronger, sustained touch in massage can have a greater effect than other forms of touch. A skilled massage therapist not only stretches and loosens muscle and connective tissue but also greatly improves blood flow and the movement of lymph fluid throughout the body. Massage speeds the removal of metabolic waste products resulting from exercise or inactivity, allowing more oxygen and nutrients to reach the cells and tissues. The release of muscular tension also helps unblock and balance the overall flow of life energy throughout the body known as qi, ki, prana, or subtle energy. In addition, massage can stimulate the release of endorphins, serotonin, dopamine, and oxytocin. The benefits of massage are described in Box 12.1.

BOX 12.1

The Benefits of Massage

Physical level
- Relieves muscle tension and stiffness
- Reduces muscle spasm and tension
- Provides relief from pain
- Speeds recovery from exertion
- Improves joint flexibility and range of motion
- Increases ease and efficiency of movement
- Improves posture
- Stimulates lymphatic circulation, which decreases edema
- Improves local circulation, which increases healing of injured tissues
- Lowers blood pressure, slows heart rate
- Promotes deeper, easier breathing
- Eases tension headaches
- Improves the health of the skin

(continued)

Mental level

- Induces a relaxed state of alertness
- Reduces mental stress, thus clearing the mind
- Increases capacity for clearer thinking

Emotional level

- Satisfies the need for caring and nurturing touch
- Increases feelings of well-being, decreases mild depression
- Enhances self-image
- Reduces levels of anxiety
- Increases awareness of mind–body connection

As an adjunct to medical treatment, massage may be helpful in relieving backaches, headaches, muscle spasm and pain, hypertension, swelling and pain from injuries or after surgery, grand mal seizures, insomnia, anxiety, and depression. Massage can be a palliative treatment for those with terminal conditions and can help maintain circulation and muscle tone in individuals who are bedridden. Even people in deep comas may show improved heart rates when their hands are held. Most comprehensive cancer treatment programs offer massage as a standard component of care. Massage can reduce agitation in persons with Alzheimer's disease, and it has been used to relieve stress at disaster sites.

Massage has been used with individuals who have psychiatric disabilities as an adjunct to conventional psychiatric interventions. Clients are given a chair massage, done with the client fully dressed and seated on a massage chair. The head, neck, back, arms, and legs are massaged for 10 to 20 minutes per session.

Some businesses provide chair massage for their employees as part of their wellness programs. The immediate effect is one of feeling better immediately. The longer range effect is an improvement in employee performance and productivity, as well as feelings of loyalty to the business.

TREATMENT

Touch is the fundamental medium of massage therapy. It is, however, more than just mechanical manipulation. Touch is a form of communication; thus, one of its most significant benefits is the comfort of human care conveyed by the therapist. Massage communicates gentleness and connection, trust and receiving, and peace and alertness.

The first massage therapy appointment begins with questions about one's physical condition, medical history, and current aches and pains. The therapist determines what a client hopes to gain from the massage. The client undresses in private and uses a sheet or blanket for draping. The individual decides whether underwear is on or off. The client lies on a cushioned table, and the therapist uncovers only that part of the body that is being massaged, using oil or lotion to help the hands move smoothly. It is recommended that clients not eat just before a massage and drink extra water afterward to clear the body of toxins released from deep tissues. At home, clients are encouraged to enjoy a salt bath as another aid in detoxifying the body. A half cup each of sea salt, Epsom salt, and baking soda is added to a tub of warm water for the salt bath.

From hour-long massages in therapists' offices to 10-minute massages at the workplace, a massage is available for practically everybody and every budget. Massage therapists offer their services in a wide variety of settings such as private practice clinics, health clubs and fitness centers, chiropractic offices, nursing homes and hospitals, salons and resorts, on site in the workplace, and even in clients' homes. There are almost as many styles of massage as there are practitioners. Most therapists combine a variety of methods in their work, which allows them to tailor each session to the specific needs of the client. Box 12.2 lists some cautions and risks associated with massage therapy.

Massage is contraindicated in the following conditions:

- Phlebitis/thrombosis
- Severe varicose veins
- Any acute inflammation of the skin, soft tissue, or joints
- Burns
- Areas of hemorrhage or heavy tissue damage
- Unregulated blood pressure
- Unstable blood sugar
- Herniated disk
- Recent fractures or sprains
- Advanced osteoporosis
- A bleeding disorder or taking blood-thinning drugs
- Some types of cancer

BOX 12.2

Cautions/Risks of Massage Therapy

Rarely can cause:
- Internal bleeding
- Nerve damage
- Temporary paralysis
- Allergic reactions to massage oils or lotions

Prenatal massage—consult health-care provider
- High-risk pregnancy
- Pregnancy-induced hypertension
- Preeclampsia
- Previous preterm labor
- Can induce labor

Swedish Massage

Peter Ling of Sweden, who integrated ancient Asian massage with a Western understanding of anatomy and physiology, developed **Swedish massage** about 150 years ago. It is the most common form of massage in the United States. Swedish massage uses a system of long gliding strokes, as well as kneading and friction techniques on the more superficial layers of the muscles, combined with active and passive movements of the joints. It is used primarily for a full-body massage to promote general relaxation, improve circulation and range of motion, and relieve muscle tension.

Swedish massage uses five basic strokes. *Effleurage*, French for "touching," is the introductory stroke. The therapist uses the whole hand in providing long, gliding strokes to relax the central nervous system and prepare the local area for the other strokes. *Petrissage* involves grasping muscle groups and lifting them, stretching them away from the bones, and then kneading or rolling them. This technique is the closest to imitating exercise because it makes the muscles contract. This stroke is used mostly on flaccid muscles that require an increase in contractile ability. Petrissage also stimulates the central nervous system and therefore is not used with clients who have cerebrovascular dysfunctions. *Friction* involves using the fingers and thumbs to press on small areas and move in a circular motion around each area. *Vibration* involves placing the hands on a muscle group and moving them back and forth quickly in a shaking motion. *Tapotement* or *percussion* involves striking the skin with the outside edges of the hands, fingers, or cupped palms to stimulate circulation (Benjamin, 2016).

Shiatsu Massage

In Japanese, *shi* means "finger" and *atsu* means "pressure." **Shiatsu massage** is the Japanese adaptation of acupressure. Like Chinese acupuncture and acupressure, shiatsu is based on the idea that life energy, *ki*, flows along invisible pathways called meridians. Health is related to a free flow of energy, and illness is caused by blockages to the flow. Blocked energy can cause physical discomforts, so the aim is to release the blocks associated with the discomfort or disease and rebalance the energy flow. Therapists use their hands, elbows, and even their feet to press for about 30 seconds on each point. Depending on the way it is done, shiatsu can be gentle or quite forceful. Done on a floor mat rather than a massage table, a typical shiatsu session lasts about an hour (Jackson & Latini, 2016).

Watsu

Harold Dull, shiatsu therapist, started Watsu, a form of aquatic rehabilitation, in 1980 at Harbin Hot Springs, California. Watsu is done in a chest-deep, warm water pool with the practitioner cradling the client in a floating position. With the client deeply relaxed, the therapist moves and stretches the client's body. Watsu increases range of motion, improves sleep, decreases anxiety, and decreases hypertonicity. It is used for neuromuscular injuries, stress, chronic pain, fibromyalgia, arthritis, lower back pain, and pregnancy discomfort (Scaer, 2014).

Sports Massage

Sports massage uses techniques of both Swedish and shiatsu massage but focuses on parts of the body that are likely to be stressed by a particular sport. It takes less time than Swedish or shiatsu and is usually more vigorous. For example, runners might need to have their hamstrings worked extensively. This technique also concentrates on reducing or eliminating factors that interfere with human performance, such as muscle spasms, tendonitis, and muscle fatigue.

Prior to an athletic event, massage loosens, warms, and readies the muscle for intensive use, especially when combined with stretching. Besides helping prevent injury, massage can improve performance and endurance. Postevent massage relieves pain, prevents stiffness, and returns the muscles to their normal state more rapidly. The use of massage in sports health care is increasing rapidly in both training and competition. Recreational athletes have also discovered the benefits of sports massage as a regular part of their workouts.

Trigger Point Massage

Trigger point massage is a type of deep massage in which the fingers are used to release knots and tender spots in muscles. Rubbing and exerting pressure on these points has been found to have a positive effect on the healing process by interrupting the cycle of spasm and pain. Techniques are similar to those used in shiatsu but are based on Western anatomy and physiology. Trigger point massage is typically a technique incorporated into Swedish or sports massage.

Myofascial Release

Myofascial release is a whole-body therapy preceded by a comprehensive evaluation and diagnostic workup. The therapist evaluates the fascial system through visual analysis and palpation of tissue and fascial layers. Normal tissue is soft and mobile in all directions. Abnormal tissue may feel hot, hard, sensitive, or somewhat stringy or crunchy. When the therapist has determined where the fascial restrictions lie, gentle pressure is applied in the direction of the restriction, which is designed to break up the collagen of the fascia. Myofascial release is effective in strains and sprains, headaches, chronic pain, temporomandibular joint (TMJ) pain, and adhesions. Myofascial release is contraindicated in malignancy, open wounds, cellulitis, febrile state, hematoma, infection, advanced degenerative changes, acute circulatory conditions, and acute rheumatoid arthritis (Benjamin, 2016).

Rolfing

Developed by the late biochemist Ida P. Rolf, **Rolfing** (also known as structural integration) is a system of whole-body manipulation in which the Rolfer uses the fingers, knuckles, and elbows to stretch the fascia, which tends to bind up because of injury, bad posture, emotional problems, or genetic weaknesses. The fascia is stretched to release patterns of tension and rigidity and return the body to a state of correct alignment. Whereas other massage therapists work by applying smooth strokes over muscles, Rolfers press deeply into muscle tissue and fascia to release them. Clients are asked to breathe deeply during the session and visualize the muscle lengthening. The current Rolfing method is gentler and far less painful than the original style of treatment. Practitioners use a broad range of touch and pressure from feather-light to deep massage. When performed with the right sensitivity, even deep and heavy pressure may not be painful.

Thai Massage

Some people call **Thai massage** "passive yoga" because the receiver is fully clothed, lies on a futon, and is deeply stretched, compressed, and gently rocked. The whole body of the therapist is used to treat the whole body of the receiver. The experience feels like a combination of yoga, shiatsu, and meditation. Point pressure and kneading of the tissues are similar to massage techniques. Yoga techniques involve positioning the client in numerous stretches similar to yoga poses, then gently rocking the person to deepen the stretch and open the joints. The gentle rocking creates an energy flow through the different stretches. Thai massage gives the person flexibility, inner organ massage, oxygenation of the blood, and quieting of the mind that comes with yoga, and because the receiver is passive, the session becomes meditative. Sometimes, the therapist stands on the recipient and gently rolls one foot on and off the body. This compression can be gentle to deep and can energize or relax the recipient.

Chinese Massage

Tui na is one of the four main branches of Traditional Chinese Medicine, the others being herbs, acupuncture, and qigong. Tui na is the forerunner of all forms of massage that exist today, but it differs from other types of massage in that it is used to treat specific illnesses as well as musculoskeletal problems. A practitioner of Tui na must be a Traditional Chinese Medicine physician to make an accurate diagnosis before instituting treatment. Tui na is often combined with qigong exercises for building up general health and strength. See Chapter 23 for information on qigong.

Bowenwork®

Bowenwork® is a type of massage that uses gentle hand movements to stretch muscles and fascia to stimulate nerve pathways. Lymph and blood movement is increased, which improves tissue repair of injuries. Bowenwork® was first introduced in Australia and has become an accredited, 2-year vocational program in Victoria, Australia. It is offered as a therapy worldwide.

Chair Massage

Chair massage is done with the client fully dressed, seated on a portable massage chair. A doughnut-shaped pillow that allows for easy breathing supports the person's face. The sessions, which last 10 to 20 minutes, involve massage of the head, neck, back, arms, and hands. This type of massage is often provided in the workplace, shopping malls, or airports. The purpose of the massage is to decrease tension, reduce stress, and enhance people's adaptive capabilities.

Pregnancy Massage

Massage is contraindicated until after the first trimester of pregnancy because of the danger of miscarriage during that time. During the second and third trimesters, massage can ease pain and provide comfort to the pregnant woman. Massage relaxes the woman and reduces the flow of stress hormones to the baby. It also nurtures the woman, which helps her nurture her baby after birth. Pregnancy massage is usually done in a side-lying position with plenty of pillows or cushions for support (see Figure 12.1). The massage usually is done to the neck, arms/hands, back, pelvis, and legs/feet. Since not all massage therapists are trained in pregnancy massage, consumers must ask about the experience and/or credentials of a particular therapist.

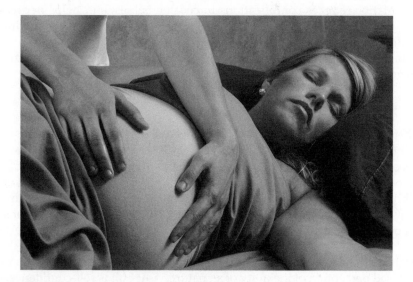

FIGURE 12.1   Pregnant Woman Getting a Massage
Source: Alwekelo/Getty Images.

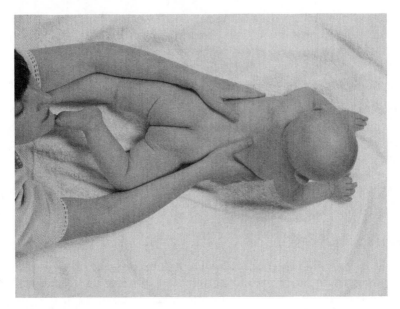

FIGURE 12.2 Baby Boy Having His Back and Side Massaged

Source: Banana Stock/Alamy Stock Photo.

Infant Massage

Infant massage is gaining in popularity in the United States (see Figure 12.2). Researchers have found that infant massage produces weight gains in premature infants, reduces complications in cocaine babies, and helps depressed mothers soothe their babies. In healthy babies, it improves parent–infant bonding, eases painful procedures such as inoculations, reduces pain from teething and constipation, reduces colic, induces sleep, and makes parents feel good (Benjamin, 2016).

Self-Massage

Self-massage is a wonderful way for people to better acquaint themselves with their entire body. It is a process in which they learn to be aware of and release tensions and inhibitions, to reclaim parts of themselves that have been neglected, and to accept themselves as they are. Self-massage increases one's ability to listen to the body and enhances one's healing journey. Getting to know and appreciate one's body through touch is an important part of self-acceptance. The more in touch people are with themselves, the more they come in touch with the reality and experience of the world around them. Heightened awareness of the unity of body, mind, and spirit often leads to an increased perception of the unity of all nature. As it builds self-confidence and self-acceptance, this awareness enables people to respond with more compassion and caring toward others.

Self-massage is done in a warm, comfortable, and quiet environment. Breath work and relaxation techniques are utilized to ground and center oneself before the experience. Self-massage often begins with gazing at oneself naked in a mirror, withholding judgment and criticism. The next step is to stretch like a cat and pay attention to how the body feels. If there is an area that is stiff or tender, the person slowly moves, gently holds, or massages that part. Then the person finds a position that is relaxing and comfortable. Without a set route or sequence, individual senses guide self-massage. Sometimes one may explore and massage the whole body, and at other times one may feel like spending the whole time on one part, such as the face and head. Self-massage is done slowly and rhythmically with the eyes closed so that one's whole attention can be focused on the sensation (Benjamin, 2016).

RESEARCH

During the past half century, numerous reports on clinical trials have been published in health-care literature. These reports have documented the benefits of massage therapy for the treatment of pain, inflammation, lymphedema, nausea, muscle spasm, various soft-tissue dysfunctions, grand mal seizures, anxiety, depression, and insomnia. Randomized controlled trials are somewhat difficult, since therapists individualize treatment approaches for each client.

- A systematic review and meta-analysis found that massage therapy was effective for relief from cancer pain compared to no massage treatment and conventional care (Lee, Kim, Yeo, Kim, & Lim, 2015).
- A systematic review and meta-analysis found that massage was effective in reducing pain in people with osteoarthritis of the knee (Field, 2016).
- A Joanna Briggs Institute evidence summary found that
  - massage therapy may be useful for reducing anxiety and blood pressure (Grade B)
  - massage therapy may be beneficial for people with subacute and chronic low back pain, especially when combined with exercise and education
  - massage can be recommended for improving quality of life and immune function for people with HIV/AIDS (Grade B)
  - massage is recommended for women who are in labor (Grade B)
  - there is insufficient evidence to recommend massage for mechanical neck pain and for people with intellectual disability (Slade, 2012).
- A controlled pilot study found that Watsu significantly decreased stress and pain and improved mood for women in their third trimester of pregnancy (Schitter, Nedeljkovic, Baur, Fleckenstein, & Raio, 2015).
- A controlled clinical trial studied the effect of myofascial massage on stress responders and stress nonresponders. The stress responders experienced a significantly better response to myofascial massage (Diaz-Rodriguez et al., 2016).

INTEGRATED NURSING PRACTICE

Massage provides a valuable tactile approach that when combined with verbal approaches communicates nurses' care and compassion. Back rubs, lasting 3 to 5 minutes, offer physiological and mechanical benefits to clients in a variety of settings. A back rub is usually given after the bath, but you may also find that giving one in the evening will help clients relax and fall asleep. Massage the back in a slow, rhythmical, and relaxed manner. Tightness through the shoulder and neck muscles from an uncomfortable resting position can be relieved with friction or petrissage. Gently rubbing the skin over bony areas increases circulation and helps prevent skin breakdown. If you are caring for someone who is in bed a great deal of the time, offer massage each time the person's position is changed. Observe for areas of redness, especially over the sacrum and the back of the heels, elbows, and knees. Stroking toward the pressure areas encourages capillary dilation.

People who are self-conscious about full-body or even back massage may accept and benefit from hand and foot massage. Figure 12.3 illustrates the procedure for a hand massage. These same steps can be adapted for a foot massage. By stimulating the circulation, massage eases stiffness and pain in persons with arthritis and helps drain lymph and decrease fluid retention in persons with dependent edema.

Childbirth nurses and *nurse midwives* have long advocated massage during pregnancy. A light, natural oil such as tangerine, almond, or safflower is used. Essential oils are not added because they may have ill effects on the fetus. The benefits of massage during pregnancy (Benjamin, 2016) are as follows:

- *Relaxes.* Massage helps reduce tension in the neck and shoulders and, in the later stages of pregnancy, in the lower back.
- *Uplifts.* Massage minimizes fatigue and improves the flow of energy and induces a general feeling of well-being.
- *Improves circulation.* Massage may help prevent varicose veins that may accompany pregnancy.
- *Stimulates lymphatic drainage.* Massage helps reduce fluid retention in the ankles and feet that often occurs during the later stages of pregnancy.
- *Tones muscles.* Massage helps relieve the pain of distended ligaments and decreases the tendency to cramp that may occur toward the fifth month of pregnancy.
- *Maintains skin tone.* Massage increases the skin's suppleness and elasticity and may help prevent stretch marks.

Midwives and *maternal child nurses* incorporate massage during labor and delivery. During contractions, deep massage of the lower back and hips provides counterpressure that many women find helpful. In between contractions, massage of the shoulders, back, hands, and feet increases comfort and relaxation. If contractions are lagging, a light massage of the breasts may stimulate activity. After delivery, gentle heat may be applied to the breasts followed by a firm massage around the breast toward the nipple to assist in milk letdown.

If you practice nursing in *newborn nurseries* and neonatal intensive care units, you should advocate infant massage and incorporate it as a basic nursing intervention. Most premature and drug-exposed infants given three massages a day are more alert, active, and responsive than nonmassaged infants. Massaged infants are also able to calm themselves, sleep more deeply, and have fewer episodes of apnea.

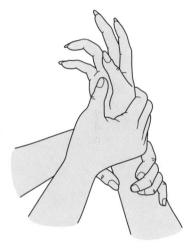

While holding the client's hand, place massage oil or lotion on the hand. Gently bend the hand backward and forward to limber the wrist. Grasp each finger and do range-of-motion exercises.

A

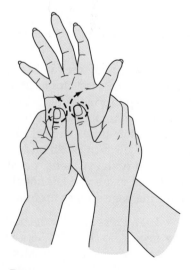

With the client's elbow resting on the table, hold the hand upright and massage the palm of the hand with the cushions of your thumbs, using circular movements in opposite directions.

B

FIGURE 12.3 Procedure for Hand Massage

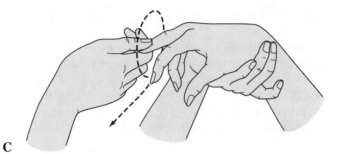

C

Massage each finger from the base to the tip, along all surfaces of the finger.

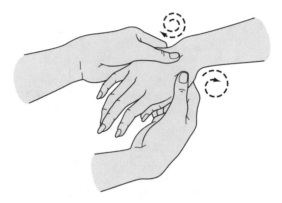

D

Use your thumbs to massage the wrist and top of the
hand, using circular movements. Repeat three times.
Repeat the entire procedure on the other hand.

FIGURE 12.3 Procedure for Hand Massage (*Continued*)

Whether you are massaging a newborn or teaching parents infant massage, the process lasts for as little as a few minutes or as long as a half hour but
should be performed only when a baby is willing. If a baby is crying, hiccup-
ping, or turning the head to the side, the massage should be discontinued and
tried another time. The oil for infant massage should be a light-textured,
unscented oil such as almond, coconut, or safflower oil. Infants should not be
massaged with synthetic, petroleum-based products because they have no
nutritional value and are not absorbed into the skin. The following are some
gentle massage strokes for infants:

- *Foot.* Press all over the bottom of the foot using the thumbs.
- *Leg.* Hold the leg like a baseball bat and move the hands up the leg,
  squeezing slightly and turning in opposite directions.
- *Stomach.* Make scooping strokes, one hand following the other.
- *Chest.* Begin with both hands at the center and gently push out to the
  sides along the rib cage.

- *Back.* With fingers spread apart, "comb" the back from the neck to the buttocks.
- *Hand.* Roll each finger between your finger and thumb; press gently all over the palm, using the thumbs.
- *Face.* Make small circles around the jaw using the fingertips.

If you are a *hospice* nurse, an important part of your care might be massage, which often helps manage pain and symptom distress. As well as integrating it into your routine nursing care, you can easily teach it to family members. Touch is a primal need, even during the process of dying. Being able to communicate caring through massage makes the process a little easier for all concerned.

You may wish to expand your expertise in massage by becoming a massage therapist and combining that practice with your practice of nursing. Contact the National Association of Nurse Massage Therapists (see the Resources section) for appropriate programs.

TRY THIS

Massage

One-Minute Massage

Revive your hair and your spirits with a simple scalp massage you can do anytime and almost anywhere. With your fingertips, rub the entire scalp using small circular motions. Massage stimulates the scalp oils that bring out the natural shine in hair. It is also an all-over energy booster.

Two-Minute Massage

Mix a tablespoon each of wheat germ, olive oil, and sunflower oil. Rub on your shoulders and neckline. After 2 minutes, rinse and pat dry. Lavish the damp skin with lotion.

Partner Massage

- Set the mood with scented candles and soft music in a dimly lit room.
- Lay folded quilts on the floor rather than using your bed, so you can easily move around your partner.
- Remove jewelry to avoid catching hairs as you work.
- Comfort your partner by covering her or him with a sheet and placing a pillow under the knees when lying faceup and under the ankles when lying facedown.
- Massage works best when strokes are lubricated. Any vegetable oil will work, but scented massage oils can add to the sense of relaxation and sensuality.
- Begin with both of you breathing slowly and deeply to center and ground yourselves.

(continued)

- Warm the oil by rubbing it between your hands before applying it.
- Begin with light strokes and proceed to deeper pressure only after the muscles in the area have relaxed and warmed up.
- Your partner should tell you if any strokes feel uncomfortable: too light, too deep, or on a tender spot.
- Take your time: ideally 2 to 3 minutes per foot, 10 minutes per leg, 15 to 20 minutes for the back, and 15 minutes for the front, including 5 minutes on the face.
- Stroke toward the heart instead of against the flow of blood returning to the heart.
- Never press directly on the spinal column, just on the muscles on either side of it.
- The best massage comes from using your whole body, not just your arms.

Sources: Benjamin (2016); Bligny (2011); Salvo (2015).

CONSIDERING THE EVIDENCE
Hand Massage with Essential Oils

Prichard, C., & Newcomb, P. (2015). Benefit to family members of delivering hand massage with essential oils to critically ill patients. *American Journal of Critical Care,* 24(5): 446–449.

What Was the Approach of the Research?

Primary research: Quasi-experimental pilot study.

What Was the Aim/Purpose/Objective(s) of the Research as Related to Complementary and Alternative Therapies?

To determine the feasibility of teaching family members a simple intervention combining hand massage with essential oils in a trauma intensive care unit.

How Was the Study Done?

All family members agreeing to participate in the study were asked to complete the Hospital Anxiety and Depression Scale (HADS) on the day of study enrollment. Fifteen family members were assigned to engage in a 5-minute hand massage with essential oils for six sessions (twice a day for 3 days). Each study participant in the treatment group received written instructions for hand massage and a bottle of 5% bergamot oil mixed in almond oil. Participants were instructed in hand massage according to M Technique® (a method using repetitive strokes in a structured sequence). Additionally, 15 family members were assigned to the control group and did not participate in the intervention after completion of the HADS. All participants (both treatment and control groups) completed the HADS after completion of the study (day 4).

What Were the Significant Findings of the Research?

The improvement (positive direction) in anxiety scores within the treatment group was significantly greater than that in the control group. Younger participants experienced greater relief from anxiety than older family members. Effects on depression were not statistically significant.

What Additional Questions Might I Have?

What would be the findings with using a larger sample size? Would the findings be statistically different if a randomized controlled trial was implemented? Would the use of other oils alter the findings? Would altering the design of the study to a mixed method approach and the addition of interview reveal other findings related to hand massage performed by family members? What were the patient's perspectives regarding hand massage on their anxiety?

What Is the Clinical Significance of This Study?

This study could have considerable value for nurses working in both intensive care units and other care units such as hospice. Families frequently express "feeling useless" in visiting their loved ones and not knowing what to do or how to help. Teaching and encouraging hand massage may assist in allowing families to understand that it is acceptable to touch their loved one and in doing so they can promote comfort.

References

Benjamin, P. J. (2016). *Tappan's Handbook of Massage Therapy* (6th ed.). Boston, MA: Pearson.

Bligny, Y. (2011). *Bioharmonic Self-Massage*. Rochester, VT: Healing Arts Press.

Colt, G. H. (1997). The magic of touch. *Life*, 8: 52–62.

Delany, J. (2015). Massage, bodywork, and touch therapies. In M. S. Micozzi (Ed.), *Fundamentals of Complementary and Alternative Medicine* (5th ed., pp. 247–274). St. Louis, MO: Elsevier/Saunders.

Diaz-Rodriguez, L., Fernandez-Perez, A. M., Galiano-Castillo, N., Cantarero-Villanueva, I., Fernandez-Lao, C., Martin-Martin, L. M., & Arroyo-Morales, M. (2016). Do patient profiles influence the effects of massage? A controlled clinical trial. *Biological Research for Nursing*. doi: 10.1177/1099800416643182

Dzobo, N. K. (1973). *African Proverbs: Guide to Conduct: The moral Value of Ewe proverbs*. University of Cape Coast, Department of Education.

Field, T. (2016). Knee osteoarthritis pain in the elderly can be reduced by massage therapy, yoga and tai chi. *Complementary Therapies in Clinical Practice*. doi: 10.1016/j.ctcp.2016.01.001

Hippocrates. (1983). *Hippocratic Writings* Vol. 451). Edited by G. E. R. Lloyd, J. Chadwick, & W. N. Mann. Penguin Books Limited.

Jackson, C., & Latini, C. (2016). Touch and hand-mediated therapies. In B. M. Dossey & L. Keegan (Eds.), *Holistic Nursing* (7th ed., pp. 299–319). Burlington, MA: Jones & Bartlett Learning.

Lee, S. H., Kim, J. Y., Yeo, S., Kim, S. H., & Lim, S. (2015). Meta-analysis of massage therapy on cancer pain. *Integrative Cancer Therapies*. doi: 10.1177/1534735415572885

Rose, M. K. (2012). *Comfort Touch: Massage for the Elderly and the Ill.* Baltimore, MD: Lippincott Williams & Wilkins.

Salvo, S. G. (2015). *Massage Therapy.* St. Louis, MO: Elsevier/Saunders.

Scaer, R. (2014). *The Body Bears the Burden: Trauma, Dissociation, and Disease* (3rd ed.). New York, NY: Routledge.

Schitter, A. M., Nedeljkovic, M., Baur, H., Fleckenstein, J., & Raio, L. (2015). Effects of passive hydrotherapy

WATSU (WaterShiatsu) in the third trimester of pregnancy: Results of a controlled pilot study. *Evidence-Based Complementary & Alternative Medicine.* doi: org/10.1155/2015/437650

Slade, S. (2012). Massage therapy: Various conditions. Joanna Briggs Institute Evidence Summary. Retrieved from http://connect.jbiconnectplus.org/ViewDocument.aspx?0=6747

Resources

American Massage Therapy Association
500 Davis St., Suite 900
Evanston, IL 60201-4695
877.905.2700
www.amtamassage.org

American Organization for Bodywork
Therapy of Asia
P.O. Box 343
West Berlin, NJ 08091
856.809.2953

Associated Bodywork & Massage
Professionals
25188 Genesee Trail Road, Suite 200
Golden, CO 80401
800.458.2267
www.abmp.com

Australian Association of Massage
Therapists
Level 6, 85 Queen St.
Melbourne, VIC 3000
www.aamt.com.au

Federation of State Massage
Therapy Boards
150 4th Avenue North, Suite 350
Overland Park, KS 66224
913.681.0380
www.fsmtb.org

International Association of Infant
Massage
Unit 10, Marlborough Business Centre
South Woodford, London E18 1AD
020.8989.9597
www.iaim.org.uk

National Association of Nurse
Massage Therapists
28 Lowry Drive
P.O. Box 232
West Milton, OH 45383
800.262.4017
www.nanmt.org

Rolf Institute of Structural
Integration
5055 Chaparral Ct., Suite 103
Boulder, CO 80301
303.449.5903
www.rolf.org

Touch Research Institute
University of Miami School
of Medicine
P.O. Box 016820
Miami, FL 33101
305.243.6781
www6.miami.edu/touch-research

13

Pressure Point Therapies

*Let parents then bequeath to their children
not riches but the spirit of reverence.*

PLATO

A cupuncture, acupressure, Shonishin, Jin Shin Jyutsu, Jin Shin Do, and reflexology are different forms of the same practice of stimulating points on the body to balance the body's life energy. Jin Shin Jyutsu, Jin Shin Do, and reflexology are forms of acupressure, and in this chapter the term *acupressure* includes all the forms. **Acupuncture** and **acupressure** are based on the theory that applying pressure or stimulation to specific points on the body, known as *acupuncture points*, can relieve pain, cure certain illnesses, and promote wellness. Acupuncture uses needles, whereas acupressure uses finger pressure. Although the older of the two techniques, acupressure is not as powerful and could be considered the over-the-counter version of acupuncture. Acupressure is easy to learn and convenient for self-care, whereas acupuncture requires training to use the needles. Frequently, these practices are part of a holistic approach to wellness and are combined with diet, herbs, massage, mind–body techniques, and spiritual therapies. Used with great success on humans for thousands of years, acupuncture and acupressure are now available for cats, dogs, and horses through veterinarians trained in Traditional Chinese Medicine.

BACKGROUND

Acupuncture and acupressure started in China several thousand years ago. The practice spread to Korea around 300 A.D. and to Japan and Europe in the 17th century. In the late 19th century, a

203

Canadian physician, Sir William Osler, became interested in acupressure techniques, but they remained largely unknown in North America until the 1970s. Accompanying President Richard Nixon on his trip to China in 1972, James Reston, a reporter for the *New York Times*, wrote about his experience with acupuncture for relief of pain following abdominal surgery in China. This article began the upsurge of interest in these therapies in the United States. At the present time, acupuncture and acupressure are practiced widely in Asia, the former Soviet Union, and Europe and are gaining in popularity in North America (Hunts, 2012).

Jin Shin Jyutsu (pronounced "jin-shin jit-soo") and **Jin Shin Do** are Japanese phrases meaning "the way of the compassionate spirit." They are ancient practices that fell into relative obscurity until they were dramatically revived in the early 1900s by Master Jiro Murai in Japan. Dying from a terminal illness, he turned in desperation to Jin Shin Jyutsu and meditation. Within a week, he was completely well. He spent the remaining 50 years of his life researching and sharing his knowledge of this healing art, which he referred to as the art of happiness, the art of longevity, and the art of benevolence. After World War II, a Japanese American, Mary Burmeister, studied with Master Murai for many years and eventually returned to the United States with the "gift" of Jin Shin Jyutsu and Jin Shin Do. Today, thousands of students throughout the United States and around the world study and practice Jin Shin Jyutsu and Jin Shin Do (Riegger-Krause, 2014).

Reflexology, an associated ancient practice, limits the use of acupressure points, or reflexes, to the feet, hands, and ears. William Fitzgerald, an American physician, introduced reflexology to the West in 1913. He noted that there was less postoperative pain when pressure was applied to people's feet and hands just before surgery. In spite of Fitzgerald's work, it was Eunice Ingham, a physical therapist, who expanded and refined Fitzgerald's observations and found that reflexology not only reduced pain but provided other health benefits as well. Ingham mapped the specific reflex zones on the feet, hands, and ears that reflexologists use today. This work gave her the distinction of being the founder of modern reflexology in the West (Keet, 2009).

PREPARATION

The United States has 56 schools and colleges of acupuncture approved by the Council of Colleges of Acupuncture and Oriental Medicine. The graduate-level program of 2,625 hours or 146 credits covers Oriental medicine, acupuncture theory, Chinese herbs, and biomedicine theory and includes 1,330 hours of clinical practice. The master's level program for practitioners seeking licensure only as an acupuncturist is for a minimum of 3 years and 1,905 hours or 105 credits. There is also an herb certificate program of 450 hours of didactic instruction and 210 hours of clinical training in the use of Chinese herbs for those practitioners who already have a master's degree in acupuncture. Forty-four states plus the District of Columbia require passing a national board exam as a prerequisite for licensure. In addition, each state has its own eligibility requirements.

An estimated 7,000 to 8,000 U.S. doctors now include acupuncture in their practice following 300 hours of study. Most are family physicians, anesthesiologists, orthopedists, and pain specialists. Few physicians are certified by the National Certification Commission for Acupuncture and Oriental Medicine (NCCAOM), but most are certified by the American Academy of Medical Acupuncture (AAMA) instead. Even though acupuncture is used in China to treat many conditions, in the United States, conventional physicians have taken the technique out of context, basing it more on a biomedical model of diagnosis and treatment. Nationally, an estimated 15,000 nonmedical professionals practice acupuncture, including nurses, naturopathic physicians, and chiropractors.

Professionals using acupressure are usually physical therapists or massage therapists with special training in this field. Some nurses are trained in acupressure and use it to help clients sleep and to reduce levels of anxiety. Midwives may use acupressure techniques to promote relaxation during labor and reduce breast engorgement after delivery. No specific license or certification is needed to practice any of the forms of acupressure, although practitioners of reflexology have the option to become certified by the American Reflexology Certification Board.

CONCEPTS

Meridians

Acupuncture, acupressure, Jin Shin Jyutsu, Jin Shin Do, and reflexology are treatments rooted in the traditional Eastern philosophy that *qi*, or life energy, flows through the body along pathways known as **meridians**. Like major power lines, the meridians connect all parts of the body. As vital energy flows through the meridians, it forms tiny whirlpools close to the skin's surface at places called *hsueh*, which means "cave" or "hollow." In Traditional Chinese Medicine, these are acupuncture points; in India, *marma* points. These pressure points function somewhat like gates to moderate the flow of qi. Acupuncture needles inserted into these points or pressure on these points releases blocked energy and improves the circulation of qi in the body (Yoga Journal, 2016).

In addition to the major meridians, the body has 360 to 365 classic points through which qi can be accessed. Most practitioners, however, focus on 150 points. The points themselves are metaphors for a person's journey through life, with names such as "Spirit Gate," "Great Esteem," "Joining the Valleys," and "Inner Frontier Gate." Meridians are associated with internal organs after which they are named: stomach, spleen, heart, small intestine, bladder, kidneys, gallbladder, liver, lungs, and large intestine. The triple-warmer meridian is associated with the thyroid and adrenal glands, the governing meridian with the spine, and the central meridian with the brain. Chapters 2 and 4 present more detailed information regarding energy and meridians.

Microsystems

The meridians converge at many points in the body, called **microsystems**, which are reflexes to distant parts of the body. These microsystems are small, local representations of the whole body and are located on the feet, hands, and ears. In other words, each individual part of the body has an associated reflex on the ear, the hand, and the foot. The reflexes are symmetric in that the organs on the right side of the body are reflected in the right foot, and the left organs are reflected in the left foot. The reflexes also correspond in descending order: the brain reflexes are in the tips of the toes, the eyes and ears under the toes, the shoulders and lungs on the ball of the foot, the stomach and pancreas on the instep, the intestines and colon toward the heel, and the hips on the heel. See Figures 13.1A, B, and C for reflexology maps.

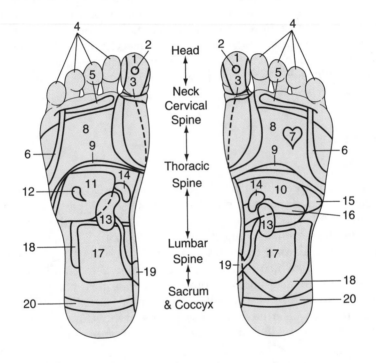

1. Head and brain
2. Pituitary and pineal glands
3. Throat and thyroid gland
4. Sinus
5. Eyes and ears
6. Shoulder
7. Heart
8. Lungs and thymus gland
9. Diaphragm and solar plexus
10. Stomach
11. Liver
12. Gallbladder
13. Kidney
14. Adrenal gland
15. Spleen
16. Pancreas
17. Small intestine
18. Large intestine
19. Bladder
20. Sacrum and sciatic nerve

FIGURE 13.1A Foot Reflexology Points

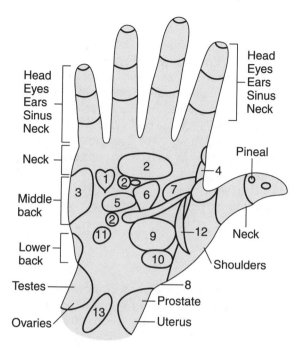

1. Heart (left hand) and thymus gland
2. Lungs
3. Liver (right hand) and shoulders
4. Solar plexus
5. Pancreas
6. Kidneys and adrenals
7. Stomach
8. Large intestine
9. Small intestine
10. Bladder
11. Appendix
12. Thyroid
13. Sacrum and pelvis

FIGURE 13.1B   Hand Reflexology Points

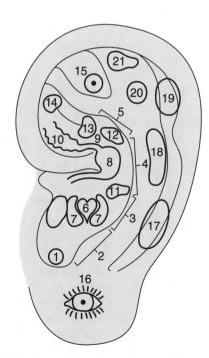

1. Endocrine glands and hormones
2. Head and brain
3. Neck
4. Upper and middle back
5. Lower back
6. Heart and thymus gland
7. Lungs
8. Stomach
9. Small intestine
10. Large intestine
11. Spleen
12. Liver
13. Kidney
14. Bladder
15. Nervous system and spirit
16. Eyes and face
17. Shoulders
18. Arm and elbow
19. Hand
20. Leg and knee
21. Foot

FIGURE 13.1C   Ear Reflexology Points

Mind–Body Connections

In the pressure point tradition, the mind, body, spirit, and emotions are never separated. Thus, the heart is not just a blood pump, but it also influences one's capacity for joy, one's sense of purpose in life, and one's connectedness with others. The kidneys filter fluids, but they also manage one's capacity for fear, one's will and motivation, and one's faith in life. The lungs breathe in air and breathe out waste products, but they also regulate one's capacity to grieve, as well as one's acknowledgment of self and others. The liver cleanses the body, and it also influences one's feeling of anger as well as that of vision and creativity. The stomach has a part in digestion of food and influences one's ability to be thoughtful, kind, and nurturing as well. These are just a few of the mind–body connections recognized by pressure point practitioners (Ergil & Ergil, 2015).

VIEW OF HEALTH AND ILLNESS

Health is viewed as a state of harmony, or balance, of the opposing forces of nature, both internal and environmental. The body requires balanced *yin* and *yang* energy to function properly and to utilize its natural ability to resist disease. It is believed that everything needed to maintain and restore health already exists in nature and that pressure point therapies free up energy and restore balance, thus enabling individuals to maintain or regain their health.

Symptoms are caused by an imbalance of yin and yang in some part of the body, leading to excesses or deficiencies of life energy throughout the body. When the flow of energy becomes blocked or congested, people experience discomfort or pain on a physical level, may feel frustrated or irritable on an emotional level, and may experience a sense of vulnerability or lack of purpose in life on a spiritual level. When the flow of energy is interrupted, the area cannot nourish or cleanse. If not corrected, these blocks and imbalances in energy channels can result in disease and eventually illness.

The goal of care is to recognize and manage the disruption before illness or disease occurs. Qi can be thrown out of balance in a number of ways, including genetic vulnerability, accident or trauma, diet, lifestyle, emotional upset, spiritual distress, climate, or noxious agents. Pressure point practitioners bring balance to the body's energies, which promotes optimal health and well-being and facilitates people's own healing capacities.

DIAGNOSTIC METHODS

The initial consultation involves a holistic assessment because no part of the self is considered a neutral bystander when the body is in a state of imbalance. A detailed medical history is an important part of the diagnostic process. Special attention is paid to the connection between body, mind, emotions, and spirit.

Palpation is the major diagnostic method of pressure point therapies within the context of Traditional Chinese Medicine. Reading the pulses provides a remarkable amount of information about the person's condition. Imbalances in the body can be detected through palpating microsystems on the feet, hands, and ears. If something feels unusual in the microsystems, the corresponding organ is examined in more detail. Chapter 4 discusses the diagnostic process of Traditional Chinese Medicine in greater detail.

TREATMENT

Pressure point therapies consider symptoms to be an expression of the condition of the person as a whole. Thus, sessions focus on not only relieving pain and discomfort but also responding to disruptions before they develop into illnesses.

Acupuncture

To restore the flow of energy, acupuncturists insert sterile, hair-thin needles at points along the meridians. The needles are rotated, twirled, or accompanied by a weak electrical current and are often left in several minutes or longer. Acupuncturists also may apply heat or use finger pressure to alter the flow of qi. Clients feel little, if any, pain (see Figure 13.2). Some people experience sensations of warmth, tingling, relaxation, heaviness, or a dull ache.

Western medical explanations of evidence now indicate that, in addition to restoring the flow of energy within the meridians, acupuncture reduces pain by triggering the release of endogenous opioids. Many of the analgesic

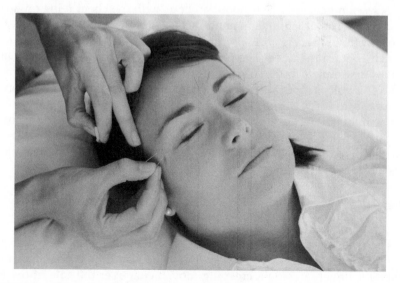

FIGURE 13.2 Sense of Ease During Acupuncture Treatment

Source: Tyler Olson/Shutterstock.

effects of acupuncture can be partially or completely blocked by the use of opioid antagonists such as naloxone. Acupuncture also stimulates the nervous system to release adrenocorticotropic hormone (ACTH), a chemical that aids in fighting inflammation; prostaglandins, which help wounds heal more quickly; and other substances that may promote nerve regeneration. Antiemetic effects apparently stem from the increase in endorphins and ACTH, which inhibits the chemoreceptor trigger zone and the vomiting center in the brain. Acupuncture also calms the upper gastrointestinal tract. Research has found that acupuncture is effective for nausea from morning sickness, motion sickness, postoperative nausea, and chemotherapy-induced nausea. Unlike drugs and surgery, acupuncture has virtually no side effects (Ergil & Ergil, 2015).

Shonishin

Shonishin is Japanese noninvasive pediatric acupuncture. A very fine needle is used to gently prick but not insert the acupuncture sites. This has a relaxing effect that is especially good for infants and children. The younger the child, the faster she/he will respond to treatment (Wernicke, 2014).

Jin Shin Jyutsu and Jin Shin Do

Jin Shin Jyutsu and Jin Shin Do can be applied as self-help and also by a trained practitioner, who places the fingertips over clothing on designated pressure points to harmonize and restore the energy flow. Rather than doing something to the body, Jin Shin encourages the body to "let go," which is seen as the path to awakening one's awareness of harmony within the self and with the universe.

A session generally lasts about an hour with the client lying on a table fully clothed. The practitioner's hands act as "jumper cables" to "kick start" the correct flow of energy. A spot on the shoulder may be held at the same time as a spot on the knee. The practitioner uses special sequences of hand positions to stimulate the circulation of energy. The touch is gentle and steady, and never involves force. It is generally pain free; any tenderness in a particular area is caused by a blockage and tends to dissipate as the area is held. Some people may feel hot or cold or feel a sensation in another part of the body than the one where the practitioner is working. Most people experience a sense of deep relaxation with Jin Shin Jyutsu and Jin Shin Do (Riegger-Krause, 2014).

Reflexology

Most commonly, reflexologists manipulate the reflex zones on the feet, but the hands or ears may also be manipulated. A session usually lasts about 45 minutes with the client sitting comfortably in a chair and the practitioner using thumb and fingers in small, creeping movements over the sole of the foot. This manipulation prompts the nervous system to speed up the body's response to an afflicted area by stimulating the flushing of toxins from the area. Side effects of reflexology are usually mild and include sore or achy feet, slight swelling in legs, feet, arms, and hands, and emotional reactions when energy blocks are cleared.

Uses

Pressure point therapies are widely used around the world to treat many conditions, including addiction, allergies, bronchitis, cerebral palsy, depression, diabetes, hemorrhoids, hepatitis, herpes, infertility, irritable bowel syndrome, nausea, premenstrual syndrome, stroke, and ulcers. In the United States, reduction of pain is a major therapeutic use, including pain from dental work, temporomandibular joint (TMJ) syndrome, migraine headaches, osteoarthritis, low back pain, sciatica, carpal tunnel syndrome, and sports injuries. Acupuncture can provide symptomatic relief from the pain of bursitis and is much safer than anti-inflammatory drugs and injections of steroids (Cross, 2014; Tse, 2016).

Contraindications

Pressure point therapy is not appropriate for every ailment. It is not indicated for an acute or infectious illness or fever or if surgery is needed. Foot injuries need to heal before reflexology is used on the foot. If someone has a pacemaker, practitioners avoid stimulating the left chest zone. Recent myocardial infarction is a contraindication. If someone has gallstones or kidney stones, the gallbladder and kidney points are avoided. If the person is pregnant, uterine points are avoided. Needling is not done on scar tissues, open wounds, lipomas, cysts, or on persons having psychotic tendencies.

RESEARCH

In 1997, the National Institutes of Health (NIH) assembled a panel of experts in a scientific court known officially as a consensus conference. A panel of 12 experts was drawn from a variety of backgrounds, including biomedical research scientists, physicians, and others. The panel's task was to listen to as much evidence as the acupuncture/pressure point research community could present in the first half of the 3-day conference. The panel's conclusions included the following statement: "There is sufficient evidence of acupuncture's value to expand its use into conventional medicine and to encourage further studies of its physiology and clinical value" (NIH, 1998). The panel determined that acupuncture was clearly effective for nausea and vomiting in pregnancy, motion sickness, chemotherapy, and anesthesia, and for postoperative pain from dental surgery. The panel also noted "other situations such as addiction, stroke rehabilitation, headache, menstrual cramps, tennis elbow, fibromyalgia, myofascial pain, osteoarthritis, low back pain, carpal tunnel syndrome, and asthma where acupuncture may be useful as an adjunct treatment or an acceptable alternative or be included in a comprehensive management program" (NIH, 1998). This panel focused only on data collected by means of randomized controlled clinical trials and therefore did not review data on technique, cost benefit, patient preference, or practitioner education. The following is a small sample of findings of pressure point therapies:

- A systematic review and meta-analysis of Chinese herbal medicine as an adjunctive therapy for people with senile vascular dementia found improved cognitive response and quality of life (Zeng et al., 2015). A systematic review and meta-analysis of acupuncture in patients with Alzheimer's disease found similar results (Zhou, Peng, Xu, Li, & Liu, 2015).
- A systematic review and meta-analysis of ear acupuncture for primary insomnia found a positive effect on insomnia but the evidence is not yet strong enough to support it as a primary management tool (Lan et al., 2015).
- A systematic review and meta-analysis studied acupuncture for shoulder pain during the subacute phase in stroke patients. Combined with rehabilitation treatment, it appeared to increase the effectiveness of rehabilitation (Lee & Lim, 2016).
- A systematic review and meta-analysis considered acupuncture for symptom management in people with cancer. Acupuncture reduced pain more quickly and for a longer period of time compared with conventional medicine. Acupressure reduced fatigue when compared with sham acupressure. There was no evidence that acupuncture was effective for anorexia, constipation, or paresthesia (Lau et al., 2016).
- A systematic review and meta-analysis found that acupuncture demonstrated an improvement in sleep disturbances for women in menopause (Chiu, Hsieh, & Tsai, 2016).

INTEGRATED NURSING PRACTICE

If you are interested in incorporating pressure point therapies into your nursing practice, you may want to attend a weekend or weeklong program on reflexology, Jin Shin Jyutsu, or Jin Shin Do. Even without further education, you can incorporate hand, foot, or ear massages into your practice. This type of massage is easy to learn and nonintrusive. The procedure for a hand massage is shown in Figure 12.3. These procedures can be modified for an ear massage. The hands, feet, and ears are fairly small. If you simply massage them, focusing on any tender spots you find, you are bound to send qi or energy to all parts of the body. Few people object to this type of massage. Even if the recipient has no particular physical complaint, this type of massage is wonderfully relaxing.

You can teach clients about a number of pressure points as you advocate self-help. Box 13.1 describes this process for nausea, headaches, hiccups, and carpal tunnel syndrome. To ease tension and restore energy, try this pressure point: Hold your left palm in front of you, fingers together. The fleshy spot between your thumb and index finger is a key pressure point. Using your right thumb, massage this spot in a circular motion for a slow count of 15. Then, switch hands and repeat the process. You can also teach clients several finger holds to improve their general level of well-being. Explain that they should gently hold the appropriate finger on either hand while imagining the negative emotions melting away and physical symptoms easing.

- **Thumb.** Corresponds to worrying, depression, and anxiety. Physical symptoms may include stomachaches, headaches, skin problems, and nervousness.
- **Index finger.** Corresponds to fear, mental confusion, and frustration. Physical symptoms are digestive problems and muscle problems such as backaches.
- **Middle finger.** Corresponds to anger, irritability, and indecisiveness. Physical symptoms are eye or vision problems, fatigue, and circulation problems.
- **Ring finger.** Corresponds to sadness, fear of rejection, grief, and negativity. Physical symptoms are digestive, breathing, or serious skin problems.
- **Little finger.** Corresponds to insecurity, effort, overdoing it, and nervousness. Physical symptoms are sore throat and bone or nerve problems.

BOX 13.1

Self-Help: Pressure Points

The following are several examples of how you can use pressure points to relieve discomfort or pain. Once you think you have located one of the appropriate points, probe the area with a fingertip or pencil eraser in a tight circular motion in the general location. Points often feel tender, sore, or tingling. Press the point for 1 minute, then stop for a few seconds, and press again. Work the point for 5 to 20 minutes. If you are experiencing a headache, hiccups, or symptoms of carpal tunnel syndrome, experiment for yourself and find which points work best for you. Remember, only some of the points need to be worked to achieve relief. There is only one point for nausea.

Nausea

Point	Hold your hand open, palm up. This point is 2 inches toward the elbow from the wrist crease and is centered in the groove between the two large tendons. Using the thumb and a finger, press firmly on this point on both sides of the wrist. Wrist bands can also be purchased that apply pressure to the correct spot. This procedure is safe during pregnancy and also helps with other types of nausea.

Headache

Point 1	Hold your hand open, palm down, and find the point in the center of the fleshy webbing between the thumb and index finger.
Point 2	Find the point on the top of the foot in the valley between the big toe and the second toe.

(continued)

Point 3   This point is at the base of the back of the skull in the hollow above the two large vertical neck muscles.

Point 4   This point is in the hollow above the inner eyes, where the bridge of the nose meets the ridge of the eyebrows.

Point 5   Find the point between the eyebrows in the indentation where the bridge of the nose meets the forehead.

Point 6   This point is two finger-widths above the webbing of the fourth and fifth toes in the groove between the bones.

Hiccups

Point 1   Find the point in the indentation behind each earlobe.

Point 2   This point is located at the base of the throat in the center of the collarbone.

Point 3   Find this point on the center of the breastbone three thumb-widths up from the base of the bone.

Point 4   This point is located three finger-widths below the base of the breastbone in the pit of the abdomen. If you are healthy, do not press this point for more than 2 minutes. If you are not healthy, do not press this point at all.

Carpal Tunnel Syndrome

Point 1   Find the point in the middle of the inner side of the forearm, two and a half finger-widths below the wrist crease.

Point 2   This point is located in the middle of the inside of the wrist crease.

Point 3   Find the point on the outside of the forearm, midway between the radius and ulna, two and a half finger-widths below the wrist crease.

Sources: Alexander (2015); Keet (2009); Tse (2016).

TRY THIS

Foot Massage

When your feet ache, your whole body suffers. Here are instructions for a 10- to 15-minute foot massage to relax and soothe your feet and perhaps your entire body.

- Sit in a comfortable, quiet place where you will not be disturbed. You may want to have soothing music in the background.
- Pour a small amount of nongreasy lotion or massage oil into your hands and rub them together.
- Begin massaging one foot, stroking each toe in an up-and-down motion. Then, massage the entire foot using kneading, wringing motions until the lotion is absorbed.

- Holding your foot firmly in one hand, press the thumb of the other hand (slightly bent) on the sole of the foot near the heel. Apply even pressure with the thumb and "walk it" forward, little by little. Press one spot, move forward, press again, move forward, and so on.
- When you get to the toes, go back to the heel and trace another line from heel to toe. Continue this process until the entire sole of the foot has been worked.
- Repeat the entire process with the other foot.

Sources: Cross (2014); Riegger-Krause (2014); Tanner (2012).

Clients can be taught acupressure for relief of nausea from a variety of causes. The pericardium 6 point is located in the midline of the inner wrist between two and three finger-widths up toward the elbow from the crease where the hand joins the wrist. People can stimulate this point using their own finger or apply an acupressure wristband to the point.

CONSIDERING THE EVIDENCE
Reflexology (Pressure Point Therapy)

Marvis, B., & Bhattacharya, C. (2013). A comparative study to assess the effectiveness of reflexology and two minute relaxation technique on fatigue reduction and relaxation in clients undergoing haemodialysis in selected setting. *International Journal of Nursing Education*, 5(2): 34–38.

What Was the Approach of the Research?

Primary research: Pre- and postintervention.

What Was the Aim/Purpose/Objective(s) of the Research as Related to Complementary and Integrative Therapies?

1. To determine the level of relaxation and fatigue among clients undergoing hemodialysis before and after introduction of reflexology.
2. To determine the level of relaxation and fatigue among clients undergoing hemodialysis before and after introduction of 2-minute relaxation technique.
3. To compare the effectiveness of reflexology and 2-minute relaxation technique on fatigue reduction and relaxation.
4. To determine the association between selected demographic variables and fatigue reduction and relaxation.

(continued)

How Was the Study Done?

Forty patients undergoing hemodialysis for end-stage renal disease were assigned to two groups. One group was provided reflexology for four times in a 2-week period for 20 minutes; pretest fatigue scores and relaxation scores were assessed using established tools. Another group of patients was assigned to the 2-minute relaxation group and the same tools were administered prior to initiating the intervention. The research protocol consisted of a 2-minute relaxation technique for 2 to 3 minutes for 2 weeks. At the completion of the 2-week intervention period, a posttest using the same tools was completed by both groups.

What Were the Significant Findings of the Research?

Reflexology and 2-minute relaxation techniques are effective in fatigue reduction and relaxation without adverse effects.

What Additional Questions Might I Have?

What method was implemented in assigning patients to their respective groups? Would a larger study sample suggest the same results? What if both interventions were combined, would this have additional positive effects for the patients? What additional education needs to be provided to nurses in appropriately administering reflexology and relaxation techniques?

What Is the Clinical Significance of This Study?

The findings of this study provide nurses with additional interventions to assist patients experiencing fatigue without implementing pharmacological measures. The value for nurses caring for persons living with end-stage renal disease is the opportunity to enhance their quality of life as fatigue can be very debilitating. Nurses should be aware that additional research of good methodological quality is needed to strengthen the evidence and enhance confidence in implementing reflexology and relaxation techniques for selected patients based on the best available evidence.

References

Alexander, J. (2015). *Wellbeing & Mindfulness*. London: Carlton Books Limited.

Chiu, H. Y., Hsieh, Y. J., & Tsai, P. S. (2016). Acupuncture to reduce sleep disturbances in perimenopausal and postmenopausal women: A systematic review and meta-analysis. *Obstetrics & Gynecology*. doi: 10.1097/AOG.0000000000001268

Cross, J. R. (2014). *The Concise Book of Acupoints (revised ed.)*. Indianapolis, IN: Blue River Press.

Ergil, K. V., & Ergil, M. C. (2015). Classical acupuncture. In M. S. Micozzi (Ed.),

Fundamentals of Complementary and Alternative Medicine (5th ed., pp. 508–543). St. Louis, MO: Elsevier/Saunders.

Hunts, L. (2012). *History of Acupuncture*. Charleston, SC: CreateSpace.

Jowett, B. (1892). *The Dialogues of Plato (Laws, Index to the Writings of Plato, Volume 5)*. Clarendon Press.

Keet, L. (2009). *The Reflexology Bible: The Definitive Guide to Pressure Point Healing*. New York, NY: Sterling.

Lan, Y., Wu, X., Tan, H. J., Wu, N., Xing, J. J., Wu, F. S., . . . Liang, F. R. (2015). Auricular acupuncture with seed or pellet attachments for primary insomnia: A systematic review and meta-analysis. *BMC Complementary and Alternative Medicine.* doi: 10.1186/s12906-015-0606-7

Lau, C. H. Y., Wu, X., Chung, V. C. H., Liu, X., Hui, E. P., Cramer, J., . . . Wu, J. C. Y. (2016). Acupuncture and related therapies for symptom management in palliative cancer care. *Medicine.* doi: 10.1097/MD.0000000000002901

Lee, S. H., & Lim, S. M. (2016). Acupuncture for poststroke shoulder pain: A systematic review and meta-analysis. *Evidence-Based Complementary and Alternative Medicine.* doi: 10.1155/2016/3549878

National Institutes of Health. (1998). NIH consensus conference: Acupuncture. *Journal of the American Medical Association,* 280: 1518–1524.

Riegger-Krause, W. (2014). *Health Is in Your Hands.* New York, NY: Upper West Side Philosophers.

Tanner, R. (2012). *Foot Massage.* Leicester, UK: Lorenz Books.

Tse, H. (2016). *Sole Guidance: Ancient Secrets of Chinese Reflexology to Heal the Body, Mind, Heart, and Spirit.* Carlsbad, CA: Hay House.

Wernicke, T. (2014). *Shonishin: The Art of Non-Invasive Pediatric Acupuncture.* London: Singing Dragon.

Yoga Journal. (2016). *Your Guide to Reflexology.* Avon, MA: Adams Media.

Zeng, L., Zou, Y., Kong, L., Wang, N., Wang, Q., Wang, L., . . . Liang, W. (2015). Can Chinese herbal medicine adjunctive therapy improve outcomes of senile vascular dementia? Systematic review with meta-analysis of clinical trials. *Phytotherapy Research.* doi: 10.1002/ptr.5481

Zhou, J., Peng, W., Xu, M., Li, W., & Liu, Z. (2015). The effectiveness and safety of acupuncture for patients with Alzheimer disease. *Medicine.* doi: 10.1097.MD.0000000000000933

Resources

American Association of Acupuncture and Oriental Medicine
1925 W. County Rd. B2
Roseville, MN 55113
651.631.0204
www.aaaom.edu

American Academy of Medical Acupuncture
2512 Artesia Blvd, Suite 200
Redondo Beach, CA 90278
310.379.8261
www.medicalacupuncture.org

Australian Acupuncture & Chinese Medicine Association
Unit 1, 55 Clarence St.
Coorparoo, QLD 4151
617.3457.1800
www.acupuncture.org.au

British Acupuncture Council
63 Jeddo Rd.
London W12 9HQ
020.8735.0400
www.acupuncture.org.uk

Council of Colleges of Acupuncture and Oriental Medicine
P.O. Box 65120
Baltimore, MD 21210
410.464.6040

Jin Shin Do® Foundation for Bodymind Acupressure
P.O. Box 416
Idyllwild, CA 92549
951.767.3393
www.jinshindo.org

National Commission for the Certification of Acupuncture and Oriental Medicine
76 South Laura St., Suite 1290
Jacksonville, FL 32202
904.598.1005
www.nccaom.org

14

Hand-Mediated Biofield Therapies

Sheila Lewis, BScN, MHSc

Energy is the living, vibrating ground of your being, and it is your body's natural self-healing elixir, its natural medicine.

EDEN (2008, pp. 1–2)

A wide variety of alternative and integrative healing practices are emerging in popularity and are designed to balance the body's **biofield,** or energy field, and increase the flow of energy. The National Center for Complementary and Integrative Health (NCCIH, 2016) defines biofield therapy/energy healing therapy as "a technique that involves channeling healing energy through the hands of a practitioner into the client's body to restore a normal energy balance and, therefore, health. Energy healing therapy has been used to treat a wide variety of ailments and health problems, and it is often used with other alternative and conventional medical treatments" (p. 1).

People and cultures all over the world have identified and given various names to the concept of biofield, as seen in Box 14.1. Practices related to biofield therapies have been utilized cross-culturally for millennia, but it is only recently that programs of related research have emerged in the Western Hemisphere. In the 1980s, scientists in the emerging field of psychoneuroimmunology (PNI), or mind–body medicine, began to study energy medicine. Among them were Herbert Benson, MD, and Joan Borysenko, PhD, who discovered and studied the body's innate "relaxation response" as it relates to self-healing. Many of the

BOX 14.1

Some Equivalent Terms for Biofield

Ankh	Ancient Egypt
Animal magnetism	Mesmer
Arunquiltha	Aborigine (Australia)
Bioenergy	United States/United Kingdom
Biomagnetism	United States/United Kingdom
Gana	South America
Ki	Japan
Life force	General usage
Mana e	Polynesia
Manitou	Algonquian
M'gbe	Hiru Pygmy
Mulungu	Ghana
Mumia	Paracelsus
Ntoro	Ashanti
Ntu	Bantu
Oki	Huron
Orenda	Iroquois
Pneuma	Ancient Greece
Prana	India
Qi (ch'i)	China
Subtle energy	United States/United Kingdom
Sila	Inuit
Tane	Hawaii
Ton	Dakota
Wakan	Lakota

Source: Adapted from National Institutes of Health (n.d.), p. 2.

PNI researchers were influenced by Eastern traditions that view the mind, body, spirit, and health as one, and energy as something that people can deliberately nurture within themselves. Today, the field of mind–body medicine is well established and recognized, with scientific breakthroughs occurring regularly.

Three prominent therapies using the hands to balance and support the biofield and impact the healing process are *Therapeutic Touch* (TT), *Healing*

Touch (HT), and *Reiki*. All three approaches could simply be defined as the use of the hands on or near the body with the intention to support and facilitate self-healing in a heart-centered and intentional way to balance and support the energy field. Actually, the word *touch* is a misnomer, especially in TT and HT, because the practitioner need not touch the recipient to achieve the desired effects during a healing session. All these therapies require informed consent from the client, and when touch is used, the client is always fully clothed. Practitioners use their hands with gentle, light, or near-body touch to clear, balance, energize, and support another's energy system. These therapies are modern interpretations of several ancient healing practices, traditionally known as the "laying on of hands." TT, HT, and Reiki, however, must not be confused with faith healing because the context in which they are practiced is not religious but scientific, although some clients may experience them spiritually.

The goals of these hand-mediated therapies are to facilitate self-healing and well-being. Relaxation and stress reduction may result as well (Henneghan & Schnyer, 2015; Midilli & Eser, 2015; Thrane & Cohen, 2014). All three are forms of treatment and are not designed to diagnose physical conditions but are to be used in conjunction with other recognized therapies. This means that these therapies are not meant to replace conventional surgery, medicine, or drugs in treating organic disease.

BACKGROUND

Healing Touch is an international multilevel educational program that is taught through two different programs, either Healing Beyond Borders or Healing Touch Program. Healing Touch was developed by Janet Mentgen, BSN, RN, HNC, CHTP/I, a Colorado nurse, who began practicing and teaching medically based energy therapy in 1980. In 1989, her five-course sequence in HT became the first certified program offered by the American Holistic Nurses Association (AHNA). "Healing Touch is a relaxing, nurturing, heart-centered biofield (energy) therapy. Gentle, intentional touch assists in balancing physical, mental, emotional and spiritual well-being" (Healing Beyond Borders, 2017, p. 1). The goal in Healing Touch is to assist "in creating a coherent and balanced energy field, supporting one's inherent ability to heal. It is safe for all ages and works in harmony with and may be integrated with standardized medical care" (Healing Beyond Borders, 2017, p. 1).

Therapeutic Touch was developed by Dolores Krieger, PhD, RN, Professor Emeritus, New York University, who launched the TT movement in 1970 after studying with Dora Kunz, a past president of the Theosophical Society in America and a natural healer. TT refers to the Krieger–Kunz method of Therapeutic Touch (Kreiger, 1979; Kunz, 1991), which was originally developed as an energy field interaction between nurse and client. The Therapeutic Touch education program involves a basic program consisting of three levels followed by more advanced education learning with a variety of teachers (Therapeutic Touch International Association, n.d.). "Therapeutic Touch is based on the idea that human beings are energy in the form of a field. When you are healthy, that energy is freely flowing and balanced. In contrast, disease is a condition of energy imbalance or disorder. The human energy field extends beyond the level of the skin, and the Therapeutic Touch practitioner attunes him or herself to that energy using the hands as sensor" (Therapeutic Touch International Association, n.d., para 1). In addition, nursing scholars such as Carpenito-Moyet (2006) have defined and further developed human energy field theory through the nursing diagnosis of "energy field disturbance" as a "state in which a disruption of the flow of energy surrounding a person's being results in a disharmony of the body, mind, and/or spirit" (p. 289).

Reiki (pronounced "ray-kee") originated in Japan. Reiki "is composed of two syllables: *rei*, which means universal energy, the energy that permeates the entire universe, and *ki*, the life energy of all living creatures" (Birocco et al., 2012, p. 290). The origin of Reiki can be traced to an ancient Tibetan/Buddhist practice rediscovered by Dr. Mikao Usui, a Japanese physician and monk. He first used Reiki on himself and his family and then began to share his knowledge with the public. Chujiro Hayashi, who was a student of Usui, further developed this healing practice, and Hawayo Takata, a Japanese American student of Hayashi, introduced Reiki to Western cultures between 1930 and 1940 (Thrane & Cohen, 2014). Reiki is practiced in more than 800 hospitals in the United States. In addition, a Reiki education program for BSN nursing students has successfully been integrated at the University of Maine, Augusta (Clark, 2013).

All hand-mediated biofield therapies reflect the unitary transformative perspective, which encourages each person to relate with others and his or her world as unitary "pan-dimensional" beings in a pan-dimensional universe (Newman, 1997; Rogers, 1992; Watson, 1999). Within this worldview, a unitary human being (human field) "is an irreducible, indivisible, pan-dimensional energy field identified by pattern and manifesting characteristics that are specific to the whole and which cannot be predicted from knowledge of the parts" (Rogers, 1992, p. 29). The kaleidoscopic role of nursing within this perspective is to view the client as expert with the role of the healer being one of facilitator or midwife to the client's own self-healing process. Caring–healing relationships are based on ethics of caring consciousness, presence, mutual process, pattern recognition and appreciation, and exploration of meaning (Newman, Smith, Dexheimer-Pharris, & Jones, 2008). Healing Touch, Therapeutic Touch, and Reiki reflect this unitary transformative stance, based on the idea that there is a universal energy that supports the body's ability to heal itself. In addition, each of these practices has at its core a commitment to a moral–ethical way of being and belonging.

PREPARATION

Nurses who prepare to practice hand-mediated biofield therapies take time to assess and further develop their caring–healing way of being–belonging–doing with others. As a reflective nursing practice, learning may involve study/reflective practice, such as mindfulness meditation, centering and grounding work, listening and communicating with the intent to understand others at a deeper level, considering ways to create sacred space, and connecting with nature as healer. Nurses who seek certification as HT practitioners from either of the two established Healing Touch agencies practice a variety of biofield techniques to assist the client to self-heal. They also reflect on their own development through reflective practice and activities, such as journaling and reading books about techniques, healing traditions, self-healing, and possible theoretical explanations. The preparation may take two or more years of study as practitioners meet requirements for each of the five levels prior to certification. Most programs strongly emphasize development of nurses as healers by considering the relationship they have with clients and with themselves, with a focus on "being mindful of the intention to deliver the best nursing care for the body, mind, spirit, and emotional well-being of the patient and using verbal and nonverbal communication that reflects a nurse who is caring, calm, and receptive" (Mentgen, 2001, p. 148).

A Qualified Therapeutic Touch Practitioner (QTTP) must complete the basic TT program, each level being a minimum of 8 hours taken over a 6-month period. The programs are followed by mentor guidance for 1 year. Therapeutic Touch can be learned by almost anyone who is motivated by compassion and committed to helping others. Family members can be taught how to use it effectively with their loved ones.

Both HT and TT were developed by nurses, and all nurses, regardless of clinical specialty, can use HT and TT in any setting. These are independent nursing interventions, so they do not require a physician's order, but they do require client consent. Like many other nursing practices, these interventions may also require Policy and Practice approval within the Nursing Council/Program of each institution.

Reiki is usually learned from a Reiki Master and is a spiritual practice. There are two degrees in Reiki healing, as well as a Master degree that prepares one to teach others. Most people can complete the first degree in a weekend course. The content includes historical information; the concept of energy healing; attunements to enhance the flow of Reiki energy within the person; understanding of a Reiki session, including the practitioner–client relationship; hand positions used in healing; and ethical considerations for practice. The second degree, also completed over a weekend, includes learning how to do distant healing and further enhancement of one's physical, mental, emotional, and spiritual healing abilities. The Master degree involves a training mentorship either with a Master Reiki practitioner or through Reiki sharing and Reiki practice groups or both. The American Holistic Nurses Association often approves Reiki programs for continuing education units, and such training is encouraged for all practitioners.

CONCEPTS

By any name—qi, ki, prana, or subtle energy—a life force energy is universally recognized in biofield therapies as the core of life and the driving force in healing. The belief is that all living beings are complex networks of interwoven vibratory energy systems composed of an energy field (aura), energy centers (chakras), and energy tracts (meridians) and that the energy centers control the energy flow into and out of the body. It is at this level of the subtle energy system that both health and illness originate. Many of the most sophisticated instruments widely used in conventional medicine for diagnosis and treatment are energy medicine devices. Electrocardiography (ECG), electroencephalography (EEG), and electromyography (EMG) measure heart, brain, and muscle activity, respectively, by measuring electric potentials on the surface of living tissue, while ultrasound instruments use high-frequency sound waves beyond the range of human hearing, and magnetic resonance imaging instruments use a magnetic field and radio-frequency waves to image various aspects of the body. People can detect a far greater spectrum of energies than can scientific measuring devices.

Energy field theory is based in part on laws of quantum physics. As expressed by McCormack (2009): "Drawing from quantum physics and field theory, all living things generate vibratory fields, which are interconnected by mathematical laws" (p. 45). Researchers and proponents of biofield therapies believe that conscious caring–healing intent is necessary, as well as a conscious use of self as a link between the universal life energy and the other individual. Prior to the actual intervention, practitioners focus completely on the well-being of the recipient in an act of unconditional love and compassion. Compassion, basic to all nursing intervention, involves both intention and action. Practitioners of biofield therapies always set their compassionate intention in mind first before entering and intervening in others' energy fields (Shealy, 2011).

People are open systems, so the transfer of energy is a natural, continuous event. When two people with an intent to heal are close to one another, their energy fields may overlap, and there may be a repatterning process. As they intermingle, each energy field influences the other through a process of resonance/coparticipation. In intentional healing situations, some practitioners believe that they regulate their own internal energy frequencies, thus supporting recipients as they draw on the healers' resources and energy patterns. Many other practitioners (this author included) believe that the practitioner and client/environment are in mutual process, connecting with universal life-force energy as the client accesses his or her own self-healing processes. This view is based on the assumption that each client has the innate power to self-heal and to restore his or her own state of balance and harmony. It has been found that in an intentional healing situation, with or without physical contact, a state of coherence and synchrony develops between the brain waves of the healer and the recipient, and they literally become unified in one energetic field. Thus, the client and the practitioner experience a mutual patterning process that involves resonance of the biofield and change (Shealy, 2011).

VIEW OF HEALTH AND ILLNESS

Within individuals, energy flows like a river. If it encounters no obstructions, it is smooth, gliding, and barely perceptible. People whose energy flows smoothly usually report good health and a feeling of peace with themselves and with others. Health, then, is defined as an abundance of qi and a balance or harmony of body, mind, and spirit. In addition, healthy people experience equilibrium between their own energy systems and those of the environment. If obstructions or imbalance in energy occur, such as trauma, pain, rage, sadness, or any physical, mental, emotional, or spiritual problem, the balanced stream of energy is disrupted, and illness or disease may result.

The locus of healing is within each person and cannot be "given" to a client by a biofield therapist. People must, and do, heal themselves. Healing environments are created when nurses enter into a caring relationship with clients. The nurse's caring presence provides opportunities for a spirit-to-spirit connection in which the nurse becomes a resource for nurturing the wholeness that always exists within each client. As recipients become engaged in the healing process, they often develop new insights or meaning, and the nurse acts as midwife to the unfolding process related to these patterns.

TREATMENT

Each of the biofield therapies discussed in this chapter utilizes the following treatment practices:

1. Creation of a caring–healing environment (e.g., promoting and supporting a quiet, safe, private, dignified environment with consideration of heating, ventilation, lighting, tidiness, and cleanliness of the environment; and promoting the person's comfort with appropriate positioning and attention to specific needs for order, beauty, and peace).
2. Centering before beginning the biofield practice. *Centering* is a general term for any method that people use to quiet themselves physically, mentally, and emotionally. Centering can be achieved by many methods such as deep breathing, visualization, and focusing, which allow the practitioner to relax and focus on the intent of the healing session. Being centered allows healers to operate intuitively, with awareness, and to channel energy throughout their bodies. Box 14.2 describes one centering method.
3. An interview with the client prior to caring–healing practice of Healing Touch, Reiki, or Therapeutic Touch.
4. The client may choose to sit or lie down, always fully clothed.
5. Assessment. Steps in the biofield caring–healing process include initial and ongoing assessment of the energy field. Once centered, nurses use their hands to *assess* the recipient's energy field. Some nurses are able to feel the energy field when they first learn their biofield therapy, while

BOX 14.2

How to Center

- Sit or stand comfortably and close your eyes or focus on one spot on the floor.
- Breathe in and out, slowly and deeply, concentrating on how the breath feels as it goes in and out.
- Breathe in relaxation and peace while breathing out stress and tension.
- Imagine a fairly large tree; really sense the tree as it sounds, as it smells, and according to the season.
- Get close to the tree and put your hands on the tree; lean up against the tree and put your full weight on the tree.
- Look up through the branches and feel the sun shining down; feel the sun traveling down through the tree and coming in through your head, down through your body, and out your legs.
- Focus once again on your breathing and know that you can come back to this place at any time.
- With practice and experience, you will be able to center yourself within one or two deep breaths.

Source: Therapeutic Touch video courses by Janet Quinn, PhD, RN.

others require months of practice to experience the sensations. People describe different sensations commonly characterized as heat, cold, tingling, buzzing, emptiness, or pressure. The energy field is assessed for bilateral similarities or differences in the flow of energy. A healthy energy field is symmetric with a smooth, flowing texture. Practitioners often combine both physical and nonphysical contact during the course of treatment. Clients do not have to believe in the efficacy of the biofield therapy to receive benefit. The one absolutely essential ingredient in each of these biofield therapies is the goodwill and compassion of the practitioner (see Figure 14.1).

6. The practitioner chooses specific healing interventions based on the interview findings, assessment of the energy field, and specific needs of each client. These specific techniques are carried out with a caring–healing presence and active listening process.

7. Completion and grounding. The practitioner reassesses the biofield of the client prior to "grounding" or helping the client become aware. Often, the nurse does this by gently holding the tops of both feet and shoulders for a minute or two. Another way is to brush down the arms and legs toward the ground until clients start moving their hands and feet and reconnect completely with their body. Verbal cues such as "Feel your fingers and toes and gently move them" may also be helpful.

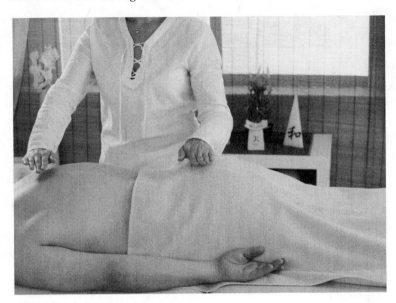

FIGURE 14.1 No Touch Energy Transfer

Source: StockLite/Shutterstock.

8. Feedback, documentation, and planning. Discharge planning begins with the first visit. The practitioner listens to what the client wishes to share about his or her experience and answers any questions the client may have. Counseling or education or both are provided in a mutual process that is based on client goals and the knowledge and skills of the nurse. Examples of areas for dialogue can include but are not limited to stress management, lifestyle, nutrition, quality of life, and self-care processes such as journaling, meditation, or exercise or yoga or both, along with other resources that the client finds helpful (i.e., need for referral to other practitioners such as a psychotherapist, massage therapist, or physician). Planning may include setting time for future visits with the nurse or teaching the client or family or both a specific biofield technique. The total number of visits with the nurse is based on the client's response to the biofield therapy. Documentation begins with the initial client interview and continues throughout the visits.

Therapeutic Touch, Healing Touch, and Reiki are used only as forms of treatment, not to diagnose physical conditions. They work in conjunction with other medical or therapeutic techniques to promote healing and to relieve side effects of conventional therapies. Indications include irritability and anxiety; lethargy, fatigue, and depression; premenstrual syndrome; nausea and vomiting; chemotherapy and radiation sickness; wound and bone healing; and acute musculoskeletal problems such as sprains and muscle spasms. These healing practices may be effective in many types of pain. Side effects of biofield therapies are temporary lightheadedness and/or a temporary sensation of heat. Very gentle, briefer treatments are used for infants, the elderly, and those experiencing a critical illness. The primary contraindication to TT, HT, and Reiki is that a person does not want it, which falls under the doctrine of informed consent (Oschman, 2016).

Practitioners believe that when they work with an individual's energy fields, they are dealing with that person as a whole, and healing may occur at many levels. Recipients may experience emotional and spiritual growth, as well as physical improvement, but in some cases the therapy may not seem to work at all. Even when these methods do not help people resolve a particular problem, the session is soothing and relaxing.

RESEARCH

The practice of biofield therapies has existed for thousands of years. Research, however, regarding the effectiveness of these therapies is relatively recent.

A Joanna Briggs Institute evidence summary found that Reiki may have positive effects on well-being (Grade B). Clinical judgment should be exercised, and patient preference should be considered when deciding on Reiki and Therapeutic Touch for older adults (Grade B; Charlton, 2012). National Center for Complementary and Integrative Health (2015) notes that Reiki "appears to be generally safe. In studies of Reiki, side effects were no more common among participants who received Reiki than among those who didn't receive it" (p. 1). The authors also note that Reiki "should not be used to replace conventional care or to postpone seeing a health care provider about a health problem" (p. 1). This caution would apply to all biofield therapies.

The following is a small sample of current studies:

- A study by Midilli and Eser (2015) investigated the effect of Reiki on pain, anxiety, and hemodynamic parameters postoperatively with 90 patients who had undergone cesarean delivery. Reiki was given for 30 minutes on the first and second days after giving birth. The authors found statistically significant differences in pain intensity, breathing rate, anxiety value, and analgesic requirements. There was no effect found on blood pressure or pulse rate.
- Henneghan and Schnyer (2015) completed a literature review to evaluate the use of biofield therapies (Therapeutic Touch, Healing Touch, and Reiki) in relation to managing symptoms associated with clients who were at the end of their life (EOL). They found these therapies to have a positive role in "relieving pain, improving quality of life and well-being, and reducing psychological symptoms of stress" (p. 90).
- A systematic review of Therapeutic Touch in patients with cancer found 17 articles that met the objectives of the study. A variety of tools were used to assess pain, fatigue, and nausea. The researchers found that Therapeutic Touch improved the health status in adults with cancer (Tabatabaee et al., 2016).

INTEGRATED NURSING PRACTICE

Hand-mediated biofield therapies of Therapeutic Touch, Healing Touch, and Reiki have been pioneered by nurses and are easily learned by them that this has been recognized for many years is evidenced by the approved nursing diagnosis of a disturbed energy field. Although many nursing curricula currently include some components of biofield therapies, most nurses did not formerly receive information about the use of hand-mediated biofield therapies in nursing school. Nurses who have not been taught any of these therapies may want to participate in courses that are shown on the websites for Healing Touch, Therapeutic Touch, and/ or Reiki.

TT, HT, and Reiki can be used in almost any clinical setting, including hospitals, nursing homes, home health care, hospice, and private practice. These hand-mediated therapies are used in Lamaze classes, labor rooms, newborn nurseries, neonatal intensive care units, pediatric units, medical surgical units, recovery rooms, palliative care, and behavioral medicine. TT, HT, and Reiki may be helpful for people with a variety of health needs. In the current health-care environment, individuals with acute and chronic disorders are rapidly discharged back to the community. Family and friends are often overwhelmed by caregiver's responsibilities. Often, they feel helpless in the face of their loved one's obvious suffering or pain. Teaching caregivers one or more biofield modalities can be a powerful nursing intervention that counteracts this sense of helplessness. As caregivers discover that biofield therapies can minimize the experience of pain and increase the sense of relaxation, they often feel they have something "worthwhile" to offer. In addition, the use of biofield therapies can be helpful to the caregiver, who is most likely exhausted from trying to carry on the normal daily routine, as well as caring for the sick or injured person. Because one of the steps of biofield therapies is centering, the process demands that caregivers take a few minutes for themselves as they concentrate on their well-being and sense of peace. As caregivers increase their self-awareness, they are quicker to recognize tension and stress in their bodies, which should encourage them to develop stress management skills. TT, HT, and Reiki produce a sense of well-being and relaxation in both the nurse and the recipient. For some nurses, it is the first time they have been given permission to be quiet, take a breath, and center during working hours. When a nurse walks into a client's room or home in a peaceful state of mind, that gentleness and compassion permeates the environment. Recipients react positively to not only the treatments but also the individual attention from nurses as they build relationships with clients, offer noninvasive nurturing touch, and reduce clients' stress and anxiety (Watson, 2011). Practicing one or more of the biofield therapies is one of the ways nurses create caring relationships and caring healing environments.

TRY THIS

Experience Your Energy Field

- Vigorously rub your hands together for 20–30 seconds.
- Hold your palms together, parallel but not touching.
- Slowly separate them a couple of inches.
- Slowly bring them close together again.
- Repeat this process several times, each time separating your palms by an additional 2 inches until they are 8 inches apart.
- You should be able to detect your energy field as you bring your palms together; you may feel a sense of bounciness, sponginess, or elasticity; some people describe it as the feeling of two magnets repelling each other.

References

Birocco, N., Guillame, C., Storto, S., Ritorto, G., Catino, C., Gir, N., . . ., Ciuffreda, L. (2012). The effects of Reiki therapy on pain and anxiety in patients attending a day oncology and infusion services unit. *American Journal of Hospice and Palliative Medicines*, 29(4): 290–294.

Carpenito-Moyet, L. J. (Ed.). (2006). *Nursing Diagnosis: Application to Clinical Practice* (11th ed.). Philadelphia, PA: Lippincott Williams & Wilkins.

Charlton, K. (2012). Reiki and Therapeutic Touch: Dementia and older adults. Joanna Briggs Institute Evidence Summary. Retrieved from http://connect.jbiconnectplus.org/ViewDocument.aspx?0=6296s

Clark, C. (2013). An integral nursing education experience: Outcomes from a BSN Reiki course. *Holistic Nursing Practice*, 27(1): 13–21.

Eden, D. (2008). *Energy Medicine for Women: Aligning Your Body's Energies to Boost Your Health and Vitality*. New York, NY: Penguin Group.

Healing Beyond Borders. (2017). The next harmonic alignment and paradigm shifts. *Perspectives in Healing: A Publication of Healing Beyond Borders*, 1st quarter. Retrieved from https://view.publitas.com/healing-beyond-borders/healing-beyond-borders-1st-quarter-2017-newsletter/page/2-3

Henneghan, A. M., & Schnyer, R. N. (2015). Biofield therapies for symptom management in palliative and end-of-life care. *American Journal of Hospice and Palliative Medicine*, 32(1): 90–100. Retrieved from http://journals2.scholarsportal.info.ezproxy.library.yorku.ca/pdf/10499091/v32i0001/90_btfsmipaec.xml

Kreiger, D. (1979). *The Therapeutic Touch: How to Use Your Hands to Help or to Heal*. New York, NY: Prentice Hall.

Kunz, D. (1991). *The Personal Aura*. Wheaton, IL: Quest.

McCormack, G. L. (2009). Using a non-contact therapeutic touch to manage post-surgical pain in the elderly. *Occupational Therapy International*, 16(1): 44–56.

Mentgen, J. (2001). Healing touch. *Nursing Clinics of North America*, 36(1): 143–157.

Midilli, T. S., & Eser, I. (2015). Effects of Reiki on post-cesarean delivery pain, anxiety, and hemodynamic parameters: A randomized, controlled clinical trial. *Pain Management Nursing*, 16(3), 388–399. doi: 10.1016/j.pmn.2014.09.005. Retrieved from http://journals2. scholarsportal.info.ezproxy.library. yorku.ca/pdf/15249042/v16i0003/ 388_eoropdparcct.xml

National Center for Complementary and Integrative Health. (2015, October). *Reiki: In Depth*. NCCIH Publication No. D315. Retrieved from https:// nccih.nih.gov/health/reiki/introduction.htm#hed2

National Center for Complementary and Integrative Health. (2016, February). *Terms Related to Complementary and Integrative Health*. Retrieved from https://nccih.nih.gov/health/providers/camterms.htm. *Note*: Terms and definitions excerpted from: Clarke, T. C., Black, L. I., Stussman, B. J., Barnes, P. M., & Nahin, R. L. (2015). *Trends in the Use of Complementary Health Approaches Among Adults: United States, 2002–2012*. National Health Statistics Report No. 79. Hyattsville, MD: National Center for Health Statistics.

National Institutes of Health. (n.d.). *Biofield therapeutics. A subsection from Alternative Medicine: Expanding Medical Horizons. A Report to the National Institutes of Health on Alternative Medical Systems and Practices in the United States* (pp. 1–20). Ad Hoc Advisory Committee to the Office of Alternative Medicine. Retrieved from http:// www.shentherapy.info/images/biofield%20therapeutics.pdf

Newman, M. A. (1997). Evolution of theory of health as expanding consciousness. *Nursing Science Quarterly*, 7: 153–157.

Newman, M. A., Smith, M. C., Dexheimer-Pharris, M., & Jones, D. (2008). The focus of the discipline revisited. *Advances in Nursing Science*, 31(1): E16–E27.

O'Mathuna, D. P., & Ashford, R. L. (2012). Therapeutic Touch for healing acute wounds. *Cochrane Database of Systematic Reviews*, (6): CD002766. doi: 10.1002/14651858.CD002766.pub2

Oschman, J. L. (2016). *Energy Medicine: The Scientific Basis* (2nd ed.). St. Louis, MO: Elsevier.

Rogers, M. E. (1992). Nursing science and the space age. *Nursing Science Quarterly*, 5(1): 27–34.

Shealy, C. N. (2011). *Energy Medicine: Practical Application and Scientific Proof.* Virginia Beach, VA: A.R.E. Press.

Tabatabaee, A., Tafreshi, M. Z., Rassouli, M., Aledavood, S. A., AlaviMajd, H., & Farahmand, S. K. (2016). Effect of Therapeutic Touch in patients with cancer: A literature review. *Medical Archives*, 70(2): 142–147. doi: 10.5455/ medarh.2016.70.142-147

Therapeutic Touch International Association. (n.d). The process of Therapeutic Touch. Retrieved from http://therapeutictouch.org/what-is-tt/history-of-tt/

Thrane, S., & Cohen, S. M. (2014). Effect of Reiki therapy on pain and anxiety in adults: An in-depth literature review of randomized trials with effect size calculations. *Pain Management Nursing*, 15(4), 897–908. doi: 10.1016/j. pmn.2013.07.008.

Watson, J. (1999). *Postmodern Nursing and Beyond*. Edinburgh, UK: Churchill Livingstone.

Watson, J. (2011). *Human Caring Science: A Theory of Nursing* (2nd ed.). Sudbury, MA: Jones & Bartlett.

Resources

American Holistic Nurses Association
100 SE 9th St., Suite 31
Topeka, KS 66612
800.278.2462
www.ahna.org

Canadian Holistic Nurses Association
www.chna.ca

Canadian Reiki Association
P.O. Box 54570, 7155 Kingsway
Burnaby, BC V5E 4J6
www.reiki.ca

Healing Touch Canada
RR2 Warsaw, ON K0L 3A0
705.652.0506
www.healingtouchcanada.net

Healing Beyond Borders
445 Union Blvd, Suite 105
Lakewood, CO 80228
www.healingbeyondborders.org

Healing Touch Program
20822 Cactus Loop, Suite 300
San Antonio, TX 78258
210.497.5529
www.healingtouchprogram.com

International Center for Reiki Training
21421 Hilltop St., Suite 28
Southfield, MI 48033
800.332.8112
www.reiki.org

Therapeutic Touch International
Association
P.O. Box 130
Delmar, NY 12054
518.325.1185
www.therapeutictouch.org

15

Combined Physical and Biofield Therapy

The art of medicine consists in amusing the patient while nature cures the disease.

VOLTAIRE

Applied kinesiology, described in this chapter, is a combination of physical and biofield interventions. Applied kinesiology is both a diagnostic method and a treatment modality using energy, acupuncture meridians, and the lymphatic, neurovascular, and muscle systems.

BACKGROUND

George Goodheart and Alan G. Beardell, American chiropractic physicians, developed **applied kinesiology** in the 1960s. In the 1970s, John Thie, also a chiropractor, took their work, simplified it for the general public, and called this modified approach Touch for Health®.

PREPARATION

Health-care professionals may go on to study applied kinesiology only after completing their basic professional education. Chiropractors, nurses, osteopaths, naturopaths, dentists, and physicians practice applied kinesiology. Interested professionals take the training in a postgraduate setting, usually in weekend classes. Prerequisites include anatomy and physiology, interpersonal communication, and nutrition. The basic course takes more than 100 hours of classroom

232

study and numerous hours of practice in the clinical setting, after which students can test for basic proficiency. Another 200 clinical hours under the guidance of a mentor are undertaken to reach the next step, in which a diplomate written and oral exam is taken. Organized courses in applied kinesiology are taught in Europe, Canada, the United States, and Australia. There is no licensure *per se*; providers of applied kinesiology practice on their professional license.

CONCEPTS

As in many alternative practices, the concept of energy is at the heart of applied kinesiology. The belief is in a life force of subtle energy that surrounds and permeates all living things, often referred to as a *biofield*. It is currently unclear whether the biofield is electromagnetic or a field in physics other than ones already known. The present hypotheses are that the biofield is a form of bioelectricity, biomagnetism, or bioelectromagnetism. The exact nature has not yet been established (Glass, Hatzel, & Albrecht, 2014).

Meridians

Practitioners of applied kinesiology work closely with the meridian system and pressure points. *Meridians* are a network of energy circuits that run vertically through the body. Each meridian passes close to the skin's surface at places called *pressure points*. Since each meridian is associated with an internal organ, the points offer surface access to the internal organ system. Each of the 14 meridians has related specific neurovascular points and neurolymphatic points (Frost, 2013).

Neurovascular Points

Neurovascular points are located mainly on the head. A few seconds after placing one's fingers on these points, a slight pulse can be felt at a steady rate of 70 to 74 beats per minute. This pulse is not related to the heartbeat but is believed to be the primitive pulsation of the microscopic capillary bed in the skin.

Neurolymphatic Points

The lymphatic system in the body flows in only one direction and acts as a drainage system for the body. It produces antibodies, makes white blood cells, and transports fats, proteins, and other substances to the blood system. Neurolymphatic reflexes, located mainly on the chest and back, regulate the energy to the lymphatic system. These reflex points act like switches that get turned off when the system is overloaded. They are usually tender spots, and those that are the sorest are in greatest need of massage.

VIEW OF HEALTH AND ILLNESS

Well-being and health are determined by the nature of the flow of energy within and outside the body. When energy flows smoothly without significant blockage or fixation, a person experiences health in an ongoing and dynamic way. Disease and pain occur when energy is blocked, fixed, or unbalanced. When someone's physical body, thoughts, and emotions are out of alignment with the energy necessary to meet a life challenge, an energy imbalance results. Within the applied kinesiology framework, one of the signs of an imbalance is a weakening of the muscles and a change in the posture. If these minor problems are not corrected, the imbalances may develop into physical, mental, and emotional discomfort or pain. Pain and discomfort are seen as signals for people to learn, change, and realign their lives.

Diagnostic Methods

An applied kinesiology exam depends on knowledge of functional neurology, anatomy, physiology, biomechanics, and biochemistry. It is combined with standard procedures, laboratory findings, X-rays, and history taking. Generally, problems can be related to a chemical imbalance, a structural imbalance, mental stress, or any combination of these states. General examination procedures are used to assess the health of the client and are followed by specific examination procedures such as testing reflexes or assessing balance (Baumgartner, Jackson, Mahar, & Rowe, 2016).

Every muscle in the body is related to a specific organ or gland through sharing lymphatic vessels or meridians. Because organs and glands have few pain and sensory fibers, people are largely unaware of energetic imbalances in these parts. Unbalanced organs or glands, however, refer pain externally to the corresponding surface meridians and muscles, indicating the cause of the problem. For example, the deltoid muscle in the shoulder shares a relationship with the lungs. If a person has abnormal lung function, such as bronchitis, pneumonia, congestion, or the flu, the problem may exhibit as a weakness in one or both deltoid muscles. When the lung problem is cleared up, the deltoid muscle returns to a normal state (Frost, 2013).

Manual muscle testing augments the other examination procedures. Goodheart and Beardall designed specific methods for testing the function of the 576 muscles of the body. Muscle weaknesses are often so subtle that physical therapists would consider the muscle strength to be within normal limits. No more than 15% difference should be discernible between the right and left sides. The testing positions are intended to isolate the muscle from the group with which it normally works, making it less strong than if it were used in the usual way. Small children, the elderly, and the frail will not be as strong as a healthy adult. It is more difficult to test a person who has great strength, such as an athlete, because the weakness cannot be distinguished by the tester (Baumgartner et al., 2016).

A number of causes result in weak muscles, including immobility, lack of exercise, poor posture, gland/organ dysfunction, dysfunction of the nerve supply, impairment of lymphatic drainage, decreased blood supply, blockage of meridians, and chemical imbalance. Testing of individual muscles combined with knowledge of the basic mechanics and physiological functioning of the body provides practitioners with information necessary to formulate a diagnosis.

TREATMENT

Applied kinesiology practitioners believe that the body, mind, emotions, and spirit are interdependent; that people are responsible for their own health; and that they can take simple steps to improve and maintain their level of wellness. The practitioner's role is to facilitate and support clients' self-healing capabilities.

Applied kinesiology uses various methods to strengthen those muscles and related organs that were found to be weak during the diagnostic phase. Improvement in the flow of energy can be measured by increased muscle strength, which is assumed to lead to an increase in energy to the corresponding organs.

Neurovascular holding points are located mainly on the head. The practitioner makes simple contact with the pads of the fingers for anywhere from 20 seconds to 10 minutes, depending on the severity of the problem. This method appears to improve the blood circulation to both the muscle and the related organ, and the weak muscle will have increased strength when retested.

Neurolymphatic points are located mainly on the chest and back. Practitioners work on the points that are related to a specific weakened muscle by a deep massage of the points for 20 to 30 seconds. This massage is believed to turn on the blocked reflexes, allowing the lymph flow to return to normal. The weak muscle will have improved strength when retested. Figure 15.1 illustrates the neurolymphatic points for the lungs.

Meridians are traced in the designated direction on both sides of the body. Practitioners use the flat of their hands to give better coverage. Meridians

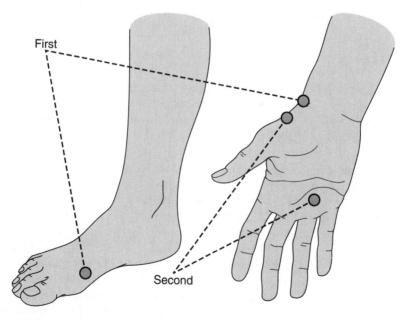

FIGURE 15.1 Lung Neurolymphatic Holding Points

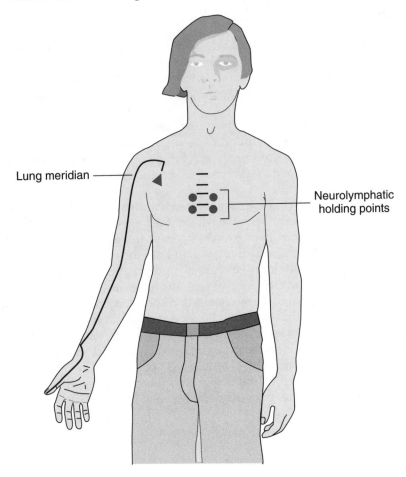

Lung meridian

Neurolymphatic holding points

FIGURE 15.2 Pressure Points for the Lungs

can be traced over clothing without actually touching the client. Tracing the meridian adds the practitioner's flow of energy to the recipient's energy in a blocked meridian and may restore the normal flow of energy. Figure 15.1 also illustrates the lung meridian.

Acupressure points are held on the same side of the body as the muscle that is weak. The first arm and leg points are held at the same time, one with each hand. Light pressure is maintained for about 30 seconds or until a pulse is felt in the leg. The hands are then moved to the second acupressure points and held, again, until a pulse is felt in the leg. Figure 15.2 illustrates the pressure points for the lungs.

Adherents of applied kinesiology believe that nutrition plays a major role in health and well-being. Kinesiology assesses people's nutritional status, including food intolerances, vitamin and mineral deficiencies, and other chemical sensitivities. Exercise is an important part of this therapy. Applied kinesiology practitioners encourage clients to walk for exercise. Walking is one of the few exercises that benefit all parts of the body. All the muscles are used when people walk with their arms swinging.

Applied kinesiology can relieve pain, stress, and muscular disorders. It is used to detect allergies, nutritional deficiencies, back or neck pain, fatigue, headache, tension, and the common cold and is believed to have some benefit for those with learning disorders.

RESEARCH

The efficacy of applied kinesiology has not yet been established in published, peer-reviewed research. Replication has been difficult because muscle testing varies in terms of duration of the test and the amount of force used by the practitioner. The International College of Applied Kinesiology expects their diplomate members to present new research. Unfortunately, these research articles are only available to members of the organization.

INTEGRATED NURSING PRACTICE

Nurses need advanced study to apply the specific techniques of applied kinesiology. Practitioners in applied kinesiology may actively intervene or make suggested changes to address food allergies, chemical imbalances, or nutritional deficiencies as determined by clinical assessment. If appropriate, they may encourage clients to take care of their physical body with moderate exercise such as walking or swimming and with good nutrition.

TRY THIS

Emotional First Aid

The next time you are upset, try this procedure to decrease your stress.

- Either hold the frontal eminences on your forehead with the first two fingers of your hands—the right and left at the same time—or place the palm of your hand flat on your forehead.
- While applying light pressure, in your mind review exactly what you are thinking and how you are feeling about the problem. Continue holding these points and going over what is bothering you for a few minutes or until you feel the emotions becoming less strong.
- Let your hands go and look around you. Mentally review the issue again. If stressful feelings are still there or have changed to other stressful feelings (fear changed to anger, for example), go back and begin the process again. After a further few minutes, release the pressure and check your feelings about the situation again.
- It is hoped that your mind will feel clearer, and the same emotions will no longer have the same stressful impact.

TRY THIS
Redirecting the Flow of Energy

Sit facing a partner, and placing both hands in the air, move your hands close to your partner's hands without touching. Experiment with distances until you can feel the energy pulsating between your hands. Imagine that your partner's energy is coming into your left hand from your partner's right hand, and your energy is flowing from your right hand into your partner's left hand. Imagine the circular circuit between the two of you as the energy flows up the left arm, across the heart, and down the right arm. Imagine how connected you feel at this given moment.

References

Baumgartner, T. A., Jackson, A. S., Mahar, M. T., & Rowe, D. A. (2016). *Measurement for Evaluation in Kinesiology*. Burlington, MA: Jones & Bartlett Learning.

Frost, R. (2013). *Applied Kinesiology* (revised ed.). Berkeley, CA: North Atlantic Books.

Glass, S., Hatzel, B. H., & Albrecht, R. (2014). *Kinesiology for Dummies*. Hoboken, NJ: John Wiley & Sons, Inc.

Voltaire. (1824). *A Philosophical Dictionary: From the French* (Vol. 3). J. and H. L. Hunt. Originally from the New York Public Library.

Resources

International College of Applied Kinesiology
www.icak.com

International Kinesiology College
www.ikc-info.org

The Kinesiology Federation (UK)
P.O. Box 10426
Newark NG24 9NF
0845.260.1094
www.kinesiologyfederation.org

Touch for Health Kinesiology Association
P.O. Box 754
Carrboro, NC 27510
919.637.4938
www.tfhka.org

Mind–Body Techniques

You yourself, as much as anyone in the entire universe,
deserve your own love and affection.

BUDDHA

16

Yoga

*Meditation is the Dissolution of thoughts
in eternal awareness or pure
consciousness without objectification,
knowing without thinking, merging
finitude in infinity.*

VOLTAIRE

Yoga, part of Ayurvedic medicine, has been practiced for thousands of years in India, where it is a way of life that includes ethical models for behavior and mental and physical exercises aimed at producing spiritual enlightenment. Although yoga developed from Hinduism, it is not a religion but rather a journey of the body, mind, and spirit on a path toward unity. It is a method for life that can complement and enhance any system of religion, or it can be practiced completely apart from religion.

The Western approach to yoga tends to be more fitness oriented, whereas the Eastern approach to yoga is to prepare people for the experience of self-realization. Most Westerners begin yoga with the goal of managing their stress, learning to relax, and increasing their vitality and well-being. After learning yoga, many become more interested in the underlying principles of physical fitness and keeping the mind focused, calm, and clear. Yoga is meant to prepare the body and mind for a useful, dedicated life.

BACKGROUND

The word *yoga* means to direct and concentrate one's attention and comes from the Sanskrit word *yuj*, meaning "to yoke" or "to join." Yoga was first described by Patanjali, an Indian sage who, thousands of years ago, wrote the *Yoga Sutra*, which recorded information that had been passed down orally for many years. This text has helped define and shape the modern practice of yoga. Over the twentieth and into the twenty-first century, yoga has become a popular practice in the Western world. In the United States, yoga is the sixth most commonly used complementary health practice among adults (National Center for Complementary and Integrative Health, 2016).

All the various methods of yoga have the same goal: to attain a state of pure bliss and oneness with the universe. *Raja yoga* emphasizes control of the intellect to attain enlightenment, accomplished through meditation, concentration, and breath control. *Kriya yoga* is the practice of quieting the mind through scripture study, breath control, mantras, and meditation. *Karma yoga* focuses on service to all beings as the path to enlightenment. *Bhakti yoga* emphasizes devotion to the divine. *Inana yoga*'s goal is wisdom and the direct knowledge of the divine. *Tantra yoga* involves the study of sacred writings and rituals. *Mantra yoga* is the study of sacred sounds. *Kundalini yoga* is the study of energy movement along the spine. *Iyengar yoga*, a form of *hatha yoga*, strives for perfection in the postures using props such as belts or ropes. *Hasyayoga*, or laughter yoga, involves prolonged voluntary laughter that increases oxygen intake, as well as a sense of playfulness with other people. *Silver yoga* and *chair yoga* are designed to accommodate those with reduced body flexibility such as older people or those with physical challenges. *Restorative yoga* is usually done in a lying or sitting position, which causes less physical strain. Props such as blankets, pillows, towels, balls, or straps support the poses and provide a gentle prolonged stretch. When combined with physical therapy, the benefits are improved strength, flexibility, and range of motion for individuals recovering from illness or injury or for those experiencing physical or emotional stress. Other contemporary styles of yoga include *doga* (practicing yoga with one's pet), *yogalates* (a combination of yoga and pilates), and Thai yoga massage (hands-on, guided yoga combined with pressure point massage) (Miles, Tait, Schure, & Hollis, 2016; Staples, 2015).

Although these many branches of yoga exist, this chapter focuses on **hatha yoga** as the form of yoga most frequently practiced by Westerners. In this particular type of yoga, the path to enlightenment is through control over the physical body as the key to control of the mind and freedom of the spirit. Physical exercises, breath control, and meditation tone and strengthen the whole person—body, mind, and spirit.

PREPARATION

No national licensure or standard certification is required for yoga instructors. Becoming a yoga instructor or yoga therapist requires much more personal dedication than that demanded by many other alternative therapy practices. To be admitted to most training programs, prospective yoga instructors must have been practicing yoga daily for 6 months to a year; must abstain from drugs, alcohol, and tobacco; and must follow a vegetarian diet.

CONCEPTS

Classical yoga incorporates *eight limbs* or *paths* that provide structure for one's daily life. These physical and psychological practices are believed to contribute to a higher level of personal development. The outer aspect of yoga consists of right living (abstinence and personal discipline), right care of the body (body control), and enhancement of vital energy (breath control). Yoga also has an inner dimension that emphasizes its key purpose. Detachment, concentration, and meditation together form a single process toward the development of pure consciousness. Box 16.1 lists the eight limbs of yoga.

Abstinences

Abstinences concern what not to do in life. The first abstinence pertains to nonviolence. Nonviolence means not only not physically hurting others but also using nonviolent words and having nonviolent thoughts. Truthfulness, the second abstinence, results in personal integrity and strength of character. Nonstealing, the third abstinence, includes not stealing others' material belongings as well as not taking credit for things one has not done, not stealing the center of attention, and so forth. The fourth abstinence, chastity or nonlust, means holding people in high esteem and loving and respecting

BOX 16.1

The Eight Limbs of Yoga: Guidelines for Living

1. Abstinences (yamas)
    Nonviolence (ahimsa)
    Truthfulness (satya)
    Nonstealing (asteya)
    Chastity or nonlust (brahmacharya)
    Nongreed (aparigraha)
2. Personal disciplines (niyamas)
    Purity (shauca)
    Contentment (samtosa)
    Self-discipline (tapas)
    Self-study (svadhyaya)
    Centering on the divine (ishvara-pranidhana)
3. Body control (asanas)
4. Breath control (pranayama)
5. Detachment (pratyahara)
6. Concentration (dharana)
7. Meditation (dhyana)
8. Pure consciousness (samadhi)

others. The fifth abstinence is nongreed, which means living simply and viewing possessions as tools to use in life. Nongreed leads to the avoidance of jealousy and envy (Staples, 2015).

Personal Disciplines

Personal disciplines concern what to do in life. Purity, the first discipline, is achieved through the practice of the five abstinences. The abstinences clear away negative ways of being, leading one straight to purity. Purity also relates to cleanliness and respect for all life. Contentment, the second discipline, means finding happiness with who one is and with what one has. The third discipline, self-discipline, means being able to make a commitment and adhere to it. The fourth discipline, self-study, means studying oneself through introspection. Centering on the divine, the fifth discipline involves devotion. These disciplines work with any religion because individuals are encouraged to focus on how the divine is in them, part of them, and all around them (Innes & Selfe, 2016).

Body Control

Body control, an important part of hatha yoga, is attained through a number of poses or **asanas.** These body positions are what most Western people think of when they hear the word *yoga* (see Figure 16.1). These poses help people learn to control their bodies, making them stronger, more flexible, better functioning, and more resistant to disease and other problems. Poses are also meant to facilitate meditation. The poses are frequently classified into the following groups: standing poses, inverted poses, twists, backward-bending poses, forward bends, and poses for restoration. Another way of classifying poses is according to balance, strength, flexibility, and relaxation. The belief in nonviolence also applies to the poses, which means that physical exercise is never done to the point of pain because pain is indicative of doing violence to the body (Meissner, Cantell, Steiner, & Sanchez, 2016).

Breath Control

Breath control teaches people to direct energy or prana for optimal physical and mental benefit. When air is inhaled, so is vital energy that flows into the body to nourish and enliven. The purpose of balancing the breath is to make respiratory rhythm more regular, which in turn has a soothing effect on the entire nervous system. It is the best antecedent to meditation because it focuses attention inward and reduces scattered thinking (Staples, 2015).

Detachment

The practice of detachment is related to the senses. It is the withdrawal of the senses from everything that stimulates them. The goal of detachment is to gain mastery over external influences. This detachment can occur during breathing exercises, during meditation, and while doing the poses. The process of detachment can also be an effective technique for pain control (Staples, 2015).

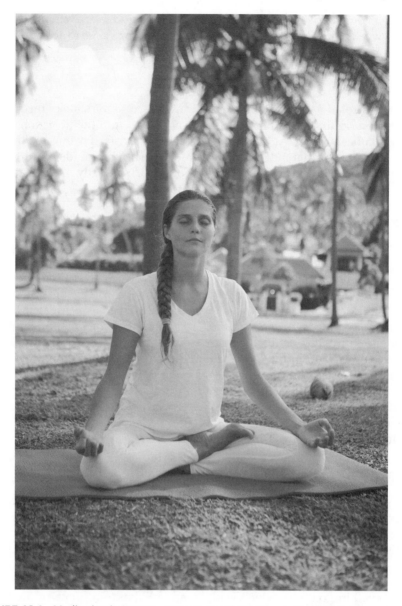

FIGURE 16.1 Meditating in Nature—Woman Practicing Yoga in Tropical Garden

Source: VetrovaMaria/Shutterstock.

Concentration

Teaching the mind to focus on one thing instead of many is the goal of concentration. Concentration means sustaining attention while quieting the mind and relaxing the breathing. Frequently, people focus on one object such as a candle flame, the figure of a circle, or a single sound. The purpose is to learn to push away many thoughts that usually float around in one's mind. Concentration works directly on the body, allowing each yoga pose to accomplish the maximum possible benefit (Kabat-Zinn, 2016).

Meditation

Breath control, detachment, and concentration lead to the state of meditation. Meditation occurs when people become absorbed into the object on which they are concentrating. At this point, nothing else exists. It is through the process of meditation that individuals are able to clear their minds of clutter and thus think more quickly and see things more clearly in daily life (Kabat-Zinn, 2016). Meditation is covered as a separate topic in Chapter 17.

Pure Consciousness

The other seven limbs of yoga lead to pure consciousness, which means a total merging with the object of meditation and thus becoming one with the universe. Generally speaking, pure consciousness is "mind without thought." Many religions throughout history include pure consciousness as part of their tradition. Christianity refers to it as "pure love," and Judaism, as the "divine nothingness" or "the naught." It is more than a mental or emotional experience. Physically, breathing slows drastically, the heart rate drops, and EEGs demonstrate unique patterns unlike those in any of the other three common states of consciousness—waking, sleeping, and dreaming. Pure consciousness is an ideal state, a state of pure bliss that is elusive for most people. A few rare and diligent yogis have been able to maintain this state for extended periods of time. Most others get occasional glimpses of it while meditating (Kabat-Zinn, 2016).

VIEW OF HEALTH AND ILLNESS

In yoga, health is related to the **five sheaths of existence.** The first sheath is the physical body; the second is the vital body, life force, or prana; the third sheath is the mind, including thoughts and emotions; the fourth sheath is the higher intellect; and the fifth sheath is bliss, filled with positive energy and inner peace. It is believed that imbalances in any of these sheaths can result in illness. For example, intense anger, a disturbance in the third sheath, disrupts one's breathing pattern, which leads to an imbalance in prana or life force. The disrupted breathing allows the invasion of a virus, leading to a disruption in the first sheath, manifesting as a cold. Living one's life in moderation is thought to keep all five sheaths in balance, which contributes to health and well-being (Staples, 2015).

Yogic thought places *food* or *ahara* on three levels. The first is the physical food that nourishes the body. The second is impressions or the sensations of sound, touch, sight, taste, and smell that nourish the mind. The third level is associations or the people who nourish the soul. Health and well-being are withdrawal from wrong food, wrong impressions, and wrong associations while simultaneously opening up to the right food, right impressions, and right associations. Just as a healthy body resists toxins and pathogens, a healthy mind resists the negative influences around it (Staples, 2015).

The yogic perspective of health and illness is related to internal and external balance. Although it is recognized that viruses, bacteria, genetics, and accidents can cause illness, disorders can also be brought on by

- insufficient prana, or life force
- blocked prana
- inappropriate diet
- lack of cleanliness
- unhappiness
- pessimism and negativity.

Healthy habits, maintenance of the body, peacefulness of mind, and calmness of spirit protect people from ill health. Yoga is a great preventive medicine. It helps the body cleanse itself of toxins by removing obstacles to the proper flow of the lymphatic system. Lymph is pumped through the body by movement—musculoskeletal movement, respiratory movement, circulatory movement, gastrointestinal movement, and so forth, all of which are part of yoga. Yoga also increases the flow of vital energy throughout the body by opening up and increasing the flexibility of body joints, considered to be minor chakras. Yoga poses and breathing techniques allow energy and lymph to flow freely throughout the entire body, resulting in a body that works better, feels better, and fights disease more effectively. Health, from a yogic perspective, can be described as the body easeful, the mind peaceful, and the life useful (National Center for Complementary and Integrative Health, 2016).

TREATMENT

Individuals can do as much or as little yoga as they wish. Some start with all three practices—poses, breath control, and meditation. Others start with the poses and may or may not develop interest in breathing and meditation.

As practiced in the United States, a typical yoga session lasts 20 minutes to an hour. Some spend 30 minutes doing poses and another 30 minutes doing breathing practices and meditation. Others spend the majority of the time doing poses and end with a short meditation or relaxation procedure. Some people practice one to three times a week in a class, while others practice daily at home. Yoga should not be done within 1 to 2 hours after a heavy meal for sake of abdominal comfort when doing the poses. Caffeine and other stimulants should be avoided because they may interfere with the goal of relaxation. Yoga should never be done under the influence of alcohol or recreational drugs because they may decrease concentration, coordination, and strength, thus increasing the risk of physical injury. Yoga is best done in comfortable, loose clothing using a nonslippery surface such as a rug, mat, or blanket. Because it is important that the process have one's full attention, the room should be void of all extraneous noise, even soft background music.

Yoga is tailored to the individual and can be done with great benefit at the beginner level as well as at the most advanced level. Participants must remember that yoga is not a competitive sport, and thus a person's level does not matter. If people are stiff and out of shape, sick, or weak, sets of easy exercises help loosen the joints and stimulate circulation. If practiced regularly, these simple exercises alone make a great difference in people's health and well-being.

Poses can be slow and careful or more vigorous. Beginning poses are used to relax tension in the muscles and joints and quiet the mind. Attention is paid to how the body feels and what it is doing. Every movement is made gently and slowly. Strain or force is to be avoided because yoga is a nonviolent approach that is done comfortably. Strength training is isometric because the muscles are tensed in opposition to each other. After assuming a pose, one holds it for as long as can be done comfortably, usually about six breaths. Each pose in a well-structured workout includes a pose and its opposite, such as a forward bend and a backward bend, so the body stays physically balanced. Breathing should be easy, fluid, and continuous and used to facilitate the poses.

Every yoga session should end with a few minutes of complete and total relaxation. This period is an important part of bringing the mind and body together to maximize the benefits. Some people end the session with chanting to reach a deeper state of relaxation. The instructor ends the session with the word *namaste:* "The divine in me bows to the divine in you."

Yoga offers a number of health benefits. The physical and psychological benefits include the following:

- Increases flexibility of muscles and joints
- Improves range of motion
- Tones and strengthens muscles
- Improves endurance
- Increases circulation
- Lowers blood pressure
- Increases lymph circulation
- Improves digestion and elimination
- Promotes deeper breathing
- Increases brain endorphins, enkephalins, and serotonin
- Increases mental acuity
- Augments alpha and theta brain wave activity
- Promotes relaxation
- Manages stress (National Center for Complementary and Integrative Health, 2016).

Yoga is not a cure-all for disease. It can help, however, to relieve symptoms, decrease pain, and improve the quality of life. It helps prevent disease by reinforcing lifestyle changes such as positive health habits and attitudes. Overall, yoga is safe. If individuals have a weak link—whether it is the lower back, knees, or shoulders, they are at higher risk of injury and need to be more careful when doing yoga. The two main causes of yoga-related injuries are unqualified teachers and overzealous students. Poorly trained instructors teach improper form. Overzealous students see yoga as a competition and push themselves beyond their physical limits.

RESEARCH

Research related to yoga has been both quantitative and qualitative looking at quality of life, physical benefits, mindfulness, and spirituality. The following is a small selection of current reported research:

- A systematic review and meta-analysis found that yoga interventions had a small improvement in balance and a medium improvement in physical mobility in people 60 years and older. Further research is necessary to determine if these gains will decrease falls in older people (Youkhana, Dean, Wolff, Sherrington, & Tiedemann, 2016).
- A Cochrane systematic review found low to moderate certainty evidence that yoga improved low back pain and function compared to nonexercise or no intervention control groups. It was unclear whether yoga was superior to other forms of low back exercise (Wieland et al., 2017).
- A systematic review and meta-analysis looked at serious adverse events in the practice of yoga. It was determined that yoga is as safe as careful exercise (Cramer et al., 2015).
- A systematic review and meta-analysis was conducted on the impact of yoga on adults with type 2 diabetes. Given some limitations, the findings suggest that yoga may have significant improvement in glycemic control, lipid levels, and weight loss. Yoga may also lower blood pressure and improve mood, sleep, and quality of life (Innes & Selfe, 2016).
- A randomized controlled trial found that there was no evidence of fetal response in women beginning the practice of yoga during their pregnancy. Therefore, yoga can be recommended for low-risk pregnant women (Babbar et al., 2016).
- A randomized controlled trial found that yoga and physical exercise were equally effective in the areas of quality of life, fatigue, mindfulness, and coping with illness in women with breast cancer receiving chemotherapy and/or endocrine therapy (Lotzke et al., 2016).

INTEGRATED NURSING PRACTICE

The regular practice of yoga builds and tones muscles, increases flexibility, improves endurance, and promotes a state of relaxation. The physiological responses are the opposite of the fight-or-flight stress response. Stretching and deep breathing bring on a profound sense of relaxation. Gentle stretching and range-of-motion joint exercises decrease muscle tension and joint stiffness. The mindful focus on awareness of self, breath, and energy minimizes anxiety associated with stress. Just getting the body down on the floor tends to clear the mind, perhaps because being on the floor is so unusual that it changes people's attitudes toward and awareness of the body (Kabat-Zinn, 2016).

Hatha yoga is designed by and for healthy, flexible people. Even when experiencing a serious illness, however, most people can work on breath control even if they do not feel up to doing the poses. The breathing exercises and relaxation response nourish the body, quiet the mind, and contribute to a more balanced state. Individuals should be encouraged to check with their primary care practitioner if they have recently had surgery, have a debilitating physical handicap, or have cancer, diabetes, epilepsy, heart disease, high blood pressure, HIV, multiple sclerosis, or any other serious condition. Yoga, combined with a low-fat diet and moderate aerobic exercise, can significantly reduce blockages in coronary arteries (Ornish, 2008). Other studies have shown yoga to be effective in treating arthritis, diabetes, mood disorders, asthma, hypertension, menstrual cramps, back pain, and chronic fatigue.

Yoga can benefit people of any age, from children to older adults. Children take naturally to yoga and usually find it to be much fun. Getting the whole family involved is one way to maintain the routine. Some adults find that yoga complements their aerobic routine, while others engage in yoga as a great nonaerobic conditioner. It is possible to learn yoga from books or compact disks (see the Resources section at the end of this chapter), but it is easier to learn from a teacher. Yoga classes are available in many places, such as health clubs, community centers, universities, and hospitals.

As a nurse, you can encourage people to utilize yoga as a way to start on the path of taking responsibility for their well-being. Consistent practice of yoga changes people's attitudes about their body and their beliefs about what they can do to take care of themselves, both of which are crucial to well-being. For some, the physical exercise may be a way to attain a specific goal such as improving flexibility, improving muscle tone, or losing weight. Others have no specific goal other than the exercise itself and becoming aware of their self, breath, and energy. The relaxation that accompanies yoga can stimulate self-healing and contribute to a sense of inner peace.

Almost anyone can be taught the Mountain Pose, which is a standing position of postural awareness. When this pose is practiced well, the body is prepared for almost all daily movement: standing, sitting, walking, and running. Like the mountain poised between heaven and earth, this pose establishes grounding through the legs and feet and encourages the lift of the spine. Instruct people to stand sideways near a full-length mirror so that they can check their alignment, which may feel strange at first (see Figure 16.2). Once people are in alignment, they should notice their physical sensations. Is weight balanced evenly between the feet? Are the

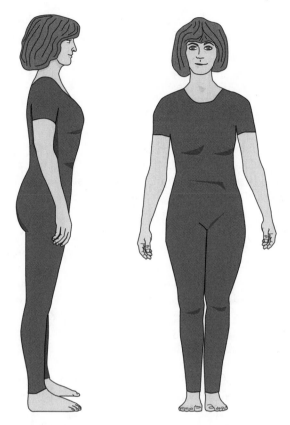

FIGURE 16.2   Mountain Pose (Tadasana)

legs firm but not tight? Are shoulders relaxed? Does the spinal cord feel light and the head feel balanced on the torso? Is breathing comfortable and easy? Encourage people to practice the Mountain Pose several times a day. Standing well reduces strain on the joints, ligaments, and muscles, especially those of the spinal column and lower extremities. It also aids respiration, digestion, and elimination. The Mountain Pose conveys a sense of poise and self-esteem.

Benefits from any fitness program, including yoga, can occur only with continued practice. Try some of these suggestions to help people develop a regular pattern:

- Encourage clients to make time for yoga practice every day, to give themselves permission to take care of themselves and take time to relax. They may find that doing a few poses before bedtime or early in the morning works best. Even if they practice for only 5 minutes, a daily practice is the foundation on which to build.

- To maintain their practice, many people find it helpful to go to a yoga class at least once a week. The support of practicing with others and the information they get from teachers help strengthen their commitment to yoga.
- Suggest that they create a dedicated yoga space. They may have to temporarily push things aside to have enough space for their practice. Or they may simply choose a place to spread their yoga mat on the floor. Having a regular space for practice helps people focus on the poses without being distracted by their surroundings.
- Have people start with the poses they like. If they like a pose, they will do it even if it is difficult. You may suggest that they take one pose they like from each class and practice it at least once a day, which takes only a few moments. They can then gradually begin to combine the poses to form their own yoga session.

One of the many applications of yoga is in pregnancy and childbirth. In fact, many of the techniques taught in childbirth classes, such as focus, relaxation, and systematic breathing, have their roots in yoga. The gentle stretching of the poses helps ease the muscle aches of pregnancy and strengthens the muscles that will be used during delivery. The breathing techniques may lessen the shortness of breath that often accompanies advanced pregnancy.

Yoga practiced while pregnant is slightly different from regular yoga in that some poses are contraindicated. These poses are the extreme stretching positions and any position that puts pressure on the uterus. Full forward bends will probably be uncomfortable for both woman and baby. Because her center of balance has shifted completely, she must be careful with balance poses. A pregnant woman should never lie on the stomach for any pose. After the 20th week, she should lie on her left side rather than her back. If any pose feels uncomfortable, the woman should stop at once. If a pregnant woman experiences dizziness, sudden swelling, extreme shortness of breath, or vaginal bleeding, she should see her midwife or doctor immediately (Babbar et al., 2016).

With midwife's or doctor's approval, most women can usually start gentle yoga poses 2 weeks after delivery or a few weeks later if they have had a cesarean section. They should start with a few poses and gradually work back to their regular routine. If their postpartum bleeding gets heavier or brighter red, they must stop and call their midwife or doctor. Filling their body with energy through breathing exercises may promote self-healing after childbirth.

As people learn yoga, they will find that each sequence of poses helps them focus on something specific; for example, one sequence can improve balance, while another may release anger and negative feelings, and some sequences will tone internal organs, increase lung capacity, or build upper-body strength. People choose the sequences that are right for them. It is most important to remind people that it is not a matter of being a beginning, intermediate, or advanced student but rather that they keep practicing, doing as much as they can whenever they can. Yoga moves at their pace, in the time they have.

TRY THIS
Heart Breathing

- Sit comfortably and close your eyes.
- Simply notice your breathing without trying to change it. Pay attention to your in-breath and your out-breath.
- Now imagine that the breath is pouring into your heart with each inhalation and flowing out of your heart with each exhalation. Just feel the breath flowing in and out of your heart. Imagine the breath is pure love.
- Do this breath awareness for 5 to 10 minutes.
- Now let your attention return to your environment, slowly open your eyes, get up, and move on.
- Think about the feeling throughout the day.

Reach for the Stars

- Notice your body posture, sitting or standing. Are you slouching?
- Reach overhead with your wrists crossed and your palms touching.
- Stretch high and feel the tension release.

Considering the Evidence

Cramer, H., Lauche, R., Klose, P., Lange, S., Langhorst, J., & Dobos, G. J. (2017). Yoga for improving health-related quality of life, mental health and cancer-related symptoms in women diagnosed with breast cancer. *The Cochrane Database of Systematic Reviews*, Art. No. CD010802. doi: 10.1002/14651858.CD010802.pu

What Was the Approach of the Research?
Systematic review of randomized clinical control trials (RCTs).

What Was the Aim/Purpose/Objective(s) of the Research as Related to Complementary and Integrative Therapies?
To assess the effects of yoga on health-related quality of life, mental health, and cancer-related symptoms among women living with a diagnosis of breast cancer who are receiving active treatment or have completed treatment for cancer.

How Was the Study Done?
The authors used a systematic review methodology to examine published and unpublished RCTs relevant to the purpose of the research. A comprehensive search strategy was implemented using selected keywords related to the phenomenon of interest and multiple

(*continued*)

databases to identify RCTs focused on the purpose of the review. Included in the review were RCTs that compared yoga interventions versus no therapy or versus any other active therapy in women with a diagnosis of non-metastatic or metastatic breast cancer, and assessed at least one of the primary outcomes on patient-reported instruments, including health-related quality of life, depression, anxiety, fatigue, or sleep disturbances. A total of 24 studies were included in the systematic review with a total of 2,166 participants.

What Were the Significant Findings of the Research?

The evidence supports that yoga was more effective in improving quality of life and reducing fatigue and sleep disturbances compared with no therapy in women living with breast cancer. Additionally, yoga reduced depression, anxiety, and fatigue more so than psychosocial or educational interventions. The researchers indicate minimal information to none was reported related to risk associated with the implementation of yoga in the study participants.

What Additional Questions Might I Have?

Are there adverse effects that can occur as a result of participation in yoga for women living with breast cancer? What would be the possible effects of combining yoga with other complementary and integrative therapies in women living with breast cancer on selected outcomes?

What Is the Clinical Significance of This Study?

This study could have value for nurses caring for women living with breast cancer. Nurses should recognize and support the incorporation of yoga in treatment plans as an effort to enhance the quality of life in women living with breast cancer. Nurses should seek to identify if the findings could be safely applied to individuals living with other types of cancer diagnosis as a strategy for improving their quality of life. Nurses may have confidence in the findings of this review as it informs their evidence-based nursing practice in caring for women living with breast cancer.

Source: Contributed by Dolores M. Huffman, RN, PhD.

References

Babbar, S., Hill, J. B., Williams, K. B., Pinon, M., Chauhan, S. P., & Maulik, D. (2016). Acute fetal behavioral response to prenatal yoga: A single, blinded, randomized controlled trial. *American Journal of Obstetrics and Gynecology.* doi: 10.1016/j.ajog.2015.12.032

Cramer, H., Ward, L., Saper, R., Fishbein, D., Dobos, G., & Lauche, R. (2015). The safety of yoga: A systematic review and meta-analysis of randomized controlled trials. *American Journal of Epidemiology.* doi: 1093/aje/kwv071

Innes, K. E., & Selfe, T. K. (2016). Yoga for adults with type 2 diabetes: A systematic review of controlled trials. *Journal of Diabetes Research.* doi: 10.1155/2016/6979370

Kabat-Zinn, J. (2016). *Mindfulness for Beginners.* Boulder, CO: Sounds True.

Lotzke, D., Wiedemann, F., Recchia, D. R., Ostermann, T., Sattler, D., Ettl, J., . . .

Bussing, A. (2016). Iyengar-yoga compared to exercise as a therapeutic intervention during (neo)adjuvant therapy in women with stage I–III breast cancer. *Evidence-Based Complementary and Alternative Medicine.* doi: 10.1155/2016/5931816

Meissner, M., Cantell, M. H., Steiner, R., & Sanchez, X. (2016). Evaluating emotional well-being after a short-term traditional yoga practice approach in yoga practitioners with an existing Western-type yoga practice. *Evidence-Based Complementary and Alternative Medicine.* doi: 10.1155/2016/7216982

Miles, C., Tait, E., Schure, M. B., & Hollis, M. (2016). Effect of laughter yoga on psychological well-being and physiological measures. *Advances in Mind–Body Medicine*, 30(1):12–20.

National Center for Complementary and Integrative Health. (2016). *Yoga: In Depth.* Retrieved from http://nccih.nih.gov/health/yoga/introduction.htm

Ornish, D. (2008). *The Spectrum: A Scientifically Proven Program to Feel Better, Live Longer, Lose Weight, and Gain Health.* New York, NY: Ballantine Books.

Silver, T. (2011). *Outrageous Openness: Letting the Divine Take the Lead.* Urban Kali Productions.

Staples, J. (2015). Yoga. In M. S. Micozzi (Ed.), *Fundamentals of Complementary and Alternative Medicine* (5th ed., pp. 332–343). St. Louis, MO: Elsevier/Saunders.

Voltaire. (1824). *A Philosophical Dictionary: From the French* (Vol. 3). J. and H. L. Hunt. Originally from the New York Public Library.

Wieland, L. S., Skoetz, N., Pilkington, K., Vampati, R., D'Adamo, C. R., & Berman, B. M. (2017). Yoga treatment for chronic non-specific low back pain. *The Cochrane Database Systematic Reviews.* doi: 10.1002/14651858.CD010671-pub2

Youkhana, S., Dean, C. M., Wolff, M., Sherrington, C., & Tiedemann, A. (2016). Yoga-based exercise improves balance and mobility in people aged 60 and over: A systematic review and meta-analysis. *Age and Ageing.* doi: 10.1093/ageing/afv175

Resources

American Yoga Association
P.O. Box 19986
Sarasota, FL 34276
941.927.4977
www.americanyogaassociation.org

The Canadian Yoga Institute
403.394.9642
www.yogacanada.org

Center for Mindfulness in Medicine,
   Health Care, and Society
University of Massachusetts
Medical School
55 Lake Ave. North
Worcester, MA 01655
508.856.2656
www.umassmed.edu/cfm

The British Wheel of Yoga
25 Jermyn St.

Sleaford, Lincolnshire NG34 7RU
01529.306.851
www.bwy.org.uk

Yoga Australia
125A Chapel St.
Windsor 3181
1300.881.451
www.yogaaustralia.org

17

Meditation

The Wise Man Believes Profoundly in Silence—the sign of a perfect equilibrium. silence is the absolute poise or balance of body, mind and spirit.

OHIYESA

Be here now. Be somewhere else later. Is that so hard?

JEWISH-ZEN SAYING

Meditation is a general term for a wide range of practices that involve relaxing the body and stilling the mind. The root word, *meditari*, means "to consider," or one could say, "to pay attention to something." *Medha*, the Sanskrit derivation, means "wisdom." The founder and director of the Stress Reduction Clinic at the University of Massachusetts Medical Center, Jon Kabat-Zinn (1994) stated, "Meditation is simply about being yourself and knowing something about who that is. It is about coming to realize that you are on a path whether you like it or not, namely, the path that is your life. . . . Meditation is the process by which we go about deepening our attention and awareness, refining them, and putting them to greater practical use in our lives" (pp. xvi–xvii).

In 1975, Dr. Herbert Benson wrote the book *The Relaxation Response*, which drew the attention of Western health-care practitioners to the physical and psychological benefits of relaxation. As Benson pointed out, the components of relaxation are quite simple: a quiet space, a comfortable position, a receptive attitude, and a focus of attention. The relaxation response involves physiological and psychological effects that appear common to many forms of focused attention in addition to meditation: prayer, yoga, biofeedback, and the presuggestion phase of hypnosis. These practices are covered in other chapters in this text. Benson (1975) described meditation as a process that anyone can use to calm down, cope with stress, and, for those with spiritual inclinations, feel as one with God or the universe. Meditation can be practiced individually or in groups and is easy to learn. It requires no change in belief system and is compatible with most religious practices.

BACKGROUND

Most meditative practices have come to the West from Eastern practices, particularly those of India, China, Japan, and Tibet. Meditative techniques, however, can be found in most cultures of the world where prayer, meditation, ritual, or contemplation are all initiated by shifting into a relaxed state. Nearly all major religions include some form of meditative practice. Christianity, Judaism, Buddhism, and Islam all use repetitive prayers, chants, or movements as part of their worship rituals. Although religious practices in the West are not typically labeled "meditative," they in fact are. The Catholic practice of using rosary beads while saying the "Hail Mary" is a familiar example. The repetition of the words combined with the movement of the beads induces a state of relaxation and a quieting of the mind.

Until recently, the primary purpose of meditation has been spiritual or religious. Since the 1970s, it has been explored as a way of reducing stress on both body and mind. Many conventional health-care practitioners recommend it for widely diverse situations, from undergoing natural childbirth to managing hypertension to controlling pain. For many years, nurses have taught clients progressive relaxation in a wide variety of clinical settings.

PREPARATION

Practicing meditation does not require a teacher, and many people learn the process through instructions from books, recordings, or compact disks. Some people, however, find that the structure of a meditation class is helpful. Many varieties of teachers and classes are available. Currently, no certification process is available for a meditation teacher. The general standard is some years of daily meditation practice before one teaches others. Both Christian and Buddhist traditions offer regular classes and retreats designed to teach meditative practices and the process of becoming a spiritual being in a material world. In the Hindu tradition, people learn meditation from a guru who is a spiritual teacher or guide. Whatever the tradition, teachers encourage self-responsibility and the practice of mindfulness in everyday life (Yates, Immergut, & Graves, 2017).

CONCEPTS

Meditative State

Meditation is about being aware of who one is in the here and now rather than about feeling a particular way. It means letting go of any expectations of the process and simply observing what happens as it unfolds. People are sometimes concerned that they do not have the skills to meditate. As Dr. Jon Kabat-Zinn (1994) stated, "Thinking you are unable to meditate is a little like thinking you are unable to breathe, or to concentrate or relax. Pretty much everybody can breathe easily. And under the right circumstances, pretty much anybody can concentrate, anybody can relax" (p. 33). All forms of meditation require regular, daily practice over a period of time to experience the many benefits.

Attention and Concentration

Basic to all meditative techniques is the intentional focus of attention on one thought, word, sound, image, or physical sensation for a sustained period of time. The mind is fully alert but not focused on the external world or events. The normal rapid series of thoughts and feelings is replaced with inner awareness and attention. Rather than allowing the mind to jump between the past and the future, a person focuses attention in the present reality. It is impossible to make the mind empty, but it is possible to focus on one thing, which helps the mind let go of the tendency to worry, plan, think, analyze, remember, or solve problems. A passive, nonjudgmental attitude is necessary during meditation. When thoughts intrude, they are noticed and then let go as the attention returns to the original focus.

In some types of meditation, the focus is on the breath, the primary purpose being to calm the mind and body. It is a process of keeping the attention on the breath while breathing deeply, slowly, and regularly. The awareness is on the breath moving in and the breath moving out and allowing all other thoughts, feelings, or sensations to pass by as this focus is maintained. Through regular meditation practice, it becomes a habit to breathe more consciously and deeply throughout the day so that in the long term the breath becomes a calming force in daily life (Seaward, 2014).

Some people use a mantra as their focus of attention. A **mantra** is a sound or sounds that resonate in the body and evoke certain energies. Mantras, such as OM, soothe the mind and awaken the senses. Another beginning mantra is OM SHANTI SHANTI SHANTI. *Shanti* means peace, and when repeated three times, it balances the body, mind, and spirit.

A mandala meditation uses an object to focus the mind through sight. A **mandala** is typically a circular geometric design that draws the eye to the center and is meant to suggest the circular patterns in the universe, such as the solar systems. Mandalas appear as **labyrinths** on the floors of some cathedrals in Europe. In a labyrinth, only one path leads to the center and back out. The faithful follow the course of the labyrinth into the center as penitence or in spiritual contemplation. Labyrinths and mandalas have recently become

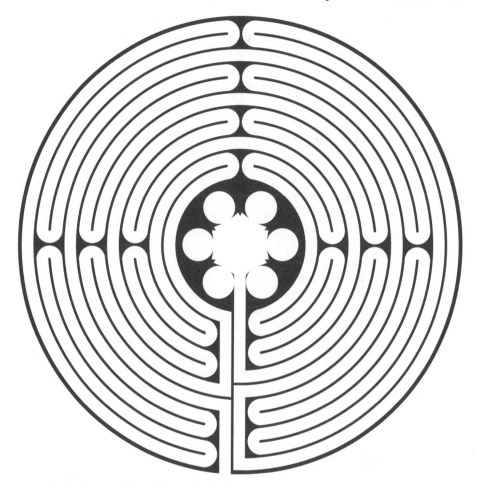

FIGURE 17.1   Mandala on the Floor of Chartres Cathedral

popular in the United States among some Christian religious groups who are renewing the contemplative aspects of their faith. Using mantras and mandalas together is an effective focus for meditation (Hume, 2015).

Figure 17.1 is the mandala on the floor of Chartres Cathedral in France. Using a pencil, trace the walking path to the center and then back to the outer world.

Researchers have used functional magnetic resonance imaging (fMRI) to assess the neurological response to meditation. Meditation activates the orbital inferior frontal gyrus, the medial anterior prefrontal cortex, and the anterior cingulate cortex, all of which are involved in focused attention, mind wandering, and emotional processing. Experienced meditators showed greater response compared to novice meditators (Garrison, Scheinost, Constable, & Brewer, 2014; Staples, 2015; Tomasino & Fabbro, 2016).

Meditation is both simple and difficult—simple because it is nothing more than maintaining focused attention, yet difficult because of the habitual, lifelong pattern of letting the mind wander wherever it wants. With extended practice, the mind tends to become better and better at staying focused. The stability and calmness that come with focused attention are the foundation of meditation.

VIEW OF HEALTH AND ILLNESS

Many disorders or diseases are aggravated or caused by stress. They are labeled as disorders of arousal, in which the limbic system of the brain has become overstimulated. In addition, overactivity of both the sympathetic nervous system and the adrenal glands is related to stress. It is thought that excessive limbic activity may inhibit immune function, which may account for the association of chronic stress and increased susceptibility to infection.

A relaxed state is the opposite of the aroused state of fight or flight. The fight-or-flight reflex increases blood pressure, heart rate, breathing, metabolism, and blood flow to the muscles. The response triggered by all the relaxing practices does the opposite and results in a lower blood pressure and slower heart rate, breathing, metabolism, and blood flow. Relaxation and meditation also decrease the production of adrenergic catecholamines, thereby decreasing limbic activity. Since a person's state of mind and emotional, attitudinal, and intellectual components initiate activities in the nervous system, individuals can consciously choose to trigger the benefits of meditation.

TREATMENT

The relaxation response can be evoked by any number of techniques, including progressive relaxation, meditation, prayer, jogging, swimming, Lamaze breathing exercises, yoga, t'ai chi, and qigong. The beauty of these techniques is their simplicity. They allow the mind to have a focus while enhancing one's vitality and well-being.

The varieties of meditation have many different names. Some are religious practices, and some are not. Some are complicated, while some are simple. Each type of meditative practice involves a form of mental focusing and the adoption of a nonjudgmental attitude toward intruding thoughts. All types appear to produce similar physical and psychological changes. People beginning the practice of meditation should look around for a form that seems comfortable, that suits them, and that does not conflict with their belief system.

Transcendental Meditation® was developed by the Indian leader Maharishi Mahesh Yogi in an effort to make the ancient practice of meditation more attainable to Westerners. TM® is a sound-focused form of meditation and is simple and easy to learn. To prevent distracting thoughts, a person is given a mantra (a word or sound) to repeat silently over and over again while sitting in a comfortable position. When thoughts other than the mantra come to mind, the person is to notice them and then gently return the focus to the mantra. It is expected that people will practice TM® for 20 minutes, once or twice a day. The trademarked Transcendental Meditation is a commercial enterprise that is a fairly expensive undertaking. Classes are typically found in Ayurvedic schools and health-care centers. Local centers may be found on the Internet at www.tm.org.

The David Lynch Foundation offers a program called Quiet Time for people living in a climate of poverty, violence, and fear, such as low-income families, veterans, homeless people, and students in urban schools. The program consists of two 15-minute periods of Transcendental Meditation® a day. The University of Chicago's Crime Lab recently began a randomized controlled study of Quiet Time with 6,800 students in Chicago and New York. Since TM® is a distinct technique, taught the same way around the world, the research results are more valid than other forms of complementary and integrative therapies.

The essence of **Buddhist meditation** is training the mind in compassion and in wisdom. The goal is to develop compassion for all living things. Meditation begins with a time of contemplation, which typically includes points such as these:

- Just as I wish to be free from suffering and experience only happiness, so do all other beings
- I am no different from any other being; we are all equal
- My happiness and suffering are insignificant when compared with the happiness and suffering of all other living beings (Mascaro, Darcher, Negi, & Raison, 2015).

Loving kindness meditation is a part of Buddhist meditation. Loving kindness is first generated for oneself, removing negative thoughts and feelings that might contaminate loving kindness for others. Next, the person creates loving kindness for someone they care about. This progresses to sending loving kindness energy to someone who is difficult or with whom one is angry. See the Try This section for a loving kindness meditation.

Mindfulness, an ancient Buddhist practice, is both a philosophy and a meditation practice. Its primary principle is "being in the moment." Most often people go through daily routines with little awareness or attention. People read while they eat, exercise while watching TV, or cook while talking to their children, and the nuances of these experiences are lost. This situation might be called living mindlessly by ignoring present moments. Mindfulness is the opposite of living on "automatic pilot." It is the art of conscious living by focusing full attention on the activity at hand. While it may be simple to practice mindfulness, it is not necessarily easy. Habitual unawareness is persistent, and mindfulness requires effort and discipline. Thus, to eat a peach mindfully would involve being actively aware of every sensation, every smell, and every taste, noticing its texture, color, and weight and how it feels on the tongue. This technique can be practiced with any activity (Kabat-Zinn, 1994).

Mindfulness meditation is a daily practice that encourages living in the moment. It begins by sitting quietly with eyes closed and focusing on breathing. The flow of thought during the meditation is observed as thoughts come and go. The key to mindfulness meditation is the ability to accept rather than judge the wandering thoughts, bringing attention back to the breathing as needed.

Mindfulness-based stress reduction (MBSR) is a structured 8-week therapy program utilizing mindfulness meditation, yoga, and group discussion. Mindfulness-based relapse prevention (MBRP) is a program focused on breathing and physical sensations as a way of coping with triggers to substance abuse relapse (Black, 2014).

Tibetan meditation is a breath-focused form of meditation. The person simply focuses attention on each in-breath and out-breath. When thoughts about anything other than the breath intrude, the person notes them by silently saying "thinking" and then returns attention to the breath. It is recognized that thoughts cannot be completely halted and that they are a natural process and are simply to be noted in a nonjudgmental way.

Sufi meditation is a worshipful meditation and a way of drawing nearer to Allah. Sufi meditation is above and beyond the traditional religious prayers. A prescribed number of verses from the Quran are recited while using prayer beads to keep count. The goal is not only to find peace but to better understand Allah, the Divine (Hall, Micozzi, & O'Leary, 2015).

Forms of **moving meditation** include the Chinese martial art t'ai chi, the Japanese martial art aikido, the Indian practice of yoga, and the walking meditation in Zen Buddhism. Instead of focusing on a word or on breathing, movement meditation uses physical sensations as the focus of concentration. In walking meditation, for example, attention is given to the feeling of each step as it is taken. Intruding thoughts are simply noticed, and attention is returned to the step. Research has found that focused walking, in contrast with unfocused walking, is associated with reduced anxiety and fewer negative thoughts. In **rhythmic meditation**, participants pay attention to their hand and body movements while their eyes are open (Henderson, 2015).

If practiced regularly, even 15 minutes twice a day, meditation produces widespread positive effects on physical and psychological functioning. The autonomic nervous system responds with a decrease in heart rate, lower blood pressure, decreased respiratory rate and oxygen consumption, and a lower arousal threshold. People who meditate say that they have clearer minds and sharper thoughts. The brain seems to clear itself so that new ideas and beliefs become available. This clearer mind may be accompanied by a cognitive restructuring in which people interpret life events in a more positive, more realistic fashion (see Figure 17.2). Meditation's residual effects— improved stress-coping abilities—are a protection against daily stress and anxiety. All other self-healing methods are improved with the practice of meditation (Sheridan, 2016).

Some adverse effects of meditation are possible. Relaxation exercises should not be practiced while driving or operating potentially dangerous machinery. Some people have been stressed so long that they are unfamiliar with deep relaxation and therefore feel threatened by it. In meditation, people

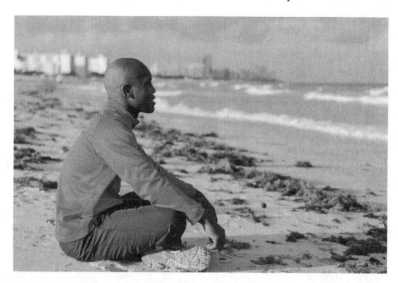

FIGURE 17.2 Meditation Provides Physical and Psychological Benefits—A Young Man in Meditation

Source: Fotoluminate LLC/Shutterstock.

are taught to accept nonjudgmentally whatever thoughts occur. Sometimes, however, extremely upsetting thoughts arise, and it is impossible to remain nonjudgmental, which could lead to disparaging thoughts about one's abilities. The adverse effects for more experienced meditators are temporary fear, anxiety, confusion, depression, and self-doubt. For an unknown reason, these kinds of thoughts are more likely to arise during the first 10 minutes of meditation. There have been rare reports that meditation worsened certain psychiatric problems such as anxiety and depression.

RESEARCH

Since the 1960s, a large body of research has been documented regarding meditation and the relaxation response. There is support for the effectiveness of meditation in dealing with a number of chronic physical disorders, reducing stress, and improving well-being and quality of life. It is possible that the effects of meditation are not linear but rather up and down depending on individuals and situations (Mascaro et al., 2015).

The following is a small sample of the research:

- A systematic review and meta-analysis of meditation programs found that there was a small but significant improvement in anxiety, depression, pain, and quality of life (Goyal, Singh, & Sibinga, 2014).
- A systematic review and meta-analysis was done on the effect of meditation on brain structure and function as measured by MRIs. Results found that meditation activated brain areas involved in self-regulation,

sensitivity to external stimuli, problem solving, and adaptive behavior (Boccia, Piccardi, & Guariglia, 2015).

- Veterans with posttraumatic stress disorder randomized to mindfulness-based stress reduction plus treatment as usual demonstrated a significant reduction in symptoms at 6-month follow-up compared with veterans who received only treatment as usual (Kearney et al., 2016).
- Mindfulness-based stress reduction, cognitive behavioral therapy (CBT), and usual care were evaluated for the effectiveness on chronic low back pain. Both MBSR and CBT groups demonstrated greater improvement than the usual care group. There was no significant difference between the MBSR and CBT groups (Cherkin et al., 2016).
- Self-help physical activity, mindfulness meditation, and heart rate variability biofeedback were compared in the effectiveness of reducing stress. It was found that all three treatments were equally effective (van der Zwan, de Vente, Huizink, Bogels, & de Bruin, 2015).
- A randomized controlled trial tested the effects of mindfulness meditation on chronic pain. Data were collected at baseline, after completion of the course/waiting period (2.5 years) and at 6-month follow-up. Researchers found a significant effect on pain, anxiety and depression, and quality of life (Cour & Petersen, 2015).

INTEGRATED NURSING PRACTICE

Progressive relaxation and meditation are used in a wide variety of clinical settings such as rehabilitation facilities, cardiac care units, postoperative units, stress management centers, behavioral counseling settings, and centers dedicated to health and wellness promotion. Thousands of hospitals, clinics, private practitioners, and universities offer training in meditation. In addition, recordings, compact disks, and books make meditation more accessible to people with busy schedules. Many individuals practice meditation to reduce stress, anxiety, anger, and other negative emotions. But increasingly, nurses are prescribing meditation as part of the treatment for a large and growing number of medical conditions.

Mindfulness-based stress reduction programs have been developed by Jon Kabat-Zinn at the University of Massachusetts Medical Center and are taught by nurses and other health-care professionals worldwide. People participate for many reasons, including job, family, or financial stress; chronic pain and illness; anxiety and panic; sleep disturbances; fatigue; hypertension; and headaches. A number of midwifery practices include MBSR as a complement to childbirth education and parenting classes. The course schedule consists of eight weekly classes and one daylong class.

Progressive relaxation is a way of decreasing muscular tension. The relaxation response can be elicited by teaching clients two common techniques: progressive relaxation and body scan. Both focus on reducing muscle tone in the major muscle groups and take about 7 to 10 minutes. If possible, help the client find a quiet place with a comfortable temperature to do the exercise, which can be done in any comfortable position. People typically do the exercise lying on their back and begin with a focus on the breath, breathing gently, slowly, and deeply. Next, instruct the client to tense a muscle group as tight as possible, hold the tension for several seconds, and then consciously relax it. Have the client repeat this sequence for each of the major muscle groups in the body, usually beginning at the toes and slowly working up the body. Progressive relaxation is designed to help people with chronic tension experience the difference between a muscle that is tense and one that is relaxed. In the body scan exercise, clients are instructed to focus their attention on body parts, one at a time, often beginning at the feet and moving toward the head, and to consciously relax each part. Box 17.1 provides directions for the body scan technique.

You can also teach clients to anchor the relaxation response with a sensory stimulus, such as an aroma of lavender or rose, or a touch, such as pressing two fingers together. The sensory anchor should be established within 30 seconds of the relaxation exercise. After performing progressive relaxation using the sensory anchor for 2 weeks, the individual should be able to instantaneously relax by re-experiencing the particular sensory trigger, be it an aroma or a physical sensation.

Meditation is the next step following the mastery of progressive relaxation and body scan. Explain the two basic steps to clients: the repetition of a word, sound, prayer, phrase, or muscular activity and the disregard of everyday thoughts that interfere with the process. The word or phrase is silently repeated with each in-breath and out-breath. Some people choose to use one word for the in-breath and another for the out-breath. Some meditators choose an object of personal significance on which to focus. Every detail of the object

BOX 17.1
Body Scan Meditation

- Lie on your back with your legs uncrossed, your arms at your sides, palms up, and your eyes closed.
- Focus on your breathing; breathe in peace and breathe out tension.
- As you begin to feel relaxed, direct your attention to your feet, paying attention to any sensations. Let your feet relax, and feel the warmth spread throughout your feet.
- Then, move your focus to your ankles. Follow the same procedure as you move up your lower legs, knees, thighs, hips, and so on all around the body.
- Pay particular attention to any areas that are painful or are the focus of any medical condition, such as the lungs or heart.
- Finish the body scan by paying particular attention to the neck and head. Experience the warmth of the relaxation.

is studied, including gradations of shape, color, texture, and so on. Flowers, candle flames, or religious statues are common choices.

Before sitting down to meditate, it is helpful to make sure that the area is clean and uncluttered, which helps keep the mind clear and fresh. No props are required for meditation, although some people may choose to include incense, candles, or religious symbols in their meditative practice. Beginners often start with 5 to 10 minutes of meditation and increase the time gradually. It is most important that time be scheduled each day, and many people find that meditating first thing in the morning, before the busy day begins, works well. Other people prefer to meditate in the evening. The key is to find a time when one is unlikely to be disturbed. It is best to wait about 2 hours after a big meal, during which time the blood flow is diverted from the brain to the gut, which makes falling asleep during meditation more likely.

All sitting meditative practices begin with finding a comfortable but erect position. The posture itself is a meditation. Slumping reflects low energy and passivity, while a ramrod-straight posture reflects tension and effort. It is easiest to meditate if the spine is straight and the body posture is symmetrical. Some people sit on the floor cross-legged using a firm cushion under their backside to support the spine. Others sit in a chair with a straight back, with both feet on the ground. The face relaxes, shoulders drop, and the head, neck, and back move into easy alignment. The eyes may be either open or closed. Hands may be resting in the lap or held with palms together. It is believed that having the palms together with the fingertips touching completes a circuit of energy extending from the heart down the arms and through the chakras in the center of the palm of each hand as well as the chakras in the fingertips. People often experiment with various ways of positioning their hands during meditation until they determine which position is best for them (Kabat-Zinn, 2011).

Once people are adept at meditation, they can be taught to use *minis*. Minis are abbreviated versions of meditation. Instruct clients to breathe deeply, releasing tension, while saying the chosen focus word, sound, phrase, or prayer. Minis are very helpful in the midst of busy, stressful times (Benson, 1997).

One type of meditation is a breathing awareness meditation. In this form, the person concentrates on the sensation of the breath as it enters the nose and fills the chest and abdomen, and then as it passes out of the body. Alternatively, one can imagine the breath coming in from the toes, up the legs, through the belly, and into the chest and out the same pathway. It is helpful to imagine healing and relaxation flowing into the body with each in-breath, and stress or pain leaving the body with each out-breath. When thoughts arise, they are noticed and then let go as attention is brought back to the breathing.

Another breathing awareness practice you can teach clients is a simple technique used in Zen meditation. Instruct clients to sit in a comfortable position with the spine straight. Ask them to gently close their eyes while breathing naturally and easily. To begin the exercise, have them count "1" to themselves as they exhale. On the next exhale, count "2," and so on, up to counting 5. Then, instruct them to begin a new cycle, counting "1" on the next exhale. Remind clients never to count higher than 5, and to count only on the exhale.

They will know their attention has wandered when they find themselves up to 8 or 10. When this occurs, have them gently refocus and restart on the count of 1. This form of meditation should be done for about 10 minutes (Weil, 1995).

Any repetitive behavior can be used as a meditative focus. One of the most universally used practices is walking meditation. In **walking meditation**, one is not walking to get to any particular place. Having no place to go makes it easier to be present in the moment. This meditation is often practiced at some place in nature, on a track, on a walking mandala, or even pushing a shopping cart through a supermarket. It can be practiced at any pace, from very slow to very brisk. The practice is to take each step as it comes and to be fully present with it. One notices the movements of each foot, how it lifts, moves forward in space, and then descends again. Just as in other forms of meditation, when thoughts intrude, they are let go, and awareness is returned to the physical sensations of walking.

An excellent book for nurses is Sherry Kahn's text, *The Nurse's Meditative Journal* (1996). This book provides step-by-step instruction in meditation and journal writing as an aid in self-exploration and growth. A nurse's ability to focus in the midst of chaos, and understand in the midst of confusion, can bring comfort to clients and inspire professional peers to find these same qualities within themselves.

There are as many ways to meditate as there are people. When people say they have tried meditation and cannot do it, they just have not found the right practice for them. One person may want to sit, one to do repetitive prayers, one to swim or run, one to walk, and one to do yoga or t'ai chi. Clients should be encouraged to explore a variety of techniques and develop the habit of meditation on a daily basis.

TRY THIS

Loving Kindness Meditation

Begin by focusing on your breathing, and take a few slow, easy breaths. Feel yourself relaxed. Imagine a white light above you and slightly in front of you, pouring a waterfall of love and light over you. Let the light enter the top of your head and wash through you. See yourself totally enclosed in a cocoon of white light, and repeat these loving kindness blessings for yourself, with all the respect and love that you would have for your only child:

May I be at peace.

May my heart remain open.

May I awaken to the light of my own true nature.

May I be healed.

May I be a source of healing for all beings.

(continued)

Next, bring one or more loved ones to mind. See them in as much detail as possible. Imagine the white light shining down on them and surrounding them. Then bless them:

May you be at peace.

May your heart remain open.

May you awaken to the light of your own true nature.

May you be healed.

May you be a source of healing for all beings.

Next, think of a person or persons whom you hold in judgment or with whom you are angry and to whom you are ready to begin extending forgiveness. Place them in the white light and see the light washing away all their negativity, just as it did for you and your loved ones. Bless them:

May you be at peace.

May your heart remain open.

May you awaken to the light of your own true nature.

May you be healed.

May you be a source of healing for all beings.

See our beautiful planet as it appears from outer space, a delicate jewel spinning in space. Imagine the green earth, the blue seas, the birds, the animals, and the fish. Earth is a realm of opposites—of day and night, good and evil, sickness and health, riches and poverty, female and male. Hold the earth as you offer these blessings:

May there be peace on earth.

May the hearts of all people be open to themselves and to each other.

May all people awaken to the light of their own true nature.

May all creation be blessed and be a blessing to all that is.

Sources: Borysenko and Borysenko (1994); Collinge (1998); Kabat-Zinn (1994).

References

Benson, H. (1975). *The Relaxation Response.* New York, NY: Morrow.

Benson, H. (1997). *Timeless Healing.* New York, NY: Fireside Books.

Black, D. S. (2014). Mindfulness-based interventions: An antidote to suffering in the context of substance use, misuse, and addiction. *Substance Use and Misuse.* doi: 10.3109/10826084.2014.860749

Boccia, M., Piccardi, L., & Guariglia, P. (2015). The meditative mind: A comprehensive meta-analysis of MRI studies. *BioMed Research International.* doi: 10.1155/2015/419808

Borysenko, J., & Borysenko, M. (1994). *The Power of the Mind to Heal.* Carlsbad, CA: Hay House.

Cherkin, D. C., Sherman, K. J., Balderson, B. H., Cook, A. J., Anderson, M. L.,

Hawkes, R. J., . . . Turner, J. A. (2016). Effect of mindfulness-based stress reduction vs cognitive behavioral therapy or usual care on back pain and functional limitations in adults with chronic low back pain: A randomized clinical trial. *JAMA.* doi: 10.1001/jama.2016.2323

Collinge, W. (1998). *Subtle Energy.* New York, NY: Warner Books.

Cour, P. L., & Petersen, M. (2015). Effects of mindfulness meditation on chronic pain: A randomized controlled trial. *Pain Medicine.* doi: org/10.1111/pme.12605

Dunn-Mascetti, M. (1996). *A Book of Zen: Sayings, Haiku, Koans* (1st ed.). Hyperion.

Eastman, C. A., (1911). *The Soul of the Indian: An Interpretation.* The Reincarnation Library. Aeon Publishing Company, LLC.

Garrison, K. A., Scheinost, D., Constable, R. T., & Brewer, J. A. (2014). BOLD signal and functional connectivity associated with loving kindness meditation. *Brain and Behavior.* doi: 10.1002/brb3.219

Goyal, M., Singh, S., & Sibinga, E. M. S. (2014). Meditation programs for psychological stress and well-being: A systematic review and meta-analysis. *JAMA Internal Medicine.* doi: 10.1001/jamainternmed.2013.13018

Hall, H., Micozzi, M. S., & O'Leary, C. A. (2015). Sufism and healing in the Middle East. In M. S. Micozzi (Ed.), *Fundamentals of Complementary and Alternative Medicine* (5th ed., pp. 581–589). St. Louis, MO: Elsevier/Saunders.

Henderson, R. (2015). *Emotion and Healing in the Energy Body.* Rochester, VT: Healing Arts Press.

Hume, U. (2015). *In the Labyrinth.* San Francisco, CA: Blue Circle Press.

Kabat-Zinn, J. (1994). *Wherever You Go, There You Are: Mindfulness Meditation in Everyday Life.* New York, NY: Hyperion.

Kabat-Zinn, J. (2011). *Mindfulness for Beginners.* Boulder, CO: Sounds True.

Kahn, S. (1996). *The Nurse's Meditative Journal.* Albany, NY: Delmar.

Kearney, D. J., Simpson, T. L., Malte, C. A., Fellerman, B., Martinez, M. E., & Hunt, S. C. (2016). Mindfulness-based stress reduction in addition to usual care is associated with improvements in pain, fatigue, and cognitive failures among veterans with Gulf War illness. *American Journal of Medicine.* doi: 10.1016/j.amjmed.2015.09.015

Mascaro, J. S., Darcher, A., Negi, L. T., & Raison, C. L. (2015). The neural mediators of kindness-based meditation: A theoretical model. *Frontiers in Psychology.* doi: org/10.3389/fpsyg.2015.00109

Seaward, B. L. (2014). *Managing Stress* (8th ed.). Burlington, MA: Jones & Bartlett.

Sheridan, C. (2016). *The Mindful Nurse.* Buffalo, NY: Rivertime Press.

Staples, J. (2015). Yoga. In M. S. Micozzi (Ed.), *Fundamentals of Complementary and Alternative Medicine* (5th ed., pp. 332–343). St. Louis, MO: Elsevier/Saunders.

Tomasino, B., & Fabbro, F. (2016). Increases in the right dorsolateral prefrontal cortex and decreases the rostral prefrontal cortex activation after 8 weeks of focused attention based mindfulness meditation. *Brain and Cognition.* doi: 10.1016/j.bandc.2015.12.004

van der Zwan, J. E., de Vente, W., Huizink, A. C., Bogels, S. M., & de Bruin, E. I. (2015). Physical activity, mindfulness meditation, or heart rate variability biofeedback for stress reduction: A randomized controlled trial. *Applied Psychophysiology and Biofeedback.* doi: 10.1007/s10484-015-9293-x

Weil, A. (1995). *Natural Health, Natural Medicine.* Boston, MA: Houghton Mifflin.

Yates, J., Immergut, M., & Graves, J. (2017). *The Mind Illuminated.* New York: Touchstone.

Resources

American Chronic Pain Association
P.O. Box 850
Rocklin, CA 95677
800.533.3231
www.theacpa.org

American Meditation Institute
P.O. Box 430
60 Garner Rd.
Averill Park, NY 12018
518.674.8714
www.americanmeditation.org

Australian School of Meditation
& Yoga
www.asm.org.au

Canadian Meditation Institute
2039-26 Ave. SW
Calgary, AB T2T IE5
403.802.0852
www.canadianmeditation.org

Jon Kabat-Zinn
Audiobook: *Guided Mindfulness Meditation Series 3*
Boulder, CO

Labyrinth Society
P.O. Box 736
Trumansburg, NY 14886
877.446.4520
www.labryinthsociety.org

The Raj—Authentic Ayurveda
Health Spa
www.theraj.com

Benson-Henry Institute for
Mind–Body Medicine
151 Merrimac St., 4th floor
Boston, MA 02414
617.643.6090
www.massgeneral.org/bhi

Upaya Zen Center
1404 Cerro Gordo Rd.
Santa Fe, NM 87501
505.986.8518
www.upaya.org

18

Hypnotherapy and Guided Imagery

Tension is who you think you should be.
Relaxation is who you are.

ANCIENT CHINESE PROVERB

Cultivate the inner self: its power
becomes real.

LAO-TZU

Hypnotherapy is the application of hypnosis in a wide variety of medical and psychological disorders. Hypnosis is a state of attentive and focused concentration during which people are highly responsive to suggestion. **Guided imagery**, a state of focused concentration, is a similar process that encourages changes in attitudes, behavior, and physiological reactions. Many people consider guided imagery to be a form of hypnosis.

Hypnotherapists and guided imagery therapists help people learn methods to take advantage of the mind–body–spirit connection through the medium of relaxation and imagination. The basic difference between meditation and hypnosis or guided imagery is that in meditation one empties one's mind of images, whereas in hypnosis or guided imagery one creates vivid mental images.

BACKGROUND

Around the world, shamans and traditional healers have used the power of suggested mental images for thousands of years.

Hypnotic trances have been used in a variety of healing practices and religious rituals such as holding sweat lodge ceremonies, drumming, and chanting. Inducing trance states and using therapeutic suggestion were central practices of the early Greek healing temples. People in the 14th century thought that illness was related to evil spirits, and evil spirits were often treated with imagery and hypnotic techniques. During the Renaissance (14th to 16th centuries), it was believed that dysfunctional imagination was the root of all pathology. It was even believed that the mother's imaginings during pregnancy could alter the growth and development of her fetus (Nash & Barnier, 2012).

Hypnotherapy originated in the late 18th century in Europe with Austrian physician Franz Anton Mesmer, who is considered the father of hypnosis. He is remembered for the term *mesmerize*, which described a process of inducing a trance through a series of passes he made with his hands and/or magnets over people. He worked with psychic and electromagnetic energies that he called *animal magnetism*. The medical community eventually discredited him despite his considerable success in treating a variety of ailments. In the mid-19th century, James Braid, an English physician, successfully used hypnosis in pain control and as an anesthetic in surgery. Even after witnessing live demonstrations of a patient undergoing painless surgery, his colleagues dismissed him as a fake. Not long afterward, the discovery of chloroform led to the near abandonment of hypnotic anesthesia.

In the late 19th and early 20th centuries, Émile Coué, a French physician, formulated the *laws of suggestion*, discussed later in this chapter and used to this day by hypnotherapists. He also discovered that giving positive suggestions when prescribing medication proved to be a more effective cure than prescribing medication alone. Sigmund Freud at first found hypnosis extremely effective in treating hysteria, but then, troubled by the sudden emergence of powerful emotions in his patients, abandoned it in favor of psychoanalysis. Carl Jung did not actively use hypnosis, but he encouraged his patients to use active imagination to change old memories. He often used the concept of the inner guide in his healing work. Milton Erickson, an American psychologist and psychiatrist, is considered the father of modern hypnotherapy. He demonstrated how traumatic amnesia and psychosomatic symptoms can be resolved with hypnotherapy, and was influential in the official acceptance of hypnotherapy by the American Medical Association in 1958 (Micozzi & Jawer, 2015).

Guided imagery is a process of using ideas, feelings, physical responses, and all the senses to relax, maintain health, and heal the body and mind. Since the 1970s, many books have been written on the use of guided imagery to improve health, expand thinking, and achieve life goals. Some are directed toward children and adolescents, some toward adults, and some toward people in old age. Motor imagery became popular in sports medicine and training in the later part of the 20th century. The same brain regions that are activated during physical movement are also activated when the same movement is simply imagined. Accordingly, motor imaging was incorporated into rehabilitation programs and activities in nursing homes (Boehm & Tse, 2013; Doidge, 2015).

PREPARATION

At present, no laws limit the use of hypnosis to clinical practitioners. Although anyone can hypnotize other people, hypnotherapy is best practiced by a healthcare professional. Nurses, physicians, dentists, psychologists, occupational therapists, social workers, and counselors are eligible to take approved professional training in hypnotherapy. The American Society of Clinical Hypnosis and the American Council of Hypnotist Examiners share in the education and accreditation of individuals who meet professional requirements. Therapists are required to follow the code of ethics established by these bodies. In addition to successfully passing an examination, certified hypnotherapists complete 200 hours of instruction, and certified clinical hypnotherapists complete 300 hours of instruction. Most practitioners do not identify themselves as hypnotists but as nurses, doctors, dentists, and others who use hypnosis as one of several modes of intervention.

The American Holistic Nurses Association and Beyond Ordinary Nursing offer a Nurses' Certificate Program in Imagery. The program consists of 84 hours of in-depth, hands-on training over a period of 9 to 12 months, to provide nurses with experience in relaxation and therapeutic imagery skills. These skills are used to reduce stress and anxiety; promote healing; decrease pain and symptoms; minimize side effects; manage chronic illness; prepare for procedures, surgery, or childbirth; respond to end-of-life issues; and access inner wisdom and resources. An overview of the program content is found in Box 18.1.

BOX 18.1

Program Content for Nurses' Certificate Program in Imagery

- Core concepts in integrative medicine, psychoneuroimmunology, and holistic healing
- Principles and theory of the guided imagery process
- Stress management strategies and self-care as an integral aspect of professional practice
- A variety of breathing and relaxation techniques
- Eight distinct integrative imagery techniques in the practicum

This program is approved for 108 continuing education hours by the American Holistic Nurses Association.

CONCEPTS

Trance

To understand hypnotic trance, one must understand the functional difference between the conscious and the subconscious mind. The *conscious mind* contains the short-term memory and the intellect. It functions like a computer, always analyzing, criticizing, and discriminating one's thoughts and perceptions. The language of the intellect is logic and reason. The *subconscious mind* contains emotions, creativity, imagination, intuition, long-term memory, and control of body functions. It also contains the habit center, where persistent habits such as nail biting or test anxiety are located. The subconscious does not respond to reason and facts, as does the intellect. The language of the subconscious is imagery and metaphor. During times of emotional turmoil or sudden trauma, people often become aware of the subconscious mind's power over body functions and intellect when they are unable to eat, sleep, or talk, and cannot think clearly. After years of ignoring feelings or "stuffing" them into the subconscious, in a hypnotic trance, people can access the subconscious mind, which allows them to tap into their creativity, access buried memories, change habits, unmask erroneous beliefs, repair self-esteem, and restore health.

A **trance state** is a form of heightened concentration. People in trance are aware of what is going on around them but choose not to focus on it and can return to normal awareness whenever they choose. The majority of people will tend to remember most of what happens in a controlled hypnotherapy or guided imagery session. Trance is not a form of sleep or stupor, as is easily determined by observing the range of activities possible by people in a hypnotic trance.

There are three levels or stages of trance. The first is a *superficial trance* in which people are very aware of their surroundings and may accept suggestions such as eating less or quitting smoking but do not necessarily carry them out. The second level, known as *alpha trance*, is significantly deeper. Heart rate, blood pressure, and respiration become slow. Hypnotic suggestions at this level are more effective. The third level, called *somnambulism*, is the level most beneficial to health and well-being. It is at this level that posthypnotic suggestions are most effective, and people can remember past events with clarity (Loupescou, 2014).

People naturally flow in and out of hypnotic trances. When driving a familiar route, people may slip into a trance. They can arrive at a destination and not be exactly sure about how they got there. During the trance, they drive appropriately, stop at stop signs, obey traffic laws, and so on, but have no conscious awareness of doing these things. Another example of hypnotic trance can be observed during movie watching. People enter the theater having set aside a specific period of time wherein they can enjoy themselves. The process of settling into theater seats relaxes moviegoers and puts them in a receptive frame of mind. The lights go down to reduce the distractions from the outside world, and the big screen becomes the most noticeable aspect of the perceptual world. Within moments, the audience is transported to another place and time. If the movie is frightening, many people experience a racing heart, rapid breathing, and muscle tension—yet, they are well aware that no physical danger exists. They are responding to images and sounds alone. Movies operate by mental mechanisms similar to those of hypnosis. First, participants decide to let go of normal concerns and open the mind to a new experience. Then, certain procedures relax the beta level of brain activity. Next, through the thoughtful use of metaphor and imagery, deeper levels of consciousness are reached. Finally, new images and perceptions can be introjected (Hamilton, March 1, 2001, personal communication).

A trance is characterized by muscle relaxation, predominating alpha brain waves, feelings of well-being, diminished ability to vocalize, and an ability to accept new ideas if they do not conflict with personal values. The perception of time is often distorted; 30 minutes may seem like 5. Feelings are more accessible while one is entranced, as well as memories from long ago. As one's awareness phases in and out, parts of the session may not be consciously remembered but are retained in the subconscious. People in trance describe their arms and legs as feeling heavy like lead or light and tingly, almost numb. Some experience slight twitches as the nervous system relaxes, and respiration shifts to abdominal breathing. Coming out of the trance, people awaken with very pleasant, almost euphoric feelings of well-being.

Laws and Principles of Suggestion

The first **law of suggestion,** as formulated by Coué, is that of *concentrated attention*. When people focus their attention repeatedly on a goal or idea, that event tends to be realized. Consequently, practitioners repeat hypnotic suggestions three or four times during a session. The law of *dominant affect* states that stronger emotions tend to take precedence over weaker ones. An effective hypnotherapist, after assessing the client's emotional state, connects the hypnotic suggestion to the dominant emotions. The *carrot principle* is applied when the practitioner interjects comments about the person's goals with the hypnotic suggestions, thus linking motivation to the suggestions. The principle of *positive suggestion* is applied to help people override existing attitudes. Dr. Coué was known for encouraging his patients to say to themselves 20 to 30 times each night before going to sleep, "Every day in every way, I am getting better and better." If someone is seeking hypnosis in an effort to lose weight, the suggestion is not, "You will not be hungry," which is unlikely and a negative rather than a positive statement. Rather, the positive suggestion might be, "You will be surprised to find how comfortable you will be. You treat your body with kindness and respect."

Memories

It is true that under hypnosis people often recall past forgotten events. It is also true that people under hypnosis often "remember" things quite vividly that never actually happened but that have great personal significance nonetheless. These might be called fantasized life events. In a deep trance state, memories and fantasies may be intense, and the two may be indistinguishable.

People are able to remember great detail of actual events and are also uniquely capable of making up details and experiencing them as if they were remembered. Recognizing the potential difficulties arising from what some call "false memory syndrome," several states in the United States now limit legal testimony to that obtained prior to any systematic hypnotic treatment. In 1985, the American Medical Association cautioned against the systematic use of hypnosis for memory recall for both its unreliability and its potential to create vivid false memories.

Imagery

Imagery is a two-way communication between the conscious and the unconscious mind and involves the whole body and all its senses. Most individuals image frequently throughout the day, and worry is the most common form of imagery that affects health. In their imagination, people react to current stressors and anticipated dangers. Their body becomes aroused and tense, and the fight-or-flight mechanism is activated. Guided imagery can help people learn how to stop troublesome thoughts and focus on images that help them relax and decrease the negative impact of stressors.

In guided imagery, the images may be created by the therapist based on the needs and desires of the client. Clients can also create the images as a way to understand the meaning of symptoms or to access inner resources. Imagery stimulates changes in many body functions such as heart rate, blood pressure, respiratory patterns, brain wave rhythms and patterns, electrical characteristics of the skin, local blood flow and temperature, gastrointestinal motility and secretions, sexual arousal, and levels of various hormones and neurotransmitters. The exercise in Box 18.2 is a helpful demonstration of the power of imagery and allows one to experience the physical response to imaging.

BOX 18.2

Sensory Imagery

- Relax and take some easy, deep breaths.
- Focus on letting the tension go out of your body.
- Imagine holding a juicy, yellow lemon. Feel its coolness, texture, and weight in your hand.
- Imagine cutting the lemon in half. Notice the cut surfaces—the bright yellow outer layer, the whiteness of the inner peel, and the pale yellow of the pulp.
- Cut one of the halves in two and pick up the freshly cut lemon quarter and imagine smelling the lemony scent.
- Now imagine biting into the lemon and sucking its sour juice into your mouth.
- What happened when you imagined biting into the lemon? Did you salivate or grimace? Did you have any other physical reaction?

TREATMENT

Hypnotherapists do not "put" people into trances. They arrange circumstances to increase the likelihood that people will shift themselves into a trance state. About 20% of the population have a high capacity for trance; these people may go under hypnosis deeply. Another 20% have a slight capacity for trance, are easily distracted, and may not respond to hypnotherapy at all. People who cannot be hypnotized include those with organic brain disease, those with low IQs, and those who do not want to be hypnotized. The remaining 60% of the population fall somewhere between these extremes (Micozzi & Jawer, 2015).

Some people seeking hypnotherapy or guided imagery ask whether the use of audio recordings would offer equal benefit. The answer to that question depends on several factors, including the nature and depth of the problem one wants to resolve. General self-hypnosis recordings will give only general results. Personalized audio recordings, created by a therapist using the person's own images, are more effective. Working with an experienced practitioner is most effective because the procedure is individualized according to the client's expectations and preferences.

The first and most important step in hypnotherapy is establishing a relationship with the client. It is a cooperative venture, and if the suggestions are to be effective, the therapist and client must work together. The relationship is one in which clients permit themselves to be as receptive as possible, and the therapist commits to working for the clients' well-being. People who benefit most from hypnotherapy are those who understand that hypnosis is not a surrender of control; it is only an advanced form of relaxation. The therapist gets to know clients, develops treatment plans, explains the hypnotic process, dispels myths and fears, answers questions, encourages positive attitudes about hypnosis, and, with people's permission, trains them in self-inductive procedures. This process is as applicable for a short-term case of test anxiety as it is for a lengthy terminal illness. A measure of trust is needed to start the process and develop the relationship.

The **induction phase** is generally a period of relaxation or focus on the breathing that disengages people from other concerns and helps them focus their attention. In other words, the induction phase is similar to meditation and elicits the same physiological response. The induction starts with "easy" suggestions, such as focusing on breathing and closing the eyes. Directions are given to relax physically and mentally and to focus on the therapist's voice and words.

Training in induction may take one or two sessions. When the client is comfortable with entering the trance experience, the **hypnotic suggestion** begins. Based on the assessment process, the practitioner suggests an image known to be pleasurable to the client and related to the desired outcome. Hypnotic communications contain cues and explicit instructions for focusing attention and imagining in line with the aims of suggestions. The imagery is intensified by incorporating the five senses: The person is asked not only to visualize the scene but also to smell the scents, touch things in the environment, hear the surrounding sounds, and even taste anything appropriate. The client is asked to focus attention on as many details about the situation as possible and is walked through the session focusing on the desired events. The suggestions of the hypnotherapist are translated by the client into ideas. These ideas then lead to corresponding behaviors in the nontrance state.

Trance removal is that time when clients are given suggestions that will return them to a nontrance state. The hypnotherapist, for example, may count to 10, asking clients to open their eyes at the count of 5, and to be fully alert at 10. Clients most commonly report that they feel relaxed during the session but may not be certain that they were hypnotized, since they could hear every word the therapist said. Many hypnotherapists provide guided audio recordings for their clients so that they can practice the therapy at home.

Hypnosis cannot make people do anything against their will. If they really do not want to change, hypnosis will be a waste of time and money. If, for example, a person seeks hypnotherapy to stop smoking at a spouse's insistence but is poorly motivated, hypnotherapy will not be effective. Occasionally, clients may demand that the hypnotherapist perform some magical incantation and remove 30 pounds or make the person never smoke again. This demand is the equivalent of insisting that their primary care provider cure them of hypertension while refusing to change their diet or follow a recommended medication schedule.

In some medical facilities, hypnosis and imagery are now routinely used with a variety of conditions, usually in conjunction with other forms of medical, surgical, psychiatric, or psychological treatment. People can better manage anxiety and pain with the use of these interventions. They are used as pre- and postoperative therapy, in labor and delivery, and in dentistry. They can be used with nonmedical clients as well, working through problems of living, situations of performance anxiety, and in changing bad habits. Depending on the complexity and seriousness of the complaint, treatment typically runs from 2 to 10 sessions.

Jeanne Achterberg (2008), well known for her use of imagery in the treatment of cancer, believes that imagery is as essential as radiation and chemotherapy and must not be thought of as a "last alternative." She believes that imagery plays an important role in the biochemical healing process. She hypothesizes that images produced in the mind are converted to biochemical messages that somehow initiate a path of cancer-cell destruction or organ-cell reconstruction. Possibly, this healing process inhibits the nervous and endocrine systems from secreting stress hormones. Of course, it is difficult to prove definitively that imagery is a direct cause of healing when it occurs, because imagery is never the sole treatment used.

Hypnotherapy and guided imagery can be used to help people gain self-control, improve self-esteem, and become more autonomous. People who are imprisoned by negative beliefs see themselves as hopeless, helpless victims. With guided imagery, they can learn how to substitute positive, empowering messages. Hypnosis and imagery can also be used as a mental rehearsal for procedures, treatments, or surgery. Clients are shown how to use their own images about the healing process, or, alternatively, they are guided through a series of images intended to distract them from painful procedures or anxiety-producing situations. The practitioner may have them imagine themselves in a state of good health or well-being, or having successfully achieved goals.

Virtual reality environments are a recent modification of guided imagery. With the use of head-mounted displays, people are immersed into a virtual world. This process is effective in reducing pain and anxiety from treatments or disease. Increasingly, interactive tools are providing successful distractions that allow people to cope more effectively with their treatment protocol (Enea, Dafinoiu, Opris, & David, 2014).

People, especially children, are often able to rid themselves of warts by visualizing their disappearance in one way or another. Hypnosis and imagery are often used as a clinical treatment for Reynaud's disease, a condition in which the capillaries of the extremities constrict, with the result that hands and feet are cold and painful. When they learn to "think warm," people may find that the circulation to their hands and feet improves, resulting in less pain. Similarly, hand-warming frequently cuts down on both the incidence and severity of migraine headaches. The use of hypnosis in promoting feelings of comfort, distraction, and dissociation through imagery in those with chronic pain has been well established. Clients are often able to change their perceptual experience of pain by substituting numbness, a sense of pressure, or other sensation for an unwanted pain. In 1995, a National Institutes of Health (NIH) panel endorsed hypnosis as a useful adjunct to conventional treatments. Current clinical studies at NIH include hypnosis for overactive bladder, ulcerative colitis, hot flashes, posttraumatic stress disorder (PTSD), and sleep disturbance.

Contraindications for hypnosis and imagery include poor motivation, such as "My husband sent me so I would lose weight," or an unwillingness even to try the treatment because of extreme fear or compelling religious objections. The procedure is unsuitable for people with active psychosis or somatic delusions. It is generally considered that these individuals are often bombarded with too many images already and are thus unable to differentiate between voluntary and involuntary images.

RESEARCH

One of the difficulties in conducting research on hypnotherapy is that it is not simply a single form of treatment. Hypnosis does not represent one standard set of suggestions, which may account for the large number of studies that favor anecdotal, rather than controlled, evidence. For hypnosis to be most effective in a clinical setting, hypnotic suggestions are best formulated on the basis of the individual person's interests, style, motivation, and receptivity to hypnosis. It is not like administering a drug, for which doses are standardized. In hypnosis, the personal and subjective experiences matter a great deal.

Numerous studies indicate that mental imagery can bring about significant physiological and biochemical changes. Some of these findings are from well-controlled studies, while others are reports of single cases or small studies that have not been replicated. Nevertheless, the overriding conclusion points to a relationship between imagery of body change and actual body change.

The following is a small sample of current studies in imagery and hypnotherapy:

- A systematic review examining the effectiveness of guided imagery for people with arthritis and other rheumatic diseases found improved sense of well-being, improved mobility, improved pain management, and reductions in anxiety (Giacobbi et al., 2015).
- A systematic review and meta-analysis considered the use of guided imagery/hypnosis for people with fibromyalgia. There was a reduction in pain and level of disability and an improvement in health-related quality of life (Zech, Hansen, Bernardy, & Hauser, 2016).
- A comprehensive review of the literature found that hypnosis significantly improved irritable bowel syndrome in children and adults. There was preliminary data that hypnosis may be helpful in other gastrointestinal disorders (Palsson, 2015).
- A two-group quasi-experimental study of guided imagery was conducted for people with fibromyalgia. There was statistically significant reduction in both pain and depression (Onieva-Zafra, Garcia, & Del Valle, 2015).
- A randomized, controlled study compared hypnosis and massage in reducing pain in hospitalized older people. Both treatments led to a decrease in pain. However, hypnosis had a longer analgesic effect than massage (Ardigo et al., 2016).

INTEGRATED NURSING PRACTICE

As a nurse, you can employ guided imagery for personal and professional development. On a regular basis, take time to envision what kind of nurse you would like to be. Envision yourself as healthy, alert, balanced, compassionate, and competent in the clinical arena. You can also use imagery to learn new procedures or techniques. After learning the goals, steps, and processes of a new activity, you can envision yourself doing the procedure safely and skillfully several times as you integrate knowledge with psychomotor skills. This "rehearsal" is a powerful tool for improving your technical nursing practice (Boehm & Tse, 2013).

Some people fear that hypnosis and guided imagery may cause them to lose control of their minds to an outside force. This fear, most likely, results from hypnosis demonstrations performed onstage. Volunteers may seem to be under the control of the stage hypnotist. In volunteering, they know they will be expected to do silly things in front of an audience, and it is a chance for

BOX 18.3

Hypnotherapy: Myths and Realities

Myth	Reality
People are asleep during hypnosis.	People are awake and aware throughout the entire process and are highly selective about where they focus their attention.
Hypnotized people have lost control and are under someone's power.	All hypnosis is self-hypnosis, since people cannot be hypnotized against their will. Hypnotized people are fully able to stop the process at any time.
People can be influenced to tell secrets.	Because the subconscious offers only information it deems appropriate and ready to contribute, people cannot be forced to reveal any secrets they would not disclose in a fully alert state.
People might get "stuck" in a hypnotic trance.	Because individuals control the situation, they can end the hypnotic trance at any time.

those with extrovert tendencies to perform, have fun, and be a star. The volunteers are often truly hypnotized and doing exactly what they want to do—giving themselves permission to be outrageous. They would not, however, do something against their moral beliefs (Lewis, 2013). Box 18.3 lists the myths and realities of hypnotherapy.

The reality of therapy is quite the opposite because the individual is always under self-control. When clients learn a technique like imagery, it is entirely within their control for use when, how, and where they want. It is a tool they can use whenever they feel particularly anxious, upset, or uncomfortable. That type of empowering, in itself, is healing because people feel better and do better when they have a sense of mastery over what is happening to them.

Hypnosis is used in many different clinical settings. Hypnosis is effective in surgery, in childbirth, and in the management of cancer, stress, weight loss, smoking withdrawal, and posttraumatic stress disorder. Some people use hypnosis to improve self-confidence and in spiritual growth.

Many kinds of imagery work well with clients. *Feeling-state imagery* is designed simply to help clients change their mood in a general way. The therapist can suggest to individuals that they let their imaginations take them to a favorite place, real or imagined. For example, some may imagine themselves at a beach and floating gently on the water while feeling peaceful and relaxed. Others may imagine themselves as a young child sitting on the lap of a beloved grandparent. Clients can use this kind of imagery to move from a feeling state of tension and fear to one of peace and calm.

With *end-state imagery*, clients imagine themselves already in the situation or circumstances that they wish to attain. It may be seeing themselves as healthy, strong, and free from disease. Others may imagine themselves as successful, happy, and well loved.

Symptoms of disease are often thought to result from blocked energy. *Energetic imagery* involves imagining the life force energy, or qi, flowing smoothly and easily throughout the body. Clients can be taught to imagine that they are pulling up energy from the earth through the soles of their feet to replenish the body's energy.

Cellular imagery relates to imagining events at the cellular level. For example, clients may be taught to imagine their natural killer cells surrounding and attacking cancer cells. Cellular imagery is usually specific and focused on exactly what needs to be fixed. Imagery does not have to be visual. Some people "hear" their imagery, others "feel" it, and some "taste" or "smell" it. Some people might choose to put a hand over the affected area and send healing images to the cells in that area.

Similar to cellular imagery, *physiologic imagery* involves the entire body. Thus, clients might be directed to imagine that their blood vessels are relaxed and wider in an effort to lower their blood pressure. People with back pain might imagine that all the muscles in their back are relaxing and softening. People with diabetes might put their hands over the abdomen and imagine insulin moving out of the pancreas to connect with hungry cells throughout the body.

Psychological imagery involves people's perception of themselves. For example, individuals who feel overly responsible may feel as though they have the weight of the world on their shoulders. Those who feel abandoned may feel the pain as heartache. In guiding the imagery, the therapist may direct clients to focus on their sensation, put their hands on the hurting places, and breathe into the pain. Psychological imagery can also be interactive. When conflict is the issue, people might imagine a dialogue with the adversary that may bring a fresh perspective and new solutions to problems.

The goal of *spiritual imagery* is to make contact with God or the Divine or to gain entrance into a larger world. Clients may use spiritual imagery to find guidance or inspiration. Some clients find it comforting to imagine that they are being held in the hands of God, where they are perfectly safe.

Eight characteristics help make imagery effective as a healing tool, especially with regard to cancer:

- Images must be personal. Images created by others appear to be less effective in the healing process.
- Images must feel right to the person and be congruent with who they are and their values. For example, combative or warlike images are not appropriate for those who see themselves as gentle and conciliatory.

- Imagery works best in a permissive, unforced atmosphere. An attitude of allowing the imagery to happen seems to be most effective.
- Images must be energetic and physical. People do best when they allow themselves to feel the sensations of their images.
- Images must be anatomically correct and accurate. The type of imagery must be chosen according to the nature of the disease and the body part and system affected.
- Skill at using imagery increases with practice, and response to imagery intensifies with use. It is suggested that clients use imagery in 5- to 20-minute blocks of time, once or twice a day.
- Imagery should have an end-stage component. Clients should be encouraged to see the imagery as a mission accomplished.
- People receiving medical treatment concurrently should include it in the imagery. Clients who incorporate their chemotherapy or radiation treatment do better than those who ignore these medical procedures in their imagery (Achterberg, 2008; Davenport, 2016; Pinson, 2015).

Prior to beginning guided imagery, you should assess a client's belief system, desired outcome, and basic understanding of the pathophysiology involved, as well as his or her understanding of the effects of medications, treatments, or surgery. This information is necessary to formulate appropriate script content. Establish a quiet, safe environment free of unwanted distractions. Prior to the induction phase, take a few moments to center yourself. Let your mind and body release tension and tightness. Focus on letting your vocal cords relax to enhance a calming pitch, volume, and tone to your voice. Ask clients to assume a comfortable position, reclining if possible, and to close their eyes. Guide them through a progressive relaxation or body scan as described in Chapter 17. Instruct them to go to a safe, comfortable place—an actual location or one conjured up in the imagination. Ask them to use all their senses to explore this place—what they see, hear, smell, taste, or feel. For example, you might ask them to identify the time of day or year, what flowers or trees they smell, the taste of any food that is around, and birds, train whistles, or any other sounds they hear.

Next, have clients focus on the problem at hand (e.g., the diagnosis of cancer, being HIV positive, wound or bone healing, or improved organ function). At this point, begin your script, directing them toward their previously discussed goals. You might say something like the following: "Imagine the broken edges of your bone. Now, bring lots of red blood cells to the area for extra nutrition and oxygen. Imagine new cells being formed and the bone edges growing together." After this type of individualized script, you should include an end-stage script, such as the following: "Imagine that your broken leg is totally healed now. You have returned to your favorite ski hill. See yourself skiing down the slope. Your leg is strong and healthy and pain free."

After this phase of guided imagery, talk with clients about the meaning of what occurred during the session, and reinforce the positive aspects of the experience. Some nurses make recordings of the individualized session to which clients may choose to listen as they practice on their own every day.

Gawain (2016) has developed an exercise from which most people can benefit. This "pink bubble" technique can be performed once or regularly over a period of time. It is best to practice the technique in the morning on awakening and/or in the evening right before sleep, as follows:

- Assume a comfortable position, breathe slowly, and go through a progressive relaxation or body scan procedure.
- Imagine something you would like to have or would like to have happened.
- Imagine that it has already happened. Picture the object or the situation as clearly as possible, with yourself in the picture.
- Surround this image with a pink bubble.
- Let go of the bubble and watch the bubble float off into the universe. See it becoming one with the higher power of the universe.

Guided imagery can be used in many different clinical settings to move toward the following outcomes:

- Induce a state of physiological relaxation
- Reduce stress
- Control habits: smoking, overeating, or nail biting
- Reduce pain
- Reduce anxiety (and test anxiety)
- Understand symptoms
- Stimulate healing responses
- Increase tolerance of nursing and medical procedures
- Enhance motivation and self-care
- Find meaning in illness
- Resolve conflicts
- Enhance self-esteem and self-confidence
- Increase problem-solving ability
- Access positive inner resources

Shames (1996) described numerous ways in which nurses can incorporate the use of imagery with nursing procedures. She suggested that people receiving intravenous fluids envision the fluid flushing out cellular toxins while simultaneously nourishing the cells. People taking antibiotics can be taught to imagine the medication attacking and destroying bacteria. Individuals experiencing illness or distress can be instructed to take a deep breath and send healing oxygen and a sense of peace to the lungs. On the out-breath, they can image all the toxins or tension leaving the body and disappearing into the air. When a specific organ or part of the body is disrupted, people can bring their awareness to that part and imagine healing resources migrating there to nourish and support the function. Individuals experiencing pain can envision the pain flowing out of the body through the feet and fingertips. Some imagine the capillaries and veins expanding to become large pipes, carrying the pain out. Similarly, people can imagine the soothing effects of pain medication on the affected area and feel the softening and relaxing of the body as the pain lessens. Shames's book *Creative Imagery in Nursing* is a wonderful resource and provides many suggestions for clinical application of guided imagery. This technique allows nurses to use their creativity, intuition, and imagination as they support others on their healing journeys. You may find Lusk's book *30 Scripts for Relaxation Imagery and Inner Healing* and Dormoy's book *Guided Imagery Work with Kids* very helpful in integrating guided imagery into your professional practice.

TRY THIS
Renovating Your Day

This exercise is designed for empowering yourself with your thoughts by transforming negative thoughts and events through visualization. Do this every day for a week, prior to bedtime. Mentally go through your day and decide what you could have changed that would have brought better results. Then, imagine that change occurring. For example, if someone said something negative to you, imagine that they said something more positive. If you did not like your test score, visualize the grade as a better one.

TRY THIS
Shrinking Antagonistic Forces

If you are angry with or intimidated by another person, shrink that person and put him or her in the palm of your open hand. Conduct a dialogue with that person, but have that person speak in a different voice, such as a high, squeaky, or cartoon voice. See that person getting smaller and smaller until the person disappears or you blow him or her off into space.

Source: Harding, M. (October 14, 2003, personal communication).

Considering the Evidence

Hasan, F. M., Zagarins, S. E., Pischke, K. M., Saiyed, S., Bettencourt, A. M., Beal, L., . . . McCleary, N. (2014). Hypnotherapy is more effective than nicotine replacement therapy for smoking cessation: Results of a randomized controlled trial. *Complementary Therapies in Medicine*, 22(1): 1–8. doi: 10.1016/j.ctim.2013.12.012

(continued)

What Was the Approach of the Research?

Primary research: randomized controlled trial.

What Was the Aim/Purpose/Objective(s) of the Research as Related to Complementary and Integrative Therapies?

To compare the effectiveness of hypnotherapy only, hypnotherapy with nicotine replacement therapy (NRT), or only conventional NRT in patients hospitalized with a diagnosis of cardiac or pulmonary illness.

How Was the Study Done?

The researchers reviewed self-reports and biochemical verification pertaining to a 7-day prevalence smoking abstinence rates at 12 and 26 weeks posthospitalization. Participants in this study were randomized to one of three treatment groups. The comparison group consisted of "self-quit" group of eligible patients who refused intervention during their hospitalization. The treatment groups were randomized to one of three groups. One group received hypnotherapy only, the second group received nicotine replacement therapy only, and the third group received both hypnotherapy and nicotine replacement therapy. All participants received self-help materials and counseling during their hospitalization, including the "self-quit" group.

What Were the Significant Findings of the Research?

The researchers reported that hypnotherapy combined with counseling was found to be more effective than nicotine replacement therapy combined with counseling in improving 12-week and 26-week smoking abstinence among patients hospitalized for a smoking-related illness.

What Additional Questions Might I Have?

Were these study participants highly motivated to abstain from smoking prior to their hospitalization and did that influence their commitment to the study therapies? How did the participants who declined to participate in the study differ in health acuity than those who were randomized to the treatment group? Was the nature/acuity of the illness at the time of hospitalization a factor in their adherence/response to treatment? What is the long-term effect of hypnotherapy for these patients living with smoking-related illnesses? Are there any adverse effects related to hypnotherapy?

What Is the Clinical Significance of This Study?

This study has clinical value for nurses in suggesting strategies/options to enhance smoking cessation in persons whose health has been impacted by smoking. Nurses must remain mindful of the strong addictive nature of nicotine and their obligation to support and recommend interventions based on the best available evidence. Nurses need to remain cognizant of the need for more research to strengthen the evidence related to hypnotherapy.

Source: Contributed by Dolores M. Huffman, RN, PhD.

References

Achterberg, J. (2008). *Intentional Healing: Consciousness and Connection for Health and Well-Being* [CD]. Louisville, CO: Sounds True.

Ardigo, S., Herrmann, F. R., Moret, V., Derame, L., Giannelli, S., Gold, G., & Pautex, S. (2016). Hypnosis can reduce pain in hospitalized older patients: A randomized controlled study. *Geriatrics.* doi: 10.1186/s12877-016-0180-y

Boehm, L. B., & Tse, A. M. (2013). Application of guided imagery to facilitate the transition of new graduate registered nurses. *Journal of Continuing Education in Nursing.* doi: 10.3928/00220124-20130115-16

Davenport, L. (2016). *Transformative Imagery.* London: Jessica Kingsley Publishers.

Doidge, N. (2015). *The Brain's Way of Healing.* New York, NY: Penguin Books.

Dormoy, M. (2016). *Guided Imagery Work with Kids.* New York, NY: Shambala, LLC.

Enea, V., Dafinoiu, I., Opris, D., & David, D. (2014). Effects of hypnotic analgesia and virtual reality on the reduction of experimental pain among high and low hypnotizables. *International Journal of Clinical and Experimental Hypnosis.* doi: 10.1080.00207144.2014.901087

Gawain, S. (2016). *Creative Visualization* (2nd ed.). Novato, CA: New World Library.

Giacobbi, P. R., Stabler, M., Stewart, J., Jaeschke, A. M., Siebert, J. L., & Kelley, G. A. (2015). Guided imagery for arthritis and other rheumatic diseases: A systematic review of randomized controlled trials. *Pain Management Nursing.* doi: 10.1016/j.pmn.2015.01.003

Lewis, S. D. (2013). *The Hypnosis Treatment Option.* Chicago, IL: Copper Ridge Press.

Loupescou, A. (2014). *Hypnotherapy and Intuitive Hypnosis.* London: Akakia Publications.

Lusk, J. (2015). *30 Scripts for Relaxation Imagery and Inner Healing* (2nd ed.). Duluth, MN: Whole Person Associates, Inc.

Micozzi, M. S., & Jawer, M. A. (2015). Mind–body therapies, stress, and psychometrics. In M. S. Micozzi (Ed.), *Fundamentals of Complementary and Alternative Medicine* (5th ed., pp. 114–140). St. Louis, MO: Elsevier/Saunders.

Morgan, H. T., & Taylor, T. C. (1944). *Chinese Proverbs: Chinese Classics in Miniature.* Los Angeles, CA: Quon-Quon Company.

Nash, M., & Barnier, A. (2012). *The Oxford Handbook of Hypnosis.* Oxford, UK: Oxford University Press.

Onieva-Zafra, M. D., Garcia, L. H., & Del Valle, M. G. (2015). Effectiveness of guided imagery relaxation on levels of pain and depression in patients diagnosed with fibromyalgia. *Holistic Nursing Practice.* doi: 10.1097/HNP.0000000000000062

Palsson, O. S. (2015). Hypnosis treatment of gastrointestinal disorders: A comprehensive review of the empirical evidence. *American Journal of Clinical Hypnosis.* doi: 10.1080/00029157.2015.1039114

Pinson, R. D. (2015). *Visualization and Imagery.* Brooklyn, NY: Iyyun Publishing.

Shames, K. H. (1996). *Creative Imagery in Nursing.* Albany, NY: Delmar.

Tzu, L. (1989). *Tao Te Ching.* Translated by Gia-Fu Feng & J. English. New York, NY: Vintage Books.

Zech, N., Hansen, E., Bernardy, K., & Hauser, W. (2016). Efficacy, acceptability and safety of guided imagery/hypnosis in fibromyalgia—A systematic review and meta-analysis of randomized controlled trials. *European Journal of Pain.* doi: 10.1002/ejp.933

Resources

Academy for Guided Imagery
  30765 Pacific Coast Hwy, #355
  Malibu, CA 90265
  424.242.6369
  www.acadgi.com

American Council of Hypnotist
  Examiners
  3435 Camino del Rio S. STE 316
  San Diego, CA 92108
  619.280.7200
  www.hypnotistexaminers.org/

American Society of Clinical Hypnosis
  140 N. Bloomingdale Rd.
  Bloomingdale, IL 60108
  630.980.4740
  www.asch.net

Australian Hypnotherapists
  Association
  www.ahahypnotherapy.org.au

IntegrativeImagery.com
  www.integrativeimagery.com

Canadian Society of Clinical Hypnosis
  604.688.1714
  www.hypnosis.bc.ca

HypnoBirthing Programme
  www.hypnobirthing.com

Simonton Cancer Center
  P.O. Box 6607
  Malibu, CA 90264
  800.459.3424
  www.simontoncenter.com

19

Dreamwork

Sometimes Dreams are Wiser Than Waking.

BLACK ELK

Dreams are Today's Answers to Tomorrow's Questions.

EDGAR CAYCE

In some ways, a great deal is known about **dreaming** because it has been important to people of all time and across all cultures. In the 20th and 21st centuries, the biology of the brain has been explored and increasingly understood. While this basic knowledge provides some facts underlying dreaming, it does not explain what dreaming is. Thus, in a sense, little is known about dreaming, and scientists cannot yet agree on the basic nature of dreaming. Some believe dreams are nothing more than random firing of neurons during sleep. Others believe dreams are symbolic stories or metaphors people tell themselves that represent personal and social mythology. The contemporary psychobiological view of the dream process blends the neuroscientific findings with psychoanalytic thought and believes that dreaming is one of the ways that people reflect on and make sense of their waking-life events. In other words, the mind exploits the brain's physiological state of dreaming to work on current life problems (Reiser, 2001).

BACKGROUND

Virtually every culture has believed that dreams carry important messages. To the ancient Greeks, dreams were great healers. People who were sick slept in special healing temples in hopes of receiving therapeutic dreams from the gods. The Talmud, the Hebrew sacred book of practical wisdom, states clearly that the Jews gave great importance both to the dream and to the dream interpreter. Muhammad began writing the Quran after an angel visited him in a dream. Tibetan Buddhists saw no distinction between dreaming and waking and considered all of life a dream.

Plato saw dreams as a release for fervent inner forces. Hippocrates thought dreams were windows on illness, and that normal dream content indicated a state of wellness and bizarre content a state of illness. Aristotle believed that the beginning of illness could be felt in dreams before actual symptoms appeared.

The most famous book on dream interpretation, *Oneirocritica*, was written by Artemidorus of Daldis, a professional diviner who lived in the second century. The dreams recorded by him are remarkably similar to contemporary ones. Genghis Khan is reported to have envisioned his battle plans in his dreams, while Hannibal attributed the origin of his battle plan to attack Rome over the Alps with elephants to a dream.

During the late Middle Ages, dreams began to fall into disfavor with Christians despite the fact that throughout the Bible, God spoke directly to people through dreams and visions. St. Francis of Assisi founded the Franciscan Order as a dream directive from Jesus Christ.

In the United States, the traditional Iroquois were (and are) a people of dreams. Children were taught that dreams were the most important source of practical and spiritual guidance. The people of an Iroquois village began each day with dream sharing. The entire village became involved in dreamwork, especially if a dream seemed to contain a warning of death or disease. "Big" dreams were thought to come about in one of two ways. During sleep, the dreamer would have an out-of-body experience and travel to many places, past, present, and future. Alternatively, the dreamer could receive a visit from a spiritual being. Dreams were considered to be central to healing by providing insight into the causes of illness, often before physical symptoms appeared. Dreams continue to be important tools for many traditional healers in the Native American population (Buhner, 2006).

In 1900, Sigmund Freud wrote *The Interpretation of Dreams* and proposed that dreaming might represent a unique avenue by which unconscious motivation could be explored. Freud's theory was that dreams were disguised wish fulfillments of infantile sexual needs, which were repressed by censors in the waking mind. Freud's protégé, Carl Jung, believed that humans were spiritual rather than instinctual and saw dreams as a compensatory mechanism whose function was to restore psychological balance. Jung said that the conscious and the unconscious minds speak entirely different languages. The conscious mind is analytical, critical, and rational, whereas the unconscious mind thinks in metaphor, simile, symbols, and intuition (Shields, Levin, Reich, Murnane, & Hanley, 2016; Vinocur Fischbein & Miramon, 2015).

Dr. Nathaniel Kleitman is considered to be the father of modern scientific dream research. In 1957, he and Eugene Aserinsky identified rapid eye movement (REM), demonstrating the activity of the brain during sleep. This active sleep stage has consequently been called **REM sleep**. Today, hundreds of sleep clinics operate in the United States, and sleep disorders constitute the second most common health complaint after the common cold (Cushway & Sewell, 2012).

PREPARATION

In a society that discounted dreams, Sigmund Freud introduced the concept of therapeutic **dreamwork**. He and his followers, however, began to associate dreams with illness rather than wellness and reserved dream interpretation for professionals who were deemed the only people competent to understand the latent content of dreams. This approach said, in effect, that individuals were not experts about their own dreams. In contrast, Carl Jung (1965) stated that he "avoided all theoretical points of view and simply helped the patients to understand the dream-images by themselves, without application of rules and theories. . . . That is how dreams are intended" (Jung, 1965, pp. 170–171). Many contemporary therapists believe that dreams belong to individuals, and they are the final authority on the meaning of their own dreams. This view-point is not intended to minimize the fact that the meaning of many dreams is obscure and that other people may be able to help unlock hidden meaning.

Among indigenous peoples, shamans are recognized as dream counsel-ors but not as "experts" in the Western sense. They are often called to their vocation by dreams. Shamans have a special relationship with the dream-world and through dreams are able to look into the future, communicate with spirits, and clarify the meaning of others' dreams (Tobert, 2017).

CONCEPTS

Biology of Dreaming

Sleep can be divided into two distinct kinds: a quiet phase and an active phase. Changes in brain waves, eye movements, muscle tone, and the pres-ence of dreams are used to define the two states. The quiet phase is divided into three substages. *Stage 1* is the transitional state between drowsy wakeful-ness and light sleep. It is characterized by slow, drifting eye movements and vivid, brief dream images. Falling dreams typically occur during this stage and are often accompanied by muscle spasms of the arms, legs, or the whole body that seem to happen just as one hits the ground in the dream. These sud-den contractions—myoclonic jerks—are common in many mammals. *Stage 2* is genuine sleep and is characterized by unique patterns called *sleep spindles*, which are waxing and waning brain waves. After 20 to 30 minutes, people sink into *Stage 3*, delta sleep, named after the regular, slow brain waves that are characteristic of this stage of quiet sleep. Delta sleep lasts about 30 to 40 minutes, during which the muscles are relaxed, although most people make major postural adjustments every 5 to 20 minutes. The dreaming that occurs during delta sleep is more poorly recalled, less vivid and visual, less emotional, and more pleasant than REM sleep dreaming. The sleep pattern then retraces the same stages in reverse order.

About 90 minutes after the onset of sleep, several abrupt physiological changes occur as the sleeper enters REM sleep, or the active phase, for the first time of the night. It is the sleep phase of vivid, memorable dreaming. Brain waves become desynchronized in a fast activity pattern that is similar to, but not identical with, that of the waking state. An accompanying profound loss of muscle tone throughout the body causes a general paralysis except for the muscles of the eyes, middle ear ossicles, and respiration. Sometimes, people awaken partially from REM sleep before the paralysis fades away, so that their body is still paralyzed, though they are otherwise awake. **Sleep paralysis**, as this state is called, can occur as people are falling asleep (rarely) or waking up (more frequently). Although the sensation may be terrifying, especially at the first occurrence, sleep paralysis is harmless.

The medial prefrontal cortex, anterior cingulate cortex, limbic region, basal forebrain, and occipital–temporal region become more active in REM sleep compared with non-REM sleep. At this time, breathing may accelerate to a panting pace, and the rhythm of the heart may speed up or slow down. Typically, men have erections and women experience vaginal lubrication during every REM cycle, regardless of dream content. It is not unusual for men to ejaculate and women to experience orgasm during REM sleep (Domhoff, 2011; Hobson & Friston, 2012).

During a typical night's sleep, the average adult alternates between periods of REM sleep and quiet sleep at regular intervals four to six times each night. After the first REM period, the intervals between REM periods decrease throughout the night, while the length of each REM period increases. REM sleep is both the deepest and lightest stage of sleep. It is the stage when people are least likely to be aroused by environmental stimuli, and it is also the stage when people are most likely to awaken spontaneously. Interestingly, during REM sleep, everyone experiences "symptoms" of mental illness. Box 19.1 describes what happens during sleep.

REM sleep is a primary means of brain development and maturation. Infants born 10 weeks prematurely spend 80% of their total sleep time in REM sleep, and those born 2 to 4 weeks prematurely spend 60% to 65% in REM sleep. Full-term newborns spend about half their sleeping time in REM sleep, which decreases to 30% to 35% by the age of 2 years. REM sleep stabilizes at about 25% by 10 years of age and shows little change until people are in their 70s or 80s, when it decreases to about 18%. The significance of the changing levels of REM sleep is unclear, but it may simply reflect maturation levels of the parts of the brain controlling non-REM sleep (Klemm, 2011).

Dreaming and REM sleep are not the same. People also have dreams in non-REM sleep. In addition, some individuals do not dream during REM sleep, notably, young children and people with certain kinds of brain injuries. Dreaming, as we know it, probably starts around age 3, with the development of language. Children under the age of 7 or 8 experience dreams in only 20%

BOX 19.1

How the Brain Goes Out of Its Mind

Experience	Psychiatric Label
We see things that are not there.	Hallucinations
We believe things that could not possibly be true.	Delusions, magical thinking
We become confused about times, places, and persons.	Disorientation
Scenes simply appear, and thoughts come and go.	Attention deficit
We think we are awake even though we are doing and seeing impossible things.	Lack of insight
We invent implausible narratives.	Confabulation, loose association
We forget almost everything on awakening.	Amnesia

Sources: Barrick (2001); Hobson (1996); Waters et al. (2016).

of their REM sleep, compared with normal adults, who experience 80% to 90% dream time during REM sleep (Klemm, 2011).

Every 80 to 90 minutes, during REM sleep, we become completely psychotic. This nocturnal madness is not only normal but probably essential to our health. Deprived of REM sleep, we become anxious and irritable and have trouble concentrating. Understanding this normal delirium may help you become more empathetic with the person experiencing those same symptoms while awake.

REM sleep is important to memory. Brain activity in the hippocampus during REM sleep consolidates experiences into long-term memory, as evidenced by experiments interrupting either REM sleep or non-REM sleep 60 times a night. When REM sleep is interrupted, there is a complete block of learning, while interruption of non-REM sleep appears to have no effect on learning. Thus, it is believed that REM sleep is critical for organizing the pieces for long-term memory. The amygdala, where emotions are encoded and retrieved, is the source of emotional content of dreams (Hobson & Friston, 2012).

Deprivation of REM sleep does not lead to psychosis, bizarre behavior, or anxiety, as was once feared. Interference with REM sleep may come from alcohol, sedatives, caffeine, drugs, anxiety, or depression. People with major depression dream considerably less than average and have limited dream recall. A sign that the depression is lifting is an increase in REM sleep and the reporting of more dreams. The most important effect of REM deprivation is a dramatic shift in subsequent sleep patterns. Reduction of REM sleep for several nights is followed by earlier onset and longer and more frequent periods of REM sleep. The longer the deprivation of REM sleep, the larger and longer the REM rebound. This compensatory mechanism suggests that REM sleep is physiologically necessary (Klemm, 2011).

Functions of Dreaming

Dreaming is a process of making broad connections. Dreams connect with recent experiences, old memories, and imagination. Dreaming makes connections not made during the waking state. The waking state tends to be guided by a specific task or goal, whereas dreaming tends to wander and form unique combinations. For example, people who are awake and thinking of a house may recall a specific house in which they lived in the past. People who are dreaming and thinking of a house may see a generic house or a combination of several houses or even a hotel. During dreaming, thoughts and memories are consolidated, and the bizarre twists and images of dreams often represent the processing and reclassifying of old information. Dream symbols bring together ordinary awareness and deeper levels of knowing. Images mean different things to different people. As Moss (1996) stated, "A dream of teeth falling out might evoke fears of death or job loss in one person, the memory of a boyhood fistfight in another, and the need for a routine dental checkup to a third. A snake might warn of a sneak attack, arouse sexual fears or energies, or signal potential for healing or transformation" (p. 79). The dominant emotion of the dreamer guides the dreaming process to choose images in the memory related to that emotional concern. Dreams can be viewed as explanatory metaphors for the emotional state of the dreamer. "I leave my children in a house somewhere, and then I can't find them" may be a metaphorical description for the emotional state of guilt. If no single dominant emotion is present at the time, dreams may seem confused and almost random (Moss, 2009; Shields et al., 2016).

Jung believed that dreams are a remarkable way to reveal insights and solutions to deal with everyday problems encountered during the awake state. Generally, the language of dreams is anything but obvious, and for this reason it is easy to ignore the messages. What is bizarre to the conscious, rational mind is not so to the unconscious mind, which is rich in symbols. People who work on remembering and understanding their dreams often report that dreams provide insights to overcoming and resolving problems and moving ahead (Omstedt, 2016).

While some dreams seem to be sequences of disconnected images, ideas, feelings, and sensations, others are storylike sequences that are dramatic and intricately detailed. They may have plots as coherent, funny, and profound as the best stories and plays. Some dreams last longer than one night, and the dream series is concluded the following night or may run for as long as a TV soap opera. It is known that dream content and process are similar to waking thought and behavior. That is, if individuals are outgoing and active, or introspective and quiet, in their waking moments, then they are usually the same in their dream lives (Hiebert, 2016).

Types of Dreams

Dreams offer nightly gauges of the dreamer's physical, emotional, and spiritual health. When disease begins to develop, dreams often provide warnings of specific problems before physical symptoms are apparent. The warning may be in the form of a broken heart, an exploding head, or limbs falling off. Such **early diagnosis dreams** are entirely natural and are reminders of how illness is related to one's entire being. It may be that when people are awake they tune out body messages, and when they are asleep their internal sensations get through more easily to the unconscious mind, which sends a message in a dream. Dreams may also give advice on preventive measures and ways to provide for one's well-being. Dreams frequently suggest specific courses of treatment for different problems. These suggestions may involve lifestyle changes, conventional medical treatments, alternative therapies, or counseling that addresses the hidden sources of disease. People may neglect the warnings, but the unconscious is highly inventive in rescripting the message in ways that make it increasingly harder to ignore (Moss, 2009).

Nightmares are terrifying dreams with complex imagery and story lines that are usually vividly recalled. The most common scripts of nightmares include being chased by a monster, being naked in public, falling through space, losing something precious, and being unprepared for an important exam. Nightmares are especially terrifying, because in dreams, anything is possible. Most typically, the dreamer is alone with no chance for escape. Around 70% of people experience occasional nightmares while 4–6% experience frequent nightmares defined as at least one per week (Carr, Blanchette-Carriere, Solomonova, Paquette, & Nielsen, 2016).

Because REM sleep becomes more physiologically intense as sleep continues, most nightmares occur in the early morning hours. Some factors that seem to contribute to nightmare frequency are fever, stress, and troubled relationships. Traumatic events can trigger a long-lasting series of recurrent nightmares for individuals with posttraumatic stress disorder. Alcohol, drugs, and some medications that suppress REM sleep also can cause an increase in nightmares. The person sleeps soundly for the first 5 or 6 hours, with little dreaming. When the effect of the substance has worn off, the brain makes up for the lost REM time. As a result, dreams are more intense than usual for the last few hours of sleep. Levodopa (L-dopa), used in the treatment of Parkinson's disease, and beta blockers, used in the treatment of cardiovascular disorders, seem to increase nightmares by increasing the activity during REM sleep (Rhudy, Davis, Williams, McCabe, & Byrd, 2008).

Night terrors awaken people with a scream as if they had just had a nightmare. Unlike a nightmare, however, the person frequently cannot remember anything except being afraid. Night terrors usually occur during non-REM sleep and are most common between the ages of 2 and 6 years. Although the cause is unknown, the incidence among adults increases with such factors as stress, lack of sleep, and alcohol and drug use (Moreno, 2015).

Rapid eye movement sleep behavior disorder (RBD) has only recently been described in the literature. In this disorder, people do not experience sleep paralysis, which allows them to act out the dream. Since these individuals often report action-filled and violent dreams, the acting out may cause self-injury or harm to others. People with neurodegenerative disorders such as Parkinson's disease and Lewy body dementia are at higher risk for RBD (Howell & Schenck, 2015; Kotagal, 2015).

Traumatic dreams are a major symptom of posttraumatic stress disorder (PTSD). People exposed to extremely dangerous and life-threatening situations such as war, terrorist attacks, physical or sexual assault, hostage situations, or natural disasters may develop PTSD. Traumatic dreams occur in all stages of sleep and tend to return the victim to the traumatic event in all its emotional horror. As the experience is gradually resolved, there is a decrease in frequency and an alteration in dream content. New stressors may reactivate the traumatic dream.

Recurrent dreams usually begin in childhood or adolescence, often at a time of significant stress. The emotional tone of recurrent dreams is negative 60% to 70% of the time, but the content of the dream does not directly reflect the original stress. Typical dreams include being attacked or chased by animals, monster, burglars, or natural forces. The dream often disappears when the original stressor or problem is resolved.

Lucid dreaming is being aware that one is dreaming during the experience. People in this unusual state of consciousness are simultaneously aware of their bodies lying on a bed, aware of the content of their dreams, and aware of watching themselves dreaming. When lucid dreaming occurs, the eye movements are more deliberate, and there is increased activity in the frontal regions of the brain compared with non-lucid REM sleep. Lucid dreaming may be triggered by various things, such as doing something impossible in the dream like flying or walking on water. Likewise, auditory signals such as a doorbell or a siren may startle people into becoming aware that they are dreaming. Individuals who wish to explore and use dreams constructively in their lives can learn techniques to increase their conscious dreaming time. Lucid dreaming has also been used successfully in the treatment of nightmares (Stumbrys, Erlacher, & Schredl, 2016).

Precognition is knowing about an event before it actually occurs. **Precognitive dreaming** involves seeing people and situations from the future and is an event in which individuals are not bound by space–time. As people learn to recall their dreams and record them in a dream journal, they often begin to recognize and work with precognitive material in their dreams. Precognitive dreams may indicate what may happen if certain courses of action are pursued, or they may reveal a precise event that cannot be altered (Sowerby, 2012).

TREATMENT

Until recently, Western societies have discouraged dreamwork and dream sharing. When dreams are recalled, the significance is often minimized. People tend to remember only bits and pieces from dreams and often jumble together parts from several dreams into a single confused story. By the time individuals are fully awake, they have forgotten 90%, if not more, of their nighttime adventures. Thus, the remembered dream is often different from the fuller dream experience.

By paying closer attention to dreams, people often gain greater access to their inner lives. Some of the world's most successful business executives never make a decision until they have a chance to let it pass through their minds during sleep, allowing solutions to come during dreams. The first step in making sense of a dream is to own it. It belongs solely to the dreamer and is a personal story. Although many books have been written about dream symbols, they are best understood by the dreamer. Dreaming about a horse may be a symbol of comfort and security because the person always had a horse when she was growing up. A horse for another person may be a symbol of terror because he was kicked by a horse as a young child. Yet another person may see a horse as a symbol of a challenge, since she has wanted to learn to ride for some time. Thus, dream dictionaries do not have the answers to people's dream symbols; they are personal images taken from one's life representing one's unique experiences.

Journaling helps mobilize intuition as people begin to understand their personal symbols. Because the dream journal is intensely personal, it should be kept private unless the dreamer chooses to share it with others. The entries should be dated so that they can be correlated with significant life events in the present or future, and recurring themes, places, and situations should be noted. Giving dreams titles or headlines like a newspaper headline often reveals a dream message that may otherwise be overlooked. People are encouraged to go back over their journals at regular intervals to note connections between dreams and waking events.

In the midst of nightmares, people who realize they are dreaming frequently choose to wake up. Many therapists believe, however, that the essential issue is to discover what elements from the past, mixed with current events, are creating the nightmare. Insight into the source of the nightmare can help people face and overcome the terror while remaining in the dream. Nightmares can be transformed into more pleasant experiences. People are encouraged to remember that nothing in their dreams can hurt them.

Conscious dreaming, as a form of mental imagery, has the potential to aid in the promotion of health and in the healing process. Evidence supports the idea that the vividness of mental imagery determines how strongly it affects physiology. Dreams are the most vivid form of mental imagery most people experience and, therefore, they are also likely to be a source of highly effective healing imagery.

Dreams can be immensely useful in gaining self-knowledge. Psychologist Ernest Rossi proposed that an important function of dreaming is integration of split-off parts of one's personality. According to Rossi (1985):

> In dreams we witness something more than mere wishes; we experience dramas reflecting our psychological state and the process of change taking place in it. Dreams are a laboratory for experimenting with changes in our psychic life. . . . This constructive or synthetic approach to dreams can be clearly stated: Dreaming is an endogenous process of psychological growth, change, and transformation. (p. 142)

RESEARCH

Persons who conduct dream research are often accused of working with biased or otherwise inadequate samples. Some question whether people who remember dreams are different from other people. Others surmise that people do not report their dreams honestly. Many studies of high and low dream recallers demonstrate only small differences between them on a variety of personality and cognitive tests. High recallers differ primarily in their interest in dreams and their motivation to recall them. In many studies, subjects provide dream reports anonymously, which reduces the tendency to misreport. Most people consider dreams as something that happens to them, so they do not view the dreams as reflecting on their self-image and are thus quite willing to report whatever they experience (Herlin, Leu-Semenescu, Chaumereuil, & Arnulf, 2015).

There are four sources of dream reports: the sleep laboratory, the psychotherapy relationship, personal dream journals, and reports written on anonymous forms in group settings. Sleep laboratories awaken individuals during REM and non-REM periods, which allows for the maximum recall of dreams. The process, however, is time consuming and expensive. Psychotherapy is a long-standing source of dream reports. The clients, however, constitute a small and unrepresentative sample of the population. Dream journals are personal documents of dreams but may have gaps or omissions. Some individuals are not willing to provide their journals for scientific analysis. The easiest way to get large samples of dreams is in the classroom, meetings, conferences, waiting rooms, and so on. People are simply asked to provide their gender, age, and the last dream they remember having.

Four general methods are used to analyze dream content: free associations, finding metaphoric meaning, searching for repeated themes, and quantitative analysis. Free association, that is, having clients say whatever comes into their minds about each part of the dream, often reveals the day-to-day waking events incorporated into the dream. In psychotherapy, people may look for metaphors, often based on their own past life experiences. Researchers may also look for repeated themes in a dream series. Usually these themes are unique to each dreamer, which makes it impossible to generalize to other people. The major task in quantitative content analysis is the creation of carefully defined categories that lead to the same results when used by different researchers. Nominal scales simply record the presence or absence of a characteristic in a dream report. For example, there could be a general category of aggression and then each type of aggression can be assigned separate categories. Hall and Van de Castle (1966) developed the most comprehensive and widely used empirical system of content analysis. They cataloged more than 10,000 dreams from normal people and found that approximately 64% were associated with sadness, apprehension, or anger. Only 18% were happy or exciting, and just 1% of dreams involved sexual feelings or acts. DreamBank, a website at the University of California, Santa Cruz, has more than 22,000 dream reports available for research regarding dream content (Domhoff & Schneider, 2008).

INTEGRATED NURSING PRACTICE

Dreams are the doorway into the unconscious, which is also a domain of healing. Just as guided imagery can be used to direct people's attention to specific areas or organs of the body, so can dreams become a healing tool. You can teach the following series of steps to clients who are interested in **cultivating healing dreams**:

- A half hour before bedtime, find a quiet place.
- Pay attention to the sounds and sensations of the outside environment as nature begins to settle down to rest.
- Spend a few minutes journaling the experiences and feelings you had during the day.
- Review your accomplishments of the day.
- Think for a moment of loving yourself and others with whom you interacted today.
- If you had conflict with others, put those thoughts and feelings away for now.
- Imagine yourself as part of the universe, and feel a connection with all living things.
- Allow one issue of present concern to come to your conscious awareness.
- Ask for answers, solutions, or healing as you sleep and dream.
- On awakening, remember what you wanted to learn from your dreams, and let the answers come to your awareness (Keegan, 1994).

A similar process is called **dream incubation**, which is a somewhat more deliberate format. Examples of the types of requests to make of dreams include these: How can I heal myself? Which path shall I choose? How can I solve (state problem)? How can I improve my relationship with (name)? How can I make (state project) a success? Should I do (state proposed action)? What shall I do now? Teach clients the following steps for dream incubation:

- Choose an important matter that you wish to explore.
- Write a short, simple question for which you need an answer.
- Meditate on the question for a few minutes. Repeat the question several times, followed by "I give thanks for the answer, which will be in a dream that I remember."
- Envision yourself awakening, remembering, and receiving an answer.
- Write the question again.
- Place the paper with the question on it beneath your pillow.
- On awakening, follow the guideline provided in the "Try This" box on improving dream recall near the end of the chapter.
- Watch for extra information that may come later during the day.
- Do not give up if success is not immediate.

Help clients understand that they need not seek professional help for bad dreams unless they frequently disrupt their sleep. Other distress signals include regular bouts of fatigue or depression on waking or consistently feeling worse than when they went to bed. Remind people that nothing in their dreams can hurt them. Suggestions for reframing nightmare themes are presented in Box 19.2. Alternatively, nightmares can be managed through a process called **dream re-entry**, which is practiced in the waking state. People begin by selecting the nightmare to relive, and then come up with alternative ways of acting in the nightmare to transform the events into a more enjoyable experience. They relive the nightmare in imagination, incorporating the new action, and continue with the dream until they see the result of their new behavior (Seda, Sanchez-Ortuno, Welsh, Halbower, & Edinger, 2015).

BOX 19.2

Reframing Nightmares

Being chased

Response: Stop running and face the chaser, which may cause it to disappear. If not, try to dialogue and reconcile with the person or animal. Alternatively, ask the adversary itself what you are running away from.

Being attacked

Response: Demonstrate your readiness to defend yourself, rather than giving in or running away. Then, try to dialogue with the attacker in a soothing manner. Alternatively, enlist friendly and cooperative dream characters to help overcome the threatening character.

Falling

Response: Rather than waking up, go with it, relax, and land gently. Think about landing in a pleasant and interesting place. Alternatively, transform falling into flying.

Trapped or paralyzed

Response: Relax and tell yourself you are dreaming. Go along with images or things that happen to the body, because none of it can be harmful in reality. Adopt an attitude of interest and curiosity about what happens.

Being unprepared for an exam or speech

Response: Leave the exam room or the lecture hall. Alternatively, answer the text questions creatively or give a spontaneous talk on any topic of interest. The key is to transform the experience into one that is fun.

Being naked in public

Response: Remember, modesty is a public convention, and dreams are private experiences. Have fun with the idea. Try having everyone else in the dream remove their clothing also.

Sources: Barrick (2001); Bulkeley (2003); Davenport (2016).

Spiritual care, in many settings, includes listening to clients' dreams. During times of transition, growth, or suffering, spiritual issues or struggles often occur and may be found in dreams as people wrestle with what is most important in their lives. Nurses have a unique opportunity to listen attentively to clients and help them work through this process. Sharing dreams with another person or with a group can provide a variety of insights into the many levels of the dream. Dream sharing also builds a sense of community as people discover that they have a great deal in common. Nurses who are sensitive and empathic and have good listening, communication, and group skills can facilitate a dream-sharing group.

To allow each member of the group to have time to work on a dream at every session, the number of participants will have to be limited to six or eight. Members should be asked to make a commitment to attend regular sessions over a set time, usually for no less than 6 weeks. A typical group session is 2 to 3 hours. Dream sharing requires mutual trust and respect. Individuals who are going to share their innermost thoughts must have the assurance that they are in a place where they are protected and supported. The dream is always honored as a topic worthy of attention and thought. Even without a full understanding of what dreams signify, we can use their stories to know ourselves better. For many people—and you can be one of them—dreams really do come true.

TRY THIS

Improving Dream Recall

1. Clearly declare to yourself the intention to remember your dreams when you lie down to sleep.
2. Have your tools, notebook and pen or tape recorder, at your bedside.
3. If you awaken during the night while dreaming, record your dream immediately. Use a penlight to see if you do not wish to disturb a partner. If you tell yourself that you can go back to sleep and catch the dreams later, you will probably find you are wrong.
4. When you awaken in the morning, at first lie quietly before getting out of bed. Then, write whatever you remember, even if it is only one word or scene.
5. If you wake up with no dream memories, move your body back into the position you were in as you began to awaken, and you will be more likely to recall your most recent dream.
6. Don't censor your dreams, and don't try to interpret them right away. Bizarre, weird, or trivial dreams may become important later.
7. Pay attention to your feelings. They are often your best guide to the dream's meaning and urgency.
8. Keep a journal for a month of the dreams you do remember. Look for important ideas or themes running through the dreams.
9. The more you practice these skills, the more dreams you will remember.

References

Barrick, M. C. (2001). *Dreams*. Corwin Springs, MT: Summit University Press.

Buhner, S. H. (2006). *Sacred Plant Medicine*. Rochester, VT: Bear & Company.

Bulkeley, K. (2003). *Dreams of Healing*. New York, NY: Paulist Press.

Carr, M., Blanchette-Carriere, C., Solomonova, E., Paquette, T., & Nielsen, T. (2016). Intensified daydreams and nap dreams in frequent nightmare sufferers. *Dreaming*. doi: org/10.1037/drm0000024

Cayce, E. (1976). *Dreams and Dreaming* (Vol. 1). Association for Research and Enlightenment.

Cushway, D. J., & Sewell, R. (2012). *Therapy with Dreams and Nightmares: Theory,* *Research, & Practice* (2nd ed.). Los Angeles, CA: Sage.

Davenport, L. (2016). *Transformative Imagery*. London: Jessica Kingsley Publishers.

Domhoff, G. W. (2011). The neural substrate for dreaming: Is it a subsystem of the default network? *Consciousness and Cognition, 20*(4): 1163–1174. doi: 10.1016/j.concog.2011.03.001

Domhoff, G. W., & Schneider, A. (2008). Studying dream content using the archive and search engine on DreamBank.net. *Consciousness and Cognition, 17*(4): 1248–1256.

Hall, C. S., & Van de Castle, R. L. (1966). *The Content Analysis of Dreams*. New York, NY: Appleton-Century-Crofts.

Herlin, B., Leu-Semenescu, S., Chaumereuil, C., & Arnulf, I. (2015). Evidence that non-dreamers do dream: A REM sleep behavior disorder model. *Journal of Sleep Research*. doi: 10.1111/jsr.12323

Hiebert, T. (2016). Lucid sleeping. *Performance Research*. doi: org/10.1080/13528165.2016.1138765

Hobson, J. A. (1996). How the brain goes out of its mind. *Harvard Mental Health Letter*, 12(8): 3–5.

Hobson, J. A., & Friston, K. J. (2012). Waking and dreaming consciousness: Neurobiological and functional considerations. *Progress in Neurobiology*, 98(1): 82–98. doi: 10.1016/j.pneurobio.2012.05.003

Howell, M. J., & Schenck, C. H. (2015). Rapid eye movement sleep behavior disorder and neurodegenerative disease. *JAMA Neurology*. doi: 10.1001/jamaneurol.2014.4563

Jung, C. G. (1965). *Memories, Dreams, Reflections*. Edited by A. Jaffe and translated by R. Winston & C. Winston. New York, NY: Vintage Books.

Keegan, L. (1994). *The Nurse as Healer*. Albany, NY: Delmar.

Klemm, W. R. (2011). Why does REM sleep occur? A wake-up hypothesis. *Frontiers in Systems Neuroscience*, 5: 1–12. doi: 10.3389/fnsys.2011.00073

Kotagal, S. (2015). Rapid eye movement sleep behavior disorder during childhood. *Sleep Medicine Clinics*. doi: 10.1016/j.jsmc.2015.02.004

Moreno, M. A. (2015). Sleep terrors and sleepwalking: Common parasomnias of childhood. *JAMA Pediatrics*. doi: 10.1001/jamapediatrics.2014.2140

Moss, R. (1996). *Conscious Dreaming: A Spiritual Path for Everyday Life*. New York, NY: Crown Trade Paperbacks.

Moss, R. (2009). *The Three "Only" Things: Tapping the Power of Dreams, Coincidence, and Imagination*. Novato, CA: New World Library.

Neihardt, J. G., Petri, A. N., & Utecht, L. (1932). *Black Elk Speaks* (Vol. 119).

Bison Books. University of Nebraska Press.

Omstedt, A. (2016). *Connecting Analytical Thinking and Intuition*. New York, NY: SpringerBriefs.

Reiser, M. F. (2001). The dream in contemporary psychiatry. *American Journal of Psychiatry*, 158(3): 351–359.

Rhudy, J. L., Davis, J. L., Williams, A. E., McCabe, K. M., & Byrd, P. M. (2008). Physiological–emotional reactivity to nightmare-related imagery in trauma-exposed persons with chronic nightmares. *Behavioral Sleep Medicine*, 6(3): 158–177.

Rossi, E. (1985). *Dreams and the Growth of Personality* (2nd ed.). New York, NY: Brunner/Mazel.

Seda, G., Sanchez-Ortuno, M., Welsh, C. H., Halbower, A. C., & Edinger, J. D. (2015). Comparative meta-analysis of prazosin and imagery rehearsal therapy for nightmare frequency, sleep quality, and posttraumatic stress. *Journal of Clinical Sleep Medicine*. doi: 10.5664/jcsm.4354

Shields, D. A., Levin, J., Reich, J., Murnane, S., & Hanley, M. A. (2016). Creative expressions in healing. In B. M. Dossey & L. Keegan (Eds.), *Holistic Nursing: A Handbook for Practice* (7th ed., pp. 321–343). Burlington, MA: Jones & Bartlett Learning.

Sowerby, D. F. (2012). *Intuition and Dreams*. West Conshohocken, PA: Infinity Publishing.

Stumbrys, T., Erlacher, D., & Schredl, M. (2016). Effectiveness of motor practice in lucid dreams: A comparison with physical and mental practice. *Journal of Sports Science*. doi: 10.1080/02640414.2015.1030342

Tobert, N. (2017). *Cultural Perspectives on Mental Wellbeing*. London: Jessica Kingsley Publishers.

Vinocur Fischbein, S., & Miramon, B. (2015). Theoretical trajectories: Dreams and dreaming from Freud to Bion. *International Journal of Psychoanalysis*. doi: 10.1111/1745-8315.12269

Waters, F., Biom, J. D., Dang-Vu, T. T., Cheyne, A. J., Alderson-Day, B., Woodruff, P., & Collerton, D. (2016). What is the link between hallucinations, dreams, and hypnagogic-hypnopompic experiences? *Schizophrenia Bulletin.* doi: 10.1093/schbul/sbw076

Resources

International Association for the
  Study of Dreams
1672 University Ave.
Berkeley, CA 94703
209.724.0889
www.asdreams.org

DreamGate
  www.dreamgate.com

Dream Network Australia
  www.dreamnetworkaustralia.com.au

European Association for the
  Study of Dreams
ONIROS

Chitri Mont Sabot
  58190 Neuffontaines, France
  33.03.86.24.86.41
  www.oniros.fr/home

The Lucidity Institute
  www.lucidity.com

20

Intuition

Wherever the art of medicine is loved,
there is also a love of humanity.

HIPPOCRATES

A problem cannot be solved
by the same level of consciousness
that created it.

ALBERT EINSTEIN

Intuition comes from the Latin word *intueri*, which means to look within. Intuition is described as something people see, hear, or feel rather than think; a powerful form of inner wisdom; an awareness of something without conscious attention or reasoning; or knowledge from an expanded state of awareness. Some people describe it as knowing immediately without thinking. Words and phrases associated with intuition are hunch, instinct, gut feeling, sixth sense, a flash of insight, "It suddenly hit me," "Something just clicked into place," "It just feels right," and "I don't know why, but something tells me I should do this." Intuition is a skill we all possess, albeit sometimes in subtle ways. Expert intuition is a form of rapid thinking based on past experiences and familiar situations.

BACKGROUND

Intuition is as old as humankind. Scientists, inventors, and artists have credited intuition with their ability to accomplish great things. Archimedes, one of the three greatest mathematicians of all time (born 287 B.C.), was reported to have shouted

"Eureka" when he discovered his famous flotation principle. Hippocrates, the father of medicine, wrote about the value of intuition, which he called "instinct." He warned that "cold reason" could obscure one's inner vision. Albert Einstein credited intuition for many of his own inspirations. Thomas Edison used the symbols of his dreams to intuit scientific breakthroughs. Jonas Salk, who discovered the polio vaccine, wrote an entire book on intuition, maintaining that creativity was the result of the interaction of intuition and reasoning.

The late Edgar Cayce (1877–1945) was one of the most versatile and credible psychics, or medical *intuitives*, the world has ever known. Cayce, a photographer and devout religious person, was, in a sense, the father of holistic medicine. In the early 20th century, he emphasized the importance of attitudes, emotions, diet, and exercise in health and illness. He believed that the treatment of illness should be physical, mental, and spiritual. Daily, for more than 40 years of his adult life, Cayce would lie down on a couch and enter a self-induced meditative state. Then, provided with the name and location of a person anywhere in the world, he would speak in a normal voice and give information about the state of the person's mind and body and prescribe ways to generate physical and mental health. These sessions came to be called "readings," and there are over 14,000 of them on file. A copy of the reading was always sent to the individuals for their own information and use.

There are currently several well-known medical intuitives. Judith Orloff, MD, is a board-certified psychiatrist, a professor of psychiatry at UCLA, and an author and lecturer on the interrelationship of medicine, intuition, and spirituality. Her book *Second Sight* (1996) is a *memoir* about coming to terms with her intuitive abilities. Mona Lisa Schulz, MD, PhD, is a neuropsychiatrist and neuroscientist who has worked for many years as a medical intuitive. Caroline Myss, PhD, is a writer, researcher, and medical intuitive who works closely with Norman Shealy, MD, founder of the American Holistic Medical Association.

PREPARATION

The level of training and abilities varies greatly from one medical intuitive to another. Because the practice of medical intuition is not regulated, anyone can claim the title, and the education and experience vary considerably. Indications that an intuitive is *not* legitimate include claims of the only true way to heal, resistance to collaboration with primary health-care providers, giving advice or telling the client what to do, or the charging of exorbitant fees.

Courses in medical and intuitive counseling may be taken at Holos University Graduate Seminary. The American Board of Scientific Medical Intuition (ABSMI) tests and certifies people who are proficient in medical intuition and counseling intuition. The medical intuition process is a 5-day exam during which the applicant completes an Intuitive Medical Analysis on eight different individuals. For the counseling intuitive certification process, the applicant must submit 25 case summaries signed by the clients. The applicants then conduct a counseling session with a client while being observed by an ABSMI board member.

CONCEPTS

Right and Left Brain

The cerebrum makes up 80% of the weight of the brain. The cerebrum is divided into two hemispheres, right and left. Each of the hemispheres has some separate and unique functions, yet, if one hemisphere is damaged, the other hemisphere seems to be able to take on some of those functions. The corpus callosum is composed of 200 million nerve fibers that connect the left and right hemispheres, and it relays information between the two hemispheres.

The right and left hemispheres of the brain are not nearly as separate as once thought. Some functions tend to dominate in one side or the other. For example, language tends to be on the left side and attention more on the right side, but that is not absolutely true for everyone. Most skills are not encoded in small locations but rather in patterns that are generated by neurons. Neurons work in large groups and communicate electrically through widespread networks throughout the brain. These groups of neurons constantly reform into different combinations for different skills. The brain is at its best when both sides are working together (Doidge, 2015).

Problem Solving

It is important to most individuals that they make good decisions. Intuition can help people make everyday decisions and improve their problem-solving skills. Sometimes, people simply get a gut feeling about a particular course of action. More often, however, intuition is the result of a four-step process. The first step involves *preparation and analysis*. People collect facts and information and study the situation. The second step is *incubation*. During this phase, the problem is put on the "back burner" by letting the brain move on to another subject. People often increase slow brain waves during this phase by listening to music, meditating, or engaging in movements such as dancing, t'ai chi, or yoga. The third step in *insight*. The intuitive answer may arrive in the form of images, verbal messages, physical sensations, emotions, environmental cues, or just a pervasive sense of knowing. The fourth and last step is *validation*. Once the insight is a conscious thought, the brain checks whether the intuitive message answers the question or solves the problem (Peirce, 2013).

Intuition and Dreams

Intuition is the language of dreams. Dreams offer nightly gauges on the dreamer's physical, emotional, and spiritual health. When disease begins to develop, dreams often provide warnings of specific problems before physical symptoms are apparent. Body cells may send chemical signals to a part of the brain. The warning may be in the form of dreams of a broken heart, an exploding head, or limbs falling off. Such *early diagnosis dreams* are entirely natural and are reminders of how illness is related to one's entire being. It may be that when people are awake they tune out body messages, and when they are asleep their internal sensations get through more easily to the intuitive mind, which sends a message in a dream. Intuition in the form of dreams may also give advice on preventive measures and ways to provide for one's well-being. Dreams frequently suggest specific courses of treatment for different problems. These suggestions may involve lifestyle changes, conventional medical treatments, alternative therapies, or counseling that addresses the hidden sources of disease. People may neglect the warnings, but intuition is highly inventive in rescripting the message in ways that make it increasingly harder to ignore (Dillard, 2015). See Chapter 19 for more information on dreams.

TREATMENT

It would be comforting to believe that primary health-care providers easily make medical diagnoses and treatment decisions. However, even with the technological advances of modern science, misdiagnoses are made, and treatments may cause more problems than the disease itself. Many health-care practitioners rely on their intuition to enhance their scientific understanding. More than 5,000 medical tests are currently in use. How would practitioners know which ones to order if they did not use intuition as well as their knowledge and deductive reasoning? Thus, medical intuition is an essential tool for every biomedical and integrative health-care provider.

Medical Intuitives

A **medical intuitive** is someone who has skill and/or training in reading the human energy system. Some practitioners are born with this ability, and some learn it through training and practice. Medical intuition is not a healing modality but rather a tool to provide information about what is going on in a person's body, mind, and spirit.

Medical intuitives may or may not meet their clients in person, but they will work only with the client's explicit consent. The intuitive makes it clear that it is not a physician–patient relationship, and there will be no diagnoses or treatment prescriptions. The intuitive will instead tell the person about problematic energetic and emotional factors they detect and may suggest having certain areas checked out by a regular health-care provider. Medical intuition is an empowering tool when clients use the information to make changes for the better in their health and lives.

Medical intuition presupposes that body, mind, and spirit are one unified reality and is based on the belief that the body is animated by an integrated energy called the **life force.** The life force sustains the physical body, but it is also a spiritual entity that is linked to a higher being or infinite source of energy. When the energy flows freely throughout the body, a person experiences optimal health and vitality. When the life force is blocked or weakened, organs, tissues, and cells are deprived of the energy they need to function at their full potential, and illness or disease results.

After quieting or grounding their own energy, medical intuitives tune in to their clients' mind–body–spirit energy. They pay attention to the energy without censoring, questioning, or analyzing. Some intuitives are *clairvoyant*, which means that intuition comes to them visually, and they see pictures of the inner parts of the body. They are able to see energy or qi as it flows through the body and are able to detect where this energy has become blocked. Some intuitives are *clairsentient*, which means that they are able to feel the energy or emotions in the body. They may experience actual sensations in their own bodies or they may scan clients' bodies seeking out changes in the energy field of the body. Some intuitives are *clairaudient*, which means that they receive intuitive information through sound. This may be random and dissociated words or a sentence or even an in-depth conversation (Shealy, 2010).

In a sense, biomedical health-care providers work from the outside in and look at the symptoms of the physical body. Medical intuitives work from the inside out and are more interested in spiritual, emotional, and psychological issues that create the environment for illness and disease to occur. Many medical intuitives work with (or are) medical doctors.

Self-Healing

Some individuals believe that curing their illness or disease is something that must be done to them or for them. They have lost their intuitive understanding of what is not functioning properly and why, and they often ignore symptoms or numb their pain. They have little understanding of how they set the internal scene for their illness or disease. With this mind-set, people become disconnected from their ability to heal themselves and feel like victims of their own body processes.

People interested in self-healing recognize that dysfunction and disease are ways the body communicates. All people have the ability to intuit what their bodies are saying. They can learn to trust and use their inner intelligence to tell them what is right and wrong, what's good and should be strengthened, and what's unhealthy and needs to be changed. Intuition may tell a person when to exercise, when to rest, or when to see a health-care provider. Self-healers also understand that intuitions do not heal in and of themselves. To heal, the persons must act on the intuitive information.

Thoughts trigger biochemical responses, and biochemical responses trigger thoughts. Thoughts, words, and beliefs are the link between people's inner experiences and the directions their lives take. Many individuals have long-standing negative tapes playing in their heads much of the time. This

negative self-talk includes statements such as these: I'm bad; I'm fat and ugly; No one likes me; I have no control; I'm no good; It's hopeless; I'm never going to feel better; I'm always sick; I'm all alone in this life; The world is a dangerous place; I might as well give up; and so on. The unconscious mind "hears" these thoughts and words and begins to treat them as reality. Thus, one's expectations become a self-fulfilling prophecy, and people become driven by negativity (Orloff, 2009; Zion, 2012).

In contrast, **positive attitudes** are a part of self-healing and foster growth and adaptive change. Positive beliefs set the stage for healing to occur. Positive self-talk includes statements such as these: My body is a holy vessel; I have the ability to heal myself; I like and respect my body; My body, emotions, and spirit are all one; I am well loved; I am good to other people; I enjoy being healthy; I listen to my intuition; My body knows what it needs to get well; and so on. The unconscious takes these positive attitudes seriously, and they become a self-fulfilling prophecy for health and well-being (Orloff, 2009). An old Navajo saying illustrates this process: "If you want to see what your body will look like tomorrow, look at your thoughts today" (Chang, 2006).

Another facet of self-healing is **body scanning,** or learning to decode subtle body messages before there is pain or disease. Most people can learn to discern imbalances long before these can be medically verified. Body scanning begins with meditation. When people have a quieter conscious mind, they can more easily recognize messages coming from the body, emotions, and subconscious mind. Meditation is the amplifier of intuition. Once the mind is quiet, open, and waiting, the individual scans the entire body.

During this process, the person notes any areas that are hot or cold, and any sensations of tingling, buzzing, quivering, aching, tightness, or numbness. With practice, people can learn to understand the unique language their body uses to communicate needs and problems. With this intuitive understanding, people can take steps to create a healthier and happier life (Dillard, 2015).

RESEARCH

Although there are some compelling anecdotes about medical intuition, research into the phenomenon is in its infancy. Within biomedicine, there are "master" diagnosticians who can assess a patient's condition and prognosis with extremely subtle cues, and healers in many cultures claim to make assessments by intuition. It will be interesting to see whether medical intuition, which is subjective and metaphysical, will in the future be understood from an objective, scientific viewpoint.

There are a number of studies on intuition in nursing practice, and tools have been developed to measure intuition in both experienced and novice nurses. These qualitative studies began in the mid-1980s and continue today. Nursing intuition does not lend itself to randomized blinded studies. According to Effken (2007, p. 188): "The value of intuition for clinical practice has been well documented; but because it cannot easily be measured, it can be denigrated in today's evidence-based research and practice environment."

INTEGRATED NURSING PRACTICE

Intuition in Patient Care

Nursing practice is based on more than scientific understanding; it is also inspired by intuition. Experienced nurses are able to talk about their intuitive sense and give examples of it from their own practice but are often discouraged by a work environment that emphasizes linear deductive reasoning (Pretz & Folse, 2011).

Mona Lisa Schulz, a physician and medical intuitive, states that one of the most intuitive groups of people she knows are nurses in intensive care units. A patient may appear objectively stable, but the nurse who is caring for him or her will insist that he or she is about to "go bad" or go into a crisis state. When asked how the nurse knows, the reply is usually, "I just know." It might be a smell, a slight tinge of color, a touch, or some other subtle cue that alerts the nurse. When science and medical knowledge say one thing, and a nurse's gut feeling says something else, it is important to look at the situation again (Schulz, 1998).

Patricia Benner has studied nurses and intuition for some time. She describes the intuitive process of nurses as "skilled pattern recognition." Benner believes that nursing intuition is based on previously acquired knowledge, memory, and experience. She has also found that intuitive nurses do not always trust what they are experiencing when they cannot provide the "proof" that others demand of them. Benner suggested that nurses and others might more readily accept intuition if it is called skilled pattern recognition instead (Benner & Tanner, 1987).

Novice nurses do not have the broad-based experience that underlies expert intuition. They need the guidance and support of expert nurses in developing this skill. There are three components to expert intuition. It is a quick perceptual process (1) that is mostly unconscious, (2) that is based on knowledge and experience, and (3) that results in an appropriate action for the best outcomes for our clients (Payne, 2015; Price, Zulkosky, White, & Pretz, 2016; Zander, Horr, Bolte, & Volz, 2016).

McCutcheon and Pincombe (2001) believe that nursing intuition is based on "a complex interaction of attributes, including experience, expertise and knowledge, along with personality, environment, acceptance of intuition as a valid 'behavior' and the presence or absence of a nurse/client relationship" (p. 345). Their study acknowledges that nurses acting on intuition can positively affect client care and that ignoring intuition can have a negative impact on that care.

Nyatanga and de Vocht (2008) and Gobet and Chassy (2008) believe that simple decisions are better processed by the conscious mind, while complex decisions are better processed by the unconscious mind. It is thought that the unconscious mind is able to detect familiar patterns, since more information is stored as unconscious thought. Pretz and Folse (2011, p. 287) believe that "experienced clinicians can identify relevant information and quickly detect subtle changes or unanticipated patient response to a treatment. . . . Even before objective evidence is available, nurses can use intuition to anticipate changes in patients' conditions, potentially improving the quality of care and patient outcomes."

Intuitive Leadership

Business executives have understood for some time that intuition is an important part of successful leadership. Just as businesses are doing, nurse managers can turn to experts in the field of intuition to shape decisions, assess professional relationships, and decide on courses of action. Respecting intuition is part of the environment in which innovation and new ideas naturally emerge. Intuitive leaders are able to look past their preconceptions and assumptions long enough to anticipate new possibilities. This creativity can result in new ideas for nursing research, new systems of care, and new health-care products. As individuals are able to broaden their awareness and see new options, they will also see improved professional relationships and teamwork. Greater innovation and workable strategies mean more motivated employees and decreased nursing "burnout."

TRY THIS

Positive Affirmations

Positive affirmations are a way of purposefully changing your inner reality. They are always stated in the present tense, as if they have already occurred. For a week, think about and jot down changes you would like to see in your life. Formulate several affirmations for each of these changes. For example, if you are struggling and would like your financial situation to improve, you might develop these affirmations: I have all the money I need and want; I am financially secure; money comes in as I need it; I pay my bills easily; and I am very comfortable about money. Affirmations about your career might include the following: I am an excellent nurse; I make sound and wise decisions; I care about my clients; my clients respond to my care of them; I am respected by other professionals; and I really like being a nurse.

- Write out affirmations in a number of areas such as career, health, parenting, and personal relationships.
- Make a recording of your affirmations, pausing several seconds after each one.
- Several times a day, when driving or during some other quiet time, play your affirmation recording. After each recorded affirmation, repeat the affirmation aloud.
- Pay attention to how things begin to change in your life. Remember, the thoughts you have become the reality of your life. Make that a positive process.

TRY THIS

Practice Intuition

Intuitive abilities improve with attention and practice. Try the following:

- Think of something specific to which you would like an answer.
- Do a relaxation exercise or move into a meditative state.
- Allow any answers to come into your awareness.
- Don't make any judgments about any of the answers or question where they came from.
- Jot down the answers to consider and review when you return to a normal state of consciousness.
- If you received no answers, try a different question or seek an inner guide or teacher to help you find the answer.

References

Benner, P., & Tanner, C. (1987). How expert nurses use intuition. *American Journal of Nursing*, 87(1): 23–31.

Chang, L. (2006). *Wisdom for the Soul: Five Millennia of Prescriptions for Spiritual Healing*. Gnosophia Publishers.

Dillard, S. (2015). *Develop Your Medical Intuition*. Woodbury, MN: Llewellyn Publications.

Doidge, N. (2015). *The Brain's Way of Healing*. New York, NY: Penguin Books.

Effken, J. A. (2007). The informational basis for nursing intuition: Philosophical underpinnings. *Nursing Philosophy*, 8: 187–200. Copyright John Wiley & Sons.

Einstein, A. (1983). *Albert Einstein, The Human Side: New Glimpses from His Archives*. Edited by H. Dukas & B. Hoffmann. Princeton University Press.

Gobet, F., & Chassy, P. (2008). Towards an alternative to Benner's theory of expert intuition in nursing. *International Journal of Nursing Studies*, 45: 129–139.

Hippocrates. (1983). *Hippocratic Writings* (Vol. 451). Edited by G. E. R. Lloyd, J. Chadwick, & W. N. Mann. Penguin Books Limited.

McCutcheon, H. H. I., & Pincombe, J. (2001). Intuition: An important tool in the practice of nursing. *Journal of Advanced Nursing*, 35(5): 342–348.

Nyatanga, B., & de Vocht, H. (2008). Intuition in clinical decision-making: A psychological penumbra. *International Journal of Palliative Nursing*, 14(10): 492–496.

Orloff, J. (1996). *Second Sight*. New York, NY: Three Rivers Press.

Orloff, J. (2009). *Emotional Freedom: Liberate Yourself from Negative Emotions and Transform Your Life*. Prospect, KY: Harmony House.

Payne, L. K. (2015). Intuitive decision making as the culmination of continuing education: A theoretical framework. *Journal of Continuing Education in Nursing*. doi: 10.3928/00220124-20150619-05

Peirce, P. (2013). *Leap of Perception*. New York, NY: Atria Books.

Pretz, J. E., & Folse, V. N. (2011). Nursing experience and preference for intuition in decision making. *Journal of Clinical Nursing*, 20: 2878–2889. doi:10.1111/j/1365-2702.2011.03705.x

Price, A., Zulkosky, K., White, K., & Pretz, J. (2016). Accuracy of intuition in clinical decision-making among novice clinicians. *Journal of Advanced Nursing.* doi: 10.1111/jan.13202

Schulz, M. L. (1998). *Awakening Intuition.* New York, NY: Three Rivers Press.

Shealy, C. N. (2010). *Medical Intuition.* Virginia Beach, VA: 4th Dimension Press.

Zander, T., Horr, N. K., Bolte, A., & Volz, K. G. (2016). Intuitive decision making as a gradual process. *Brain and Behavior.* doi: 10.1002/brb3.420

Zion, T. M. (2012). *Become a Medical Intuitive* (2nd ed.). AuthorHouse.

Resources

American Board of Scientific Medical Intuition
5607 S. 222nd Rd.
Fair Grove, MO 65648
888.242.6105
www.absmi.com

Holos University Graduate Seminary
P.O. Box 297
Bolivar, MO 65613
888.272.6109
www.holosuniveristy.org

Institute of Noetic Sciences
707.775.3500
www.noetic.org

International Association of Medical Intuitives
www.medical-intuitives.net

21

Music as a Therapeutic Tool

Leslie Rittenmeyer, PsyD, CNS, CNE, RN

*Music washes away from the soul
the dust of everyday life.*

BERTHOLD AUERBACH

*Music gives soul to the universe, wings to
the mind, flight to the imagination, a
charm to sadness, and life to everything.*

ATTRIBUTED TO PLATO

The focus of this chapter is to explore the use of music as a therapeutic tool to complement clinical practice. The reader should be aware that there is an academic discipline called music therapy. **Music therapy** is the clinical and evidence-based use of music interventions to accomplish individualized goals within a therapeutic relationship by a credentialed professional who has completed an approved music therapy program (American Music Therapy Association, n.d.). Music is used to promote wellness or improve the quality of life for those with disabilities or illness. For more information on music therapy, the reader is referred to *Defining Music Therapy* (3rd ed.), by Kenneth Bruscia.

BACKGROUND

It is generally believed that the utilization of music for healing dates to ancient times. The *I Ching, Chinese Book of Wisdom*, one of the oldest books in Chinese culture, references music as a powerful healing force. Thousands of years ago, humans were playing primitive instruments, and most known primitive societies had some form of music. The Greek philosopher Pythagoras believed that music contributed to health, and he prescribed music to restore harmony (White, 2001). In the mid-1800s, Florence Nightingale (1859/1992) acknowledged the benefits of music in aiding the healing process in soldiers wounded during the Crimean War. She observed that wind instruments with continuous sound seemed to have a beneficial effect, whereas those instruments that did not produce continuous sound had the opposite effect. During World Wars I and II, music was used in the Veterans Administration hospitals as a way to address traumatic war injuries. Doctors and nurses began to notice the effect music had on veterans' psychological, physiological, cognitive, and emotional state. Music was first used in the general hospital in the first half of the 1990s by health-care practitioners in conjunction with anesthesia and analgesia. Many concentration camp survivors also used music as a survival tool (Frankl, 1963).

CONCEPTS

Music and the Brain

Ways in which the brain processes music and the effect of music on the brain are of great interest, particularly in the field of neuroscience. The publication of the work *Pourquoi Mozart* (1991) by the French researcher Tomatis piqued interest in something called the *Mozart effect*. Tomatis was particularly interested in the physiological effects of music on healing and believed that the music of Mozart had the greatest effect. A seminal study by Rauscher, Shaw, and Ky (1993) demonstrated that 10 minutes of listening to a Mozart sonata improved the spatiotemporal intelligence, that is, the ability to mentally manipulate objects in three-dimensional space. Results also showed that IQ scores of college students improved by 8 to 9 points, which started a popular notion that listening to music made people smarter. Unfortunately, this was not quite so. The improvement was not permanent (nor did the researchers claim it was) and, in fact, lasted only about 10 to 15 minutes. Despite the controversy surrounding this theory, the term "Mozart effect" has been popularized to reflect the healing power of music in general.

Although the perception of music by the brain is not fully understood, it seems that there is not a single area of the brain that can be called the "music center." More than likely, listening to and perceiving music is a comprehensive experience. Sacks (2007) posited that musical powers are made possible because the brain uses systems that have already been developed for other purposes. He stated, "This might go with the fact that there is no single music center in the human brain, but the involvement of a dozen scattered networks throughout the brain" (Sacks, 2007, p. xi). Some scientists believe that the brain is hardwired for music, while others believe that this is not so. Pinker (1997) is one of the neuroscientists who believe there is no evolutionary basis for supposing that music, or any of the arts, is adaptive and hardwired in the brain. In essence, he bases this belief on the notion that if music vanished tomorrow, from an adaptive perspective, nothing would change biologically. Other scientists, such as Levitin (2006), disagree and point to the universality of music in cultures and the apparent ability of infants to perceive music early on.

In considering the role of the brain, Levitin (2006) identifies the cumulative experience of perceiving music. The motor cortex allows for movement such as foot tapping, dancing, and playing an instrument; the sensory cortex allows for tactile feedback; the auditory cortex allows for the perception and analysis of tones and sounds; the prefrontal cortex allows for the creation of expectations and satisfaction of expectations; the visual cortex allows for reading music and looking at others' and one's own movements; the hippocampus allows for memory for music and musical experiences; the amygdala allows for the emotional reaction to music; and last, the cerebellum allows for movement and the emotional reaction to music. It is unclear exactly how music affects the brain and healing, but it is fairly certain that it does, as supported by both scientific and anecdotal evidence (Sacks, 2007).

Quality of Life

In addition to affecting the brain, music therapy is also capable of affecting individual quality of life. *Quality of life (QoL)* is a broad concept that can be defined contextually; that is, quality of life for a person dying of cancer might be defined differently than for a person dealing with an anxiety disorder, and someone experiencing severe chronic pain might define quality of life differently than someone recovering from a hurtful divorce. Victor Frankl (1963) contended that quality of life is tied to a person's perception of meaning. The quest for meaning is fundamental to the human condition, and individuals are brought in touch with a sense of meaning when they reflect on that which they have created, loved, believed in, or left as a legacy. Richardson, Babiak-Vazquez, and Frankel (2008) found a connection between QoL and music suggesting that the use of it as therapeutic intervention fostered better ability to communicate sadness, fear, and other feelings while alleviating physical pain and discomfort.

RESEARCH

The body of evidence for the use of music as a therapeutic modality has been growing. Most importantly, there are now many systematic reviews on topics pertaining to music as an intervention. Please refer back to Chapter 3, which explicates the systematic review process and its importance in providing reliable evidence. The following list is not all-inclusive but provides examples of the body of literature that is available. A search in Google Scholar will yield a good starting point.

- A summary of systematic reviews based on randomized controlled trials of music interventions found that treatment improved the following: global and social functioning in schizophrenia and/or mental disorders, gait and related activities in Parkinson's disease, depressive symptoms, and sleep quality. MT may have the potential for improving other diseases, but there is not enough evidence at present. Most importantly, no specific adverse effect or harmful phenomenon occurred in any of the studies, and music as an intervention was well tolerated by almost all patients (Kamioka et al., 2014).
- A systematic review on music therapy in dementia found that recent reviews on music therapy for people with dementia have been limited to attempting to evaluate whether it is effective, but there is a need for a critical assessment of the literature to provide insight into the possible mechanisms of actions of music therapy. This systematic review uses a narrative synthesis format to determine evidence for effectiveness and provide insight into a model of action (McDermott, Crellin, Ridder, & Orrell, 2012).
- In a systematic review of music therapy and music medicine interventions with cancer patients, the authors found beneficial effects on anxiety, pain, fatigue, and quality of life (Bradt, Dileo, Magill, & Teague, 2016).
- In a systematic review of music therapy for people with dementia, the authors found significant improvement in disruptive behaviors and levels of anxiety, and a more moderate response with levels of depression and cognitive functioning (Chang et al., 2015).
- A systematic review of music therapy in the palliative setting found that patients' overall quality of life was improved, that pain and symptoms were reduced, and that mood and social interaction were improved (Leow, 2011).
- A meta-analysis of music therapy in a neonatal intensive care unit found that live music provided the greatest benefit for preterm infants (Standley, 2012).
- A qualitative study explored the impact of active participation in music therapy for persons living with cancer. Some of the benefits described included relaxation, a sense of being uplifted, connectedness to others, and evocation of particular memories (McClean, Bunt, & Daykin, 2012).
- Based on a systematic review done by Evans (2002), a best practice information sheet from the Joanna Briggs Institute (2009) made the following recommendations:
  - Use of music in the preprocedural period may reduce anxiety and decrease the amount of needed sedative medications (Grade A).
  - The use of music may reduce surgical or procedural pain but should not be used as the primary pain intervention (Grade A).

- Music may be an adjunctive intervention in the management of physiologically presented anxiety (Grade B).
- There was not sufficient evidence to recommend the use of music for the perception of well-being, the reduction of side effects of analgesic drugs, and the physiological parameters of anxiety.

INTEGRATED NURSING PRACTICE

Using music as an intervention is a client preference. Although the practice of music therapy takes specialized credentials, music can be used more generally as a complementary nursing intervention. For instance, teaching stress reduction is a common health promotion activity, and music is a very effective tool for reducing stress. Teaching clients how to perform progressive relaxation accompanied by their favorite music often reinforces the relaxation response. Some clients like to meditate, and meditating with music is effective for some. Relaxation coupled with music helps decrease the wear and tear that results when the sympathetic nervous system is stimulated by stress or when people experience anxiety or anger. Thus, music can be used to decrease the deleterious effects of any situation that is stressful or anxiety producing.

Music can also be used as a nonpharmacological intervention for pain management. It is known that muscle tension increases the pain response, so helping clients relax to music can decrease muscle tension and thereby reduce pain. The same principle can be applied with women in labor. Deep breathing, progressive relaxation, and imaging enhanced by music can be very effective in creating a positive birthing experience.

Music can also be used while caring for the older population. Many times, music helps people remember positive things about their life. Reminiscence is a developmental exercise that is healthy. The use of music is also very soothing and calming. Doing gentle exercise enhanced by music encourages increased mobility and strength.

Singing bowls are standing bells that are played by rubbing a wooden, plastic, or leather-wrapped mallet around the rim of the bowl to produce a continuous "singing" sound. A warm bell tone can be produced by striking the bowl with a soft mallet. Singing bowls are used worldwide for meditation, relaxation, and pain reduction. The vibrations lower heart and respiratory rates and relax brain wave patterns.

In 1973, Theresa Schroeder-Sheker was instrumental in creating the music intervention she called *music thanatology* (Cox & Roberts, 2013). *Thanatology*, the scientific study of death, derives from Thanatos, the personification of peaceful death in Greek mythology. Music thanatology is a subspecialty of palliative medicine; it is not for entertainment or distraction. Rather, it is prescriptive harp and voice music with its focus on the physical and spiritual care of persons with a terminal diagnosis or who are actively dying. The goal is to provide a sacred space for being with the person who is transitioning from life to death (Black, 2012).

A certified harpist conducts a vigil (a period of attentive interaction) with the client (and family) in a hospital, hospice setting, nursing home, or in a person's own home. The vigil alternates between music and silence, designed for each person according to an ongoing assessment of individual needs and symptoms. The purpose is to provide comfort and support by calming and settling, as well as reducing pain (Cox & Roberts, 2013). As Black (2012) describes it:

> Music thanatology is based on the premise that dying is a part of a larger spiritual process that affords the opportunity for growth and healing of the inner life without curing the physical body, and as such, it is part of the life cycle that can celebrate and reflect the beauty and reverence of the life lived. (p. 123)

Music-thanatology training is a 2-year nondegree program offered at Chalice of Repose Project. The curriculum includes courses in anatomy and physiology, end-of-life physical challenges, and physical, emotional, and spiritual assessment. The students also study liberal arts and spirituality. They have intense music education in both voice and harp. Following the didactic courses, students serve an internship, write a thesis, and must successfully complete comprehensive exams. A master's degree in music thanatology is a new program being offered by Chalice of Repose both as distance learning and at St. Catherine University in Minneapolis and St. Paul. The excellent book *The Harp and the Ferryman* (Cox & Roberts, 2013) brings this remarkable process to life and is a "must read" for every nurse.

TRY THIS

Music for Stress Reduction

- Keep a "bag of tricks" with you no matter the environment in which you work. What is in your bag will depend on your job, but always keep a small compact disk (CD) player with an array of CDs for stress reduction and relaxation. Then, you will be prepared when you encounter a clinical situation that calls for the use of music. Also keep a set of earphones for situations in which the music might disturb others.
- Ask clients who seem anxious whether they would like to listen to some relaxation music. Teach them how to deep breathe slowly while listening to the music. The music and the deep breathing decrease sympathetic nervous system stimulation, thereby decreasing the physiological arousal that is prevalent in anxiety.
- Use music to counteract stress. Choose and play some of your favorite music that comforts or calms you. Find a comfortable position either sitting or lying down. As you listen to the music, focus on your breathing, and let the music lead you to a relaxed state. Focus on how peaceful and calm you feel.
- Experiment with various types of music. You may want to purchase Dr. Andrew Weil's *Mind–body Tool Kit*, which is available at bookstores. Nilsson (2008, p. 803) in

a systematic review on the pain- and anxiety-reducing effects of music made the following recommendations for music interventions in clinical practice:

- Slow and flowing music, approximately 60–80 beats per minute
- Nonlyrical
- Maximum volume level of 60 decibels
- Client's own choice, with guidance
- Suitable equipment chosen for the specific situation
- Minimum duration of 30 minutes
- Measurement, follow-up, and documentation.

Considering the Evidence

Magee, W. L., Clark, I., Tamplin, J., & Bradt, J. (2017). Music interventions for acquired brain injury. *Cochrane Database of Systematic Reviews*, 1, Art. No. CD006787. doi: 10.1002/14651858.CD006787.pub3

What Was the Approach of the Research?

Systematic review of randomized clinical trials (RCTs).

What Was the Aim/Purpose/Objective(s) of the Research as Related to Complementary and Integrative Therapies?

1. To assess the effects of music interventions for functional outcomes in people with acquired brain injury (ABI).
2. Examine the efficacy of music interventions in addressing recovery in people with ABI including gait, upper extremity function, communication, mood and emotions, cognitive functioning, social skills, pain, behavioral outcomes, activities of daily living, and adverse events.
3. Compare the efficacy of music interventions and standard care with (a) standard care alone, (b) standard care and placebo treatments, or (c) standard care and other therapies.
4. Compare the efficacy of different types of music interventions (music therapy delivered by trained music therapists versus music interventions delivered by other professionals).

How Was the Study Done?

The researchers used a systematic review protocol to examine published and unpublished RCTs related to the objectives of this research. The search identified 29 new RCTs with a total of 775 participants meeting inclusion criteria. These studies were identified after a search was completed of multiple databases, including the Cochrane Stroke Group Trials Register (January 2016) and the Cochrane Central Register of Controlled Trials (CENTRAL).

(continued)

What Were the Significant Findings of the Research?

The researchers suggest that music intervention (moving to music, singing, listening to music, composing, playing musical instruments, or a combination of these) may enhance gait, the timing of upper extremity function, communication, and quality of life post stroke. A strong beat within music may be more effective as an intervention than a strong beat without music. Treatment provided by a trained therapist might be more effective than music interventions used by other professionals. The researchers were unable to identify any studies that reported adverse effects to music intervention. However, the researchers cautioned that there is a need for additional high-quality RCTs in this area.

What Additional Questions Might I Have?

Could music intervention have long-term effects on persons living with ABI? Are there specific types of music that contribute to enhanced outcomes in persons living with ABI? What type of training would be beneficial for health professionals to complete to gain competency in music intervention? Would music intervention be beneficial for persons diagnosed with neurological disorders other than ABI?

What Is the Clinical Significance of This Study?

The application of the findings of this systematic review has considerable clinical value for nurses in informing their nursing practice in caring for persons living with ABI within a variety of health-care settings. Nurses should inquire about specific training related to music intervention strategies. Nurses should recognize and incorporate music intervention in seeking to enhance the quality of life for these individuals. Additionally, nurses need to recognize the need for additional high-quality RCTs related to music intervention to strengthen the evidence and increase confidence in implementation.

Source: Contributed by Dolores M. Huffman, RN, PhD.

References

American Music Therapy Association. (n.d.). Official definition and description of music therapy. Retrieved from www.musictherapy.org

Black, B. P. (2012). Music as a therapeutic resource in end-of-life care. *Journal of Hospice and Palliative Nursing,* 14(2): 118–125. doi: 10.1097/NJH. 0b013e31824765a2

Bradt, J., Dileo, C., Magill, L., & Teague, A. (2016). Music interventions for improving psychological and physical outcomes in cancer patients. *Cochrane Database of Systematic Reviews,* Art No. CD006911. doi: 1002/14651858. CD006911.pub3

Chang, Y. S., Chu, H., Yang, C. Y., Tsai, J. C., Chung, M. H., Liao, Y. M., . . . Chou, K. R. (2015). The efficacy of music therapy for people with dementia: A meta-analysis of randomized controlled trials. *Journal of Clinical Nursing,* 24(23–24): 3425–3440. doi: 10.1111/ jocn.12976

Cox, H., & Roberts, P. (2013). *The Harp and the Ferryman.* Melbourne, Australia: Michelle Anderson.

Day, E. P. (1884). *Day's Collacon: An Encyclopaedia of Prose Quotations, Consisting of Beautiful Thoughts, Choice Extracts and Sayings, of the Most Eminent Writers of All Nations, from the Earliest Ages to* the Present Time, Together with a Comprehensive Biographical Index of Authors, and an Alphabetical List of Subjects Quoted. International Printing and Publishing Office. Originally from the University of Michigan.

Estcourt, M. J. (1857). *Music: The Voice of Harmony in Creation*. Selected and arranged by M. J. E. Longmans. Originally from the British Library.

Evans, D. (2002). The effectiveness of music as an intervention for hospital patients: A systematic review. *Journal of Advance Nursing*, 37(1): 8–18.

Frankl, V. E. (1963). *Man's Search for Meaning*. New York, NY: Pocket Books.

Joanna Briggs Institute. (2009). Music as an intervention in hospitals. (Best Practice, 13(3)), pp. 13–16.

Kamioka, H., Tsutani, K., Yamada, M., Park, H., Okuizumi, H., Tsuruoka, K., . . . Mutoh, Y. (2014). Effectiveness of music therapy: A summary of systematic reviews based on randomized controlled trials of music interventions. *Patient Preference and Adherence*, 8, 727–754. http://doi.org/10.2147/PPA.S61340

Leow, M. Q.-H. (2011). Music therapy in the palliative setting: A systematic review. *Singapore Nursing Journal*, 38(4): 14–21.

Levitin, D. J. (2006). *This Is Your Brain on Music*. New York, NY: Dutton.

McClean, S., Bunt, L., & Daykin, N. (2012). The healing and spiritual properties of music therapy at a cancer care center. *Journal of Alternative and Complementary Medicine*, 18(4): 402–407. doi: 10.1089/acm.2010.0715

McDermott, O., Crellin, N., Ridder, H., & Orrell, M. (2012). Music therapy in dementia: A narrative systematic review. *International Journal of Geriatric Psychiatry*, 28(8): 781–794. doi: 10.1002/gps.3895

Nightingale, F. (1992). *Notes on Nursing: What It Is and What It Is Not* (commemorative ed.). Philadelphia, PA: Lippincott. (Original work published in 1859.)

Nilsson, U. (2008). The anxiety- and pain-reducing effects of music interventions: A systematic review. *AORN Journal*, 87(4): 780–807.

Pinker, S. (1997). *How the Mind Works*. New York, NY: W.W. Norton.

Rauscher, F. H., Shaw, G. L., & Ky, K. N. (1993). Music and spatial task performance. *Nature*, 365: 611.

Richardson, M. M., Babiak-Vazquez, A. E., & Frankel, M. A. (2008). Music therapy in a comprehensive cancer center. *Journal of the Society for Integrative Oncology*, 6(2): 76–81.

Sacks, O. (2007). *Musicophilia: Tales of Music and the Brain*. New York, NY: Vintage Books, Random House.

Standley, J. (2012). Music therapy research in the NICU: An updated meta-analysis. *Neonatal Network*, 31(5): 311–316. doi: 10.1891/0730-0832.31.5.311

Tomatis, A. A. (1991). *Pourquoi Mozart*. Paris, France: Editions Fixot.

White, J. M. (2001). Music as intervention: A notable endeavor to improve patient outcomes. *Nursing Clinics of North America*, 36(1): 83–92.

Resources

American Music Therapy Association
8455 Colesville Rd., Suite 1000
Silver Spring, MD 20910
301.589.3300
www.musictherapy.org

Brain Music Therapy Center
330 West 58th St., Suite 202
New York, NY 10019
212.581.0821
www.brainmusictreatment.com

Chalice of Repose Project
P.O. Box 169
Mt. Angel, OR 97362
503.845.6089
info@chaliceofrepose.org

Institute of Music in Medicine
(Australia)
P.O. Box 1480
Geelong, VIC 3220
61 3 5224 1227
www.imim.com.au

Lane Community College
Music-Thanatology Training Program
4000 E. 30th Ave.
Eugene, OR 97405
541.463.3000

Music-Thanatology Association
International
www.MTAI.org

Sacred Flight, Marylhurst University
Box 6866
Portland, OR 97228
503.241.3344

Society for the Arts in Healthcare
2647 Connecticut Ave. NW, Suite 200
Washington, DC 20008
202.299.9770
www.thesah.org

22

Biofeedback

*If you are distressed by anything external,
the pain is not due to the thing itself but
to your own estimate of it; and this you
have the power to revoke at any moment.*

MARCUS AURELIUS

*We have not been informed that our
bodies tend to do what they are told, if we
know how to tell them.*

ELMER GREEN

Biofeedback is a method for learned control of physiological responses of the body. It is a relaxation technique that uses electronic equipment to amplify the electrochemical energy produced by body responses. Normally out of conscious awareness, biofeedback provides perceptible information that individuals can use to gain voluntary control over various physiological processes.

BACKGROUND

The experimental data to support the feasibility of learned control first appeared in the 1950s. In 1961, experimental psychologist Neal Miller proposed that the autonomic nervous system was trainable, contrary to beliefs about human physiology at the time. As psychologists and physiologists continued this research, it became clear that dramatic gains could be achieved by using biofeedback information to assist people living with specific conditions, including headaches, ulcers, hypertension, and many other stress-related illnesses. The result of this work was the creation of biofeedback therapy, now widely used by both conventional and alternative practitioners. With the advent of computers, the technology has become more powerful (Schwartz, Collura, Kamiya, & Schwartz, 2016).

PREPARATION

Biofeedback is a useful tool for a variety of health-care professionals including nursing, medicine, and dentistry. People utilizing biofeedback may have diverse reasons ranging from athletes to rehabilitation clients. Since 1981, all biofeedback therapists must have certification from the Biofeedback Certification International Alliance (BCIA). Applicants must hold a bachelor's degree or higher in one of the approved health-care fields. Certification requires 42 hours in didactic biofeedback education and 60 hours in clinical experience. BCIA also offers specialty certificates in neurofeedback (36 hours of didactic information and 220 hours of clinical training) and pelvic muscle dysfunction biofeedback (28 hours of didactic information and 30 hours of clinical training). When applicants meet the requirements, they are allowed to sit for a qualifying examination that consists of both written and practical assessment. The BCIA provides international directories of certified practitioners.

CONCEPTS

The nervous system has two major components: voluntary and involuntary or autonomic. In normal circumstances, the voluntary component is under a person's control. If someone decides to stand, the brain sends a message to the appropriate muscle groups, and the person stands. In contrast, the autonomic nervous system functions without conscious thought. Although individuals may be able to change their rate of respiration, for example, they are not able to consciously stop breathing indefinitely.

People continuously receive biofeedback from their body. When they do not eat, they feel hungry. When they run, they get winded. When they experience stress, their muscles tense. Other types of biofeedback are more difficult to discern. With the use of technology, however, people can learn to adjust their thought processes to control body processes such as blood pressure, temperature, muscle tension, bronchial dilation, gastrointestinal functioning, and brain wave activity. The concept is simple: If individuals can develop sensory awareness of an involuntary function, they can learn to sense it. For example, if skin temperature in the hands is converted into an audible signal, the beeps give one's ears and brain feedback. As people learn to dilate the arteries in their hands, thus raising skin temperature, the beeps speed up, providing instant feedback on what is occurring in the body. Biofeedback teaches people what it feels like to be relaxed internally so that they can recreate the feeling whenever they choose (Anselmo, 2015).

TREATMENT

Biofeedback instruments are highly sensitive electronic devices that monitor physiological processes. Signals from the body are amplified by the instruments and converted into usable information. The instruments may have meters, tones, or a computer display that presents the information to the trainee. Sensors have now been developed that are able to read physiological signals from a distance, which broadens the use of biofeedback.

Temperature or **thermal feedback** is a primary tool for general relaxation training and treatment of specific vascular diseases. Blood flow in the hands responds to stress and relaxation, and clients learn to relax by watching the rise and fall of finger temperature. Thermal feedback may be used to decrease generalized muscle tension in people with temporomandibular joint (TMJ) syndrome. Migraine headaches may be alleviated by simply raising the temperature in the hands. People with Raynaud disease can learn to dilate blood vessels in their hands.

Electrodermal response (EDR) or **galvanic skin response (GSR)** feedback devices measure sweat gland activity of the fingertips or palm. This response is highly sensitive to emotions and thoughts and is used in general relaxation training to help people reduce the impact of significant stressors and anxiety and to treat excessive sweating.

Electromyography (EMG) feedback measures muscle tension with sensors placed on the skin over appropriate muscles. EMG feedback is used for general relaxation training and insomnia due to overactivation of the autonomic nervous system. Biofeedback readings of the masseter muscle are used to treat TMJ. EMG biofeedback is able to detect muscle imbalances, allowing individuals to re-educate the involved muscles. Some people experiencing muscle spasms and back pain benefit from EMG biofeedback. People with spinal cord injuries may use biofeedback to strengthen muscles and provide the sensation of movement. An EMG device has been developed to treat kyphosis, a curvature of the spine. In addition, this type of biofeedback is the primary tool for treatment of tension headache and pain reduction.

Respiratory resistance (R_{os}) biofeedback measures the rate, volume, and rhythm of respiration and is useful in treating both asthma and the hyperventilation of anxiety and panic attacks. **Gastrointestinal biofeedback** is helpful in treating irritable bowel syndrome, colitis, heartburn, functional dyspepsia, and Crohn's disease. **Cardiovascular (EKG) feedback** is available through portable heart rate monitors to augment a person's ability to control heart rate. In addition to being used by persons with cardiac disease, many professional athletes use this system to aid their training.

Pelvic muscle dysfunction biofeedback is used for people with chronic constipation related to pelvic dysfunction. It can also successfully treat incontinence. Sensors measure and report the activity of the internal and external rectal sphincters for the treatment of fecal incontinence and the activity of the detrusor muscle for the treatment of urinary incontinence. Pelvic floor biofeedback is also used to treat sexual problems such as vaginismus, vulvodynia, or postpartum pelvic changes.

Neurofeedback, formerly called *electroencephalograph* (EEG) biofeedback, records information about brain wave activity from sensors placed on the scalp. Changes in brain waves reflect changes in attention as well as in states of arousal from sleep to alert wakefulness. This type of feedback is used for mind quieting, attention control, short-term memory improvement, mood swings, posttraumatic stress disorder, and alcohol and drug addiction. Neurofeedback is helpful in cases of insomnia related to mental or emotional problems. People with brain injuries may experience improvement of symptoms with this type of biofeedback. Other disorders treated with EEG biofeedback include autism, ADHD, Alzheimer's, anxiety, depression, and rapid cycling bipolar disorder.

After the mode of treatment is decided, electrodes are places on the identified body part(s). A computer attached to the electrodes provides feedback information to both the client and the professional via sound tones or a visual image. EEG measurements produce a kind of video game of brain waves. The human brain produces different brain waves during various states of consciousness. Beta waves are associated with normal or waking consciousness, alpha waves are produced in an altered or relaxed state of consciousness, and theta and delta waves are associated with unconscious and sleeping states. When the client produces waves associated with concentration, the game speeds up. The game slows down when brain waves associated with daydreaming are produced. This type of computer system can make learning control of body processes more interactive and fun, especially for children. Increasing health literacy and tracking physical processes are critical components in fostering health and wellness.

Smartphone features are being integrated with biofeedback technologies. There are apps to track heart rate, brain waves, skin nerve impulses, blood pressure, muscle contractions, sleep patterns, and blood oxygenation perfusion index. One example is a multimodal biofeedback system to improve balance. A smartphone is attached to clients with a belt around the waist that measures body sway and sends the data to a PC. The PC provides visual, vibrational, and tactile feedback to clients to improve postural stability (Afzal, Oh, Choi, & Yoon, 2016).

With experience and practice, clients learn to produce the desired results such as improved respiration, decreased pain or spasms, improved heart rate, better balance, improvement in depression or anxiety, mind quieting, or improved bowel function. Training usually requires 8 to 10 sessions with 20 to 30 minutes of daily practice although some people may need fewer or more sessions. Individuals eventually learn how to control the response without using the computer monitor.

A contraindication for biofeedback is that it may increase stress for some individuals who feel overwhelmed by cues and who are unable to change these cues to their desired effect. Frequent connection and focus on the machine may overstimulate the brain. The brain needs "down time" during which the default mode network stimulation allows for the development of the concept of self and for learning and memory consolidation. These unstructured mental times are a key component to mental well-being.

RESEARCH

The following is a sample of research on the effectiveness of biofeedback in a number of conditions:

- A randomized study found that biofeedback reduced postoperative pain in people undergoing total knee arthroplasty (Wang et al., 2015).
- Nursing students experiencing stress and anxiety were randomly assigned to one of three groups: biofeedback, mindfulness meditation, or control. Both the biofeedback and mindfulness meditation groups had significant reduction in anxiety and stress levels (Ratanasiripong, Park, Ratanasiripong, & Kathalae, 2015).
- Children aged 5–16 years experiencing non-neuropathic underactive bladder were randomly assigned to biofeedback and pelvic muscle exercise and standard urotherapy group or to the control group that received only standard urotherapy. There was significant improvement in the sensation of bladder fullness and contractility in the biofeedback/pelvic floor muscle exercise group compared to the control group (Ladi-Seyedian, Kajbafzadeh, Sharifi-Rad, Shadgan, & Fan, 2015).

INTEGRATED NURSING PRACTICE

Certified biofeedback therapists, many of whom are nurses, help interpret signals from monitoring devices while leading the client through physical and mental exercises to achieve the desired change in the body function being measured. As a nurse without specific training, your primary intervention is to provide information about biofeedback to appropriate clients. You can explain the types of monitoring devices and the conditions for which they are typically effective. In addition, you can help individuals find certified therapists. Explain that biofeedback creates a greater awareness of specific body parts and their functions. With training, clients can regulate these functions. Biofeedback helps people relieve or eliminate symptoms, provides an internal locus of control, and helps them reduce their own health-care costs.

TRY THIS
Mind Control of Muscular Strength

- Face your partner. Put your right hand on your partner's shoulder, palm up.
- Clench your right fist, and hold your arm straight.
- Have your partner grasp your elbow with both hands and pull down while you resist. The pull needs to be gradual until you both get a sense of how much force is needed to bend your arm.
- Imagine you are a fire engine or pump. You are rooted to the earth and are drawing water up, and it is pushing through your arm and out your fingers at high speed with tremendous force—such force that nothing can bend your arm.
- Then, place your arm again on your partner's shoulder, this time with the fingers outstretched, holding onto the feeling and the image of the pump pushing water through your arm with great force.
- Ask your partner once more to apply gradual force to bend your arm. You will need to apply a little muscle power, but will find that you can relax and hold steady with much less effort than before.

Source: Rutherford (1996).

Considering the Evidence

Sielski, R., Rief, W., & Glombiewski, J. A. (2016). Efficacy of biofeedback in chronic back pain: A meta-analysis. _International Society of Behavioral Medicine_, 24(1): 25–41. doi: 10.1007/s12529-016-9572-9

What Was the Approach of the Research?
Systematic review using a meta-analysis.

What Was the Aim/Purpose/Objective(s) of the Research as Related to Complementary and Integrative Therapies?
The aim of this meta-analysis was to review studies related to the short- and long-term efficacy of biofeedback on pain outcomes (pain intensity, disability, depression, cognitive coping, and decrease in muscle tension) in persons living with chronic back pain.

How Was the Study Done?
After a library search for relevant published research, 21 studies were identified as appropriate for this meta-analysis. The eligible studies included 23 treatment conditions and 1,062 patients living with back pain. Consistent with systematic review protocol, a literature search using PubMed, PsycINFO, and the Cochrane Library was executed. Related

reference lists from pertinent studies and review papers were manually searched for additional studies meeting the inclusion criteria. Eighteen of the 21 studies implemented EMG-based biofeedback. All included studies included biofeedback training for a minimum of 25% of the intervention time.

What Were the Significant Findings of the Research?

Biofeedback can lead to an improvement in persons living with chronic back pain on a variety of pain-related outcomes (pain intensity, reduction in muscle tension, depression, and cognitive coping) in the short and long term, as a treatment in itself or as an adjunctive intervention. Additionally, cognitive behavioral therapy or physical therapy with enhanced biofeedback may suggest greater improvement in well-being compared to standard programs. However, the researchers suggest that the results of this meta-analysis should be interpreted with caution due to the limited number of studies on this topic and a need for additional research of high methodological quality.

What Additional Questions Might I Have?

Was the duration of biofeedback a factor in improving pain outcome(s)? Would other specific additional therapies combined with biofeedback influence pain outcome(s)? Was the location or type of the back pain a significant factor in achieving pain relief from biofeedback? What interventions might be implemented related to disability in those living with chronic back pain?

What Is the Clinical Significance of This Study?

This study has clinical value for nurses caring for the myriad of persons living with chronic back pain. Nurses should recognize the benefit of biofeedback as a stand-alone therapy or incorporated with other treatments as an option for individuals with chronic back pain. Nurses should be aware that additional studies are needed to strengthen the evidence related to the efficacy of biofeedback to increase confidence in implementing an evidence-based nursing practice.

Source: Contributed by Dolores M. Huffman, RN, PhD.

References

Afzal, M. R., Oh, M.-K., Choi, H. Y., & Yoon, J. (2016). A novel balance training system using multimodal biofeedback. *BioMedical Engineering OnLine.* doi: 10.1186/s12938-016-0160-7

Anselmo, J. (2015). Relaxation. In B. M. Dossey & L. Keegan (Eds.), *Holistic Nursing: A Handbook for Practice* (7th ed., pp. 239–268). Burlington, MA: Jones & Bartlett Learning.

Aurelius, M. (1887). *The Meditations of Marcus Aurelius.* In J. Collier (Trans.) &

A. Zimmern (Ed.), *Sir John Lubbock's Hundred Books* (Vol. 3). Routledge.

Green, E., & Green, A. (1977). *Beyond Biofeedback.* A Merloyd Lawrence Book. Random House Publishing Group.

Ladi-Seyedian S., Kajbafzadeh, A. M., Sharifi-Rad, L., Shadgan, B., & Fan, E. (2015). Management of non-neuropathic underactive bladder in children with voiding dysfunction by animated biofeedback: A randomized clinical trial. *Urology.* doi: 10.1016/j.urology.2014.09.025

Ratanasiripong, P., Park, J. F., Ratanasiripong, N., & Kathalae, D. (2015). Stress and anxiety management in nursing students: Biofeedback and mindfulness meditation. *Journal of Nursing Education.* doi: 10.3928/01484834-20150814-07

Rutherford, L. (1996). *Principles of Shamanism.* San Francisco, CA: Thorsons.

Schwartz, M. S., Collura, T. F., Kamiya, J., & Schwartz, N. M. (2016). The history and definitions of biofeedback and applied psychophysiology. In M. S. Schwartz & F. Andrasik (Eds.), *Biofeedback: A Practitioners Guide* (4th ed., pp. 3–23). New York, NY: Guilford Press.

Wang, T. J., Chang, C. F., Lou, M. F., Ao, M. K., Liu, C. C., Liang, S. Y., . . . Tung, H. H. (2015). Biofeedback relaxation for pain associated with continuous passive motion in Taiwanese patients after total knee arthroplasty. *Research in Nursing & Health.* doi: 10.1002/nur.21633

Resources

Association for Applied Psychophysiology and Biofeedback
10200 West 44th Ave., Suite 304
Wheat Ridge, CO 80033-2840
303.422.8436
www.aapb.org

Biofeedback Certification International Alliance
5310 Ward Rd. Suite 201
Arvada, CO 80002
702.502.5829
www.bcia.org

Biofeedback Foundation of Europe
10 John St.
London WC1N 2EB
44 (0) 1753.56.1111
www.bfe.org

EEG Spectrum International
18017 Chatsworth St., Suite 254
Granada Hills, CA 91344
800.789.3456
www.eegspectrum.com

23

Movement-Oriented Therapies

Walking is man's best medicine.

Hippocrates

A number of therapies focus on movement, body awareness, and breathing, and their purpose is to maintain health as well as to correct specific problems. This chapter presents three Eastern movement-oriented therapies—qigong, t'ai chi, and seiki jutsu—and three Western movement-oriented therapies—the Alexander Technique, the Feldenkrais Method®, and the Trager Approach®. Common to these various approaches is the retraining of one's body to improve coordination and balance, to release and change postural faults, and to relieve structural and functional stress. A major principle is that awareness has to be experienced rather than taught verbally, which may then lead to more effective use of one's whole self.

Qigong, also spelled *Chi Kung, Chi Gong,* and *Chi Gung,* and pronounced "chee-gong," is a Chinese discipline consisting of breathing and mental exercises that may be combined with modest arm movements. Qigong is one of the four pillars of Traditional Chinese Medicine, the others being acupuncture, massage, and herbal medicine. See Chapter 4 for more information on Traditional Chinese Medicine. *Qi* is the term for "vital energy" or "life force," and *gong* means "work" or "discipline." Qigong can be translated as "mastery of qi," "cultivation of energy," "air energy," "breath work," and "energy work." People discover how to generate more energy and conserve what they have to maintain health or treat illness (Cohen, 2015).

T'ai chi, sometimes spelled *taiji,* is pronounced "teye-chee." T'ai chi arose out of qigong and is a discipline that combines physical fitness, meditation, and self-defense. Literally translated, it means "great ultimate fist" and is sometimes translated as "supreme box-ing" or "root of all motion." Although it is considered a martial art, t'ai chi is mainly practiced today as a health discipline (Cohen, 2015).

Seiki jutsu is pronounced as "say-ko ju-jit-su." Its origins are in the early eighth century in Japan. The movements are thought to increase ki or life energy that is present in all living things. The goal is to increase creativity, prevent illness, and support longevity (Keeney & Keeney, 2014).

The **Alexander Technique** is a method for improving postural and movement dysfunction that can lead to pain and disease. It is designed to reduce and eliminate body misuse in daily activities, especially with respect to the head, neck, and shoulders. The **Feldenkrais Method**® uses gentle movement and directed attention to improve movement and enhance func-tioning. The physics of body movement is combined with an awareness of the way people learn to move, behave, and interact. The **Trager Approach**® uses light, rhythmic rocking and shaking movements that loosen joints, ease movement, and release chronic patterns of tension. All three of these Western approaches are considered to be educational in nature as opposed to medical interventions.

BACKGROUND

Written records on qigong go back 4,000 years. For almost all that time, this practice remained a closely guarded family secret, available only to the elite classes in China. This discipline was handed down covertly and was not revealed until the beginning of the 12th century. In the late 1970s, the Chinese government funded several scientific studies of qigong, which had been banned during the Cultural Revolution as a superstitious practice. When a scientific basis was established, the government added qigong to the list of treatment methods offered in Traditional Chinese Medicine hospitals. T'ai chi, a modern offshoot of qigong, began in the 14th century. Some forms are practiced to enhance health, others are used for self-defense, and some are practiced as a competitive sport. T'ai chi gained popularity in the United States in the 1960s as people explored alternatives to conventional medicine. Some experts estimate that more than 800 million people practice qigong or t'ai chi internationally—nearly 20% of the world's population. A somewhat similar treatment, seiki jutsu, developed in Japan (Cohen, 2015; Keeney & Keeney, 2014).

The Alexander Technique was developed more than a century ago by F. M. Alexander, an Australian actor who had lost his voice while performing. He carefully watched himself while speaking and observed that undue mus-cular tension accounted for his vocal problem. He sought a way to eliminate that restriction, and the technique he developed focused on correcting the misuse of the neuromuscular activity of the head, neck, and spine. The Alex-ander Technique is taught in the curriculum of music conservatories, theater schools, and universities throughout the world as a foundation for improved health and creative exploration. It is also a useful tool for helping all individu-als maximize their movement potential (Lynn, 2016).

The Feldenkrais Method® was developed by Moshé Feldenkrais (1904–1984), a Russian-born Israeli physicist, mechanical engineer, and judo expert. After suffering crippling knee injuries, Feldenkrais used his own body as his laboratory and taught himself to walk again. In the process, he developed a system for accessing the power of the central nervous system to improve human functioning (Lynn, 2016).

Milton Trager developed the Trager Approach® in the early 1930s, based on his experience as a boxing trainer. He spent the next 50 years—first as a lay practitioner and later as a physician—expanding and refining his discovery. The Trager Approach® is a method of movement re-education designed to produce positive, pleasurable feelings and tissue changes by means of sensorimotor feedback loops between the mind and the muscles (Delany, 2015).

PREPARATION

For most people, qigong, t'ai chi, and seiki jutsu are personal disciplines. Most practitioners spend 30 to 60 minutes a day doing the exercises. With more intensive practice over many years, some become masters. A t'ai chi master is generally one who has exceptional skill in doing the form or in using the principles in boxing and in life. A qigong master is one who has developed the ability to emit healing energy and has achieved proven success in healing with qi. Masters may also have qualities that are generally considered supernatural in the areas of special insight and spiritual transcendence. Rarely, if ever, will a true master call herself or himself a master. Rather, they say that "the practice is the teacher" and "the qi is the teacher."

It is difficult to learn qigong, t'ai chi, or seiki jutsu from a book, audio recording, or video. While simple forms may be grasped this way, the more complex forms are nearly impossible to learn without a teacher's guidance. In the Chinese tradition, one chooses and remains devoted to a teacher. The teacher–disciple relationship is revered as the only path to advanced skill. The honor and reverence that is bestowed on the teacher is part of the belief system that empowers the disciple.

The American Society for the Alexander Technique is the certifying body for practitioners. A certified teacher must complete a 1,600-hour training program over a minimum of 3 years. The emphasis of the training is on observation and modification of human movement patterns to identify and eliminate sources of movement dysfunction.

All Feldenkrais practitioners must complete 800 hours of training over a period of 4 years. The main purpose of the training is for practitioners to develop a deep understanding of movement, to become aware of their own movement, to become skillful observers of movement in others, and to be able to teach other people to increase their awareness and improve their skills of movement.

The Trager Institute provides training and certifies Trager practitioners. The practitioner training program consists of 154 classroom hours and 180 hours of fieldwork. Students learn the relationship between various groups of muscles and organs that produce patterns of posture and movement. The focus is on the mechanics of movement, the kinesthetic interaction, and principles of neuropatterning underlying movement.

CONCEPTS

Wide Applicability

Almost anyone can participate in movement-oriented therapies. These therapies can be learned by the young and the old, by people physically challenged or physically fit, and by those in good health and those recovering from long-term injury or illness. In China, 80-, 90-, and 100-year-old people get up every morning before dawn to practice qigong or t'ai chi in parks even in the middle of winter. These Eastern practices can be done alone, in pairs, or in large groups (Figure 23.1).

Qi

Qi or ki is the invisible flow of energy that maintains physiological function and the health and well-being of individuals. Imbalance of the flow of energy can be treated in a variety of ways, including by practicing qigong and t'ai chi. The principles underlying these movement-oriented therapies are the same as those used in acupuncture. See Chapter 13 for more detailed information on acupuncture. The "forms," or sequences of movements, are specifically designed to stimulate pressure points all along the body and to encourage deep, rhythmic breathing, which fills the body with life-giving qi. The ultimate

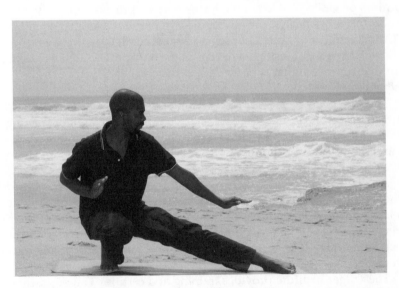

FIGURE 23.1 T'ai Chi Solo Practice by a Young African American Man in Natural Environment

Source: Michaeljung/Shutterstock.

goal is to strengthen the flow of qi through the body to promote health and well-being. When qi is flowing in balance, the body stays healthy and resistant to disease and can activate its own healing efforts.

Qigong and t'ai chi consist of soft, slow, continuous movements that are circular in nature. When practiced by a master, the movements are so slow and fluid that the person appears to be swimming in air. The softness of movements develops energy without nervousness. The slowness of movements requires attentive control that quiets the mind and develops one's powers of awareness and concentration. The continuous circular nature of the movements develops strength and endurance. Yin and yang refer to the balance of forces in the universe. T'ai chi movements are designed to express these forces in balanced form by pairs of opposites. For example, a motion that ultimately involves turning to the right often begins with a small movement to the left. In qigong, students learn to sense their qi and follow it as it moves around the body. As they become more skillful, students learn to strengthen their qi and direct it to specific areas of the body that are weak or ailing (Cohen, 2015).

Seiki jutsu uses more improvisational or spontaneous movements than qigong and t'ai chi. Movements vary from simple—rocking, swinging arms—to more complex dance-like movements. While qigong and t'ai chi are done in silence, seiki jutsu encourages participants to say whatever words, chants, or songs occur to them while moving (Keeney & Keeney, 2014).

Movement Patterns

The human body is like a remarkable instrument, capable of responding with flexibility and resilience. But as the years pass, people often develop habitual reactions, beliefs, and movement patterns that cause physical and mental strain. These habits are typically expressed by tight muscles, collapsed posture, or lack of mobility. When muscles are working overtime, people eventually feel tight, tense, heavy, or tired. The sources of these problems are many—injury, illness, or stress. Lifelong misuse of muscles arises from sitting, standing, or walking incorrectly or too much sitting and too little walking. For example, years of walking incorrectly can create back or knee problems. A knee replacement is only a temporary solution because the real problem lies not in the knee but in the way the person moves from the hip. Movement-oriented practitioners believe that the only lasting remedy is in re-educating the body to walk correctly to avoid injuring the knee. Likewise, back problems can be eliminated by learning appropriate ways of moving (Brennan, 2012).

Sensory-movement activities are used to increase people's sense of postural awareness, free them from habitual patterns, and restore the proper use of muscles. Practitioners lead students through movements to enable them to discover a more fluid range of motion. As people develop new, alternative ways of moving, they experience positive sensory feelings and learn what it is like to be freer and lighter. The goal is to teach people how to move with minimum effort and maximum efficiency through increased consciousness of how their bodies work.

TREATMENT

Qigong is an easy and nontiring exercise that contains sets of moves designed to gather qi. Most people spend 30 minutes a day doing the exercises and another 30 minutes in meditation (Figure 23.2). Some forms are quite complex. For example, Wild Goose Qigong has two sections with 64 movements in each section. Although it is difficult to learn, Wild Goose Qigong is exceptionally beautiful. In China, the goose is considered to be a marvelous creature that flies high into the clouds to gather cosmic energy and information and bring it to earth. Guo Lin Gong, a walking form of qigong, is practiced in China particularly by people with cancer. Improvements have been documented in a wide range of conditions such as stroke, hypertension, spinal cord injuries, multiple sclerosis, joint disease, cerebral palsy, headaches, and many forms of cancer (Zhang, 2008).

Yang, the most popular form of t'ai chi, was developed in the early 20th century by Yang Cheng Fu. It comprises 108 separate motions that can take 6 to 12 months to learn. When the movements are strung together, the result is a cross between slow-motion shadow boxing and dancing. Each movement has a name, such as "repulse the monkey," "the snake creeps down," "the white crane spreads its wings," or "parting the wild horse's mane," which describes what it looks like or what purpose it serves. For example, when one is trying to concentrate, monkey thoughts are distractions. As the monkey is pushed away, the person is not allowing distractions to take attention away from the process of the moment. T'ai chi also incorporates

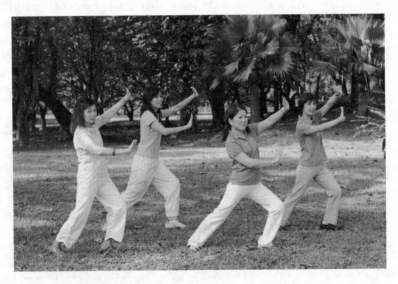

FIGURE 23.2   Qigong Group Practice by Asian Ladies in the Park

Source: Phil Date/Shutterstock.

breathing exercises for improving and strengthening the flow of qi. One form involves reversed breathing, which is contracting the stomach with the in-breath and expanding the stomach with the out-breath. The benefits of t'ai chi are seen in conditions such as hypertension, osteoporosis, and arthritis. T'ai chi can decrease stress and fatigue, improve mood, and increase energy. It is beneficial to cardiorespiratory function, balance, and flexibility (Liao, 2012).

Water t'ai chi is a combination of the principles of water exercise and t'ai chi movements. It is performed upright in chest-deep water, which allows the arms to be totally submerged and the body to be adequately stabilized. Water provides about 12 times the resistance of air, so the body naturally moves more slowly in the water. The exercises improve strength, flexibility, balance, coordination, and posture.

The Alexander Technique includes simple movements that improve balance, posture, and coordination and relieve pain. During a session, the client goes through a series of standing and seated exercises while the practitioner applies light pressure to points of contraction in the body. The techniques help people learn how to use their body with less tension and more awareness. The recommended course is 30 lessons, depending on the client's participation and initial level of functioning (Lynn, 2016).

The Feldenkrais Method® consists of two parts: awareness through movement and functional integration. They are convenient labels for doing essentially the same thing in different ways. Awareness through movement is more like conventional exercises in format, with the teacher guiding a group class verbally rather than using personal manipulation. The lessons consist of comfortable, easy movements that gradually increase in range and complexity designed for all levels of movement ability. Functional integration is a hands-on lesson that usually lasts 45 minutes to an hour and is performed with the client fully clothed and standing, sitting, or lying on a table. The practitioner touches and moves the client in gentle, noninvasive ways. The intent of this touch is to explore the person's responses to touch and movement and then to suggest alternative ways of moving.

Feldenkrais exercises are small, gentle movements, such as pelvic tilts—slowly and deliberately lifting the spine from the coccyx to the waist, one vertebra at a time. To be effective, the movements must be effortless. If exercise becomes painful, no learning takes place because the brain is too focused on how to stop doing the painful activity. Feldenkrais exercises are said to improve flexibility, posture, range of motion, relaxation, ease of movement, physical performance, vitality, and well-being. They are also said to relieve joint pain, stress, muscle tension, low back pain, neck and shoulder pain, jaw pain, and headaches (Lynn, 2016).

The Trager Approach® is a process of using motion in muscles and joints to produce particular sensory feelings. These feelings are relayed to the central nervous system, and then, through the process of feedback loops, the feelings trigger changes in the tissues. A Trager session takes 60 to 90 minutes with the client wearing a swimming suit and lying on a well-padded table. The practitioner touches in such a gentle rhythmic way that the person actually experiences the possibility of being able to move each part of the body freely and effortlessly. Because active participation of the client is discouraged, the passive body can freely learn new movements. Trager practitioners work in a meditative state they call "hook-up." This state allows the practitioner to connect deeply with the client in an unforced way, to remain continually aware of the slightest responses, and to work efficiently without fatigue (Delany, 2015).

Following this session, the client is given instruction in the use of *mentastics*, a system of simple, effortless movement sequences designed to maintain and even enhance the sense of lightness, freedom, and flexibility that was instilled during the treatment session. Mentastics, Dr. Trager's coined term for "mental gymnastics," is a powerful means of reinforcing positive changes. The Trager Approach® is said to decrease various types of chronic pain, headaches, and temporomandibular joint pain, improve muscle spasms, and aid in recovery from stroke and spinal cord injuries.

RESEARCH

A Joanna Briggs Institute evidence summary recommends that t'ai chi be used to improve the sleep status of older adults (Rathnayake, 2011). Another JBI evidence summary states there is not enough evidence to recommend the use of the Feldenkrais Method® for mobility and balance in older adults and that clinician judgment and client preference should be the determining factors (Kunde, 2012).

The following is a small sample of current studies:

- A systematic review and meta-analysis of t'ai chi and qigong in persons with Parkinson's disease showed significant improvement in motor function and balance (Yang et al., 2015).
- A systematic review and meta-analysis found that t'ai chi and qigong when practiced in conjunction with usual medications showed significant improvement in mobility and balance in persons with Parkinson's disease (Ni, Liu, Lu, Shi, & Guo, 2014).
- A systematic review and meta-analysis of traditional Chinese exercise for persons with cardiovascular disease found significant improvement in blood pressure, physical functioning, quality of life, and depression (Wang et al., 2016).
- A randomized controlled trial compared the Alexander Technique with local heat and guided imagery on pain and quality of life in people with chronic, nonspecific neck pain. Local heat and the Alexander Technique had the same outcome on pain. However, the Alexander Technique demonstrated significant improvement in the quality of life compared to the guided imagery group (Lauche et al., 2016).

- A randomized controlled trial compared seated t'ai chi to usual activities in older persons using wheelchairs. The t'ai chi group had significantly higher scores in quality of life, physical health, emotional health, and social relations and less depression compared to the usual activities group (Hsu, Moyle, Cooke, & Jones, 2016).
- A randomized controlled trial compared home-based t'ai chi with lower extremity training in older people who had a history of falls. The t'ai chi group was significantly less likely to fall during the 6-month intervention and the 6-month follow-up than the group having lower extremity training (Hwang et al., 2016).
- A controlled randomized trial found that people with Parkinson's disease demonstrated significant improvement in quality of life and level of depression when engaged in 50 sessions of Feldenkrais exercise (Teixeira-Machado et al., 2015).

INTEGRATED NURSING PRACTICE

Like most other moderate physical activities practiced on a daily basis, t'ai chi, qigong, and seiki jutsu can improve balance, stability, agility, flexibility, stamina, and muscle tone. They are good exercise for people who are already in shape, but they can also be adapted for older adults, children, or people with injury or illness. The movements are gentle and put less stress on the body than do other exercises. The breathing exercises are a form of meditation that quiets the mind and reduces the negative effects of stress.

If you and others are healthy and wish to maintain your health, learning t'ai chi or qigong is highly recommended. Experienced practitioners spend at least 20 and up to 60 minutes in daily practice. As a nurse, you can encourage your clients to consider practicing one of these forms. For those who are struggling with illness or disability, it is important that they build up stamina over a period of time. Clients who are seriously ill may be able to do only the simple breath practice as they focus on absorbing healing qi from the environment. When they can manage it, they add simple hand gestures to the breathing. As they continue to improve, they sit in a chair and do the hand motions, moving to a standing position when they feel able. Finally, they do the walking form.

When starting t'ai chi and qigong, it is best to begin with simple exercises. You can teach people a few basic principles of standing and moving so that they can begin to feel what it is like to inhabit their body with awareness. Getting the body into alignment is the most important part of these movement therapies. Instruct your clients to stand with their feet shoulder-width apart, buttocks tucked in, spine straight, shoulder relaxed, knees unlocked, and the head straight and resting lightly on top of the spine as if a string from the top of the head were gently suspending the body from above. As they are standing in this position, have them pay attention to their own breathing, inhaling deeply and exhaling completely. Also in this position, have your clients locate their *tan t'ien* (pronounced "don-tee-en"), which is the body's center of gravity and stability, located about 1½ inches below the navel and toward the center of the body. T'ai chi and qigong teach individuals to find and maintain their center through movement, whereas in meditation and yoga, they center themselves in stillness. The tan t'ien is considered to be the source of energy, and as they practice, your clients will find that all the movements begin to flow more easily as they learn to move from the tan t'ien.

Two movements in t'ai chi common to various sequences are the t'ai chi fist and the t'ai chi ball. The fist is formed by imagining a robin's egg in the center of each palm and then slowly curling one finger at a time around the egg, beginning with the little finger and ending with the thumb resting lightly on top. Throughout all the forms, frequent references are made to "picking up the ball." Have clients visualize forming a ball out of the air and picking it up and moving with it. The ball is designed to help movements flow more easily.

The tree or the horse-riding stance contributes to a sense of rootedness and stability in the body. For this posture, instruct your clients to separate their legs wider than their shoulders and bend their knees so that their thighs are parallel to the floor, thus lowering the center of gravity closer to the earth. The top part of the body feels light, while the lower half feels heavy. At first, the position may feel strenuous, because the muscles in the legs have not been used in this way. With practice, people enjoy the feeling of stability it gives them. Next, direct your clients to bring their arms up as if embracing an invisible person, joining their fingertips in front of them. Direct them to slowly turn from side to side, letting their waist initiate the movement. Their legs should feel "soft," so that they follow the movement led by the waist. Their gaze should travel slowly across an imagined horizon.

T'ai chi and qigong are popular, and lessons are available in most towns and cities. They are taught in health clubs, schools, YMCAs, community centers, hospitals, clinics, and other facilities. Explain to your clients that it is useful, in most cases, to begin with a teacher. They can ask around to find a teacher whom others like, or they can observe a class or participate in a trial class. Some people try several teachers or forms before they find the one that meets their personal preferences. Encourage clients to find general forms they like and will do regularly. If possible, they should try to find a place to learn that is convenient. If it is too far, it may become difficult for people to continue in the practice. As t'ai chi and qigong have become more popular, people can be found practicing in parks. In some cases, individuals prefer to have time alone in nature. Often, however, people are happy to have others join them, and frequently, informal groups form. These groups may develop socially as people get to know one another and socialize after the practice.

The claims for the Alexander Technique, the Feldenkrais Method®, and the Trager Approach® focus more on enhancing well-being than on healing illness. They are designed to relieve muscle tension, increase relaxation, reduce stress, and alter poor habits of posture and movement in those who are healthy. Refer clients to the appropriate associations to locate certified teachers of these techniques.

TRY THIS

Feel Your Qi

- Stand with your feet shoulder-width apart, your knees slightly bent, your spine upright, and your shoulders relaxed. Breathe easily.
- Start to flex or bounce gently at the knees.
- Still bouncing, shift your weight back and forth from your right to your left leg.
- Keep your breathing relaxed and deep.
- Begin to snap all your fingers, flipping each one past your thumb.
- Then, still bouncing and finger-snapping, twist at your waist, to the right, then to the left.
- While you are doing all this, make your exhale a sigh of relief. Do five of these sighs in a slow, relaxed manner.
- Then, stop and close your eyes and turn your attention inward. Feel the buzzing, humming, or tingling sensation that is in your hands, legs, and body. This is qi. You are literally feeling the activity of the profound medicine you have produced within yourself.

Source: Jahnke (2002).

TRY THIS

Wave Hands Like Clouds (Water T'ai Chi)

- Stand in chest-deep water with your feet several inches apart.
- Lift your arms to shoulder level.
- Step laterally with the right foot.
- Circle both arms under and out of the water—the right arm clockwise and the left arm counterclockwise.
- Repeat four times.
- Step laterally with the left foot.
- Repeat the arm sequence four times.

Considering the Evidence

Chang, W. D., Chen, S., Lee, C. L., Lin, H. Y., & Lai, P. T. (2016). The effects of Tai Chi Chuan on improving mind–body health for knee osteoarthritis patients: A systematic review and meta-analysis. *Evidence-Based Complementary and Alternative Medicine*, 2016: 1–10. doi: 10.1155/2016/1813979

What Was the Approach of the Research?

Systematic review using meta-analysis.

What Was the Aim/Purpose/Objective(s) of the Research as Related to Complementary and Integrative Therapies?

The objective of this systematic review using meta-analysis was to evaluate and summarize the evidence exploring the mental and physical effects of Tai Chi Chuan when managing knee osteoarthritis.

How Was the Study Done?

Based on the protocol used for systematic reviews, the researchers included the following databases in searching for studies meeting inclusion criteria: MEDLINE, PubMed, EMBASE, and CINAHL. Data from the identified studies were collected, and outcomes were classified using the International Classification of Functioning, Disability, and Health model. Eleven studies met the inclusion criteria for this systematic review.

What Were the Significant Findings of the Research?

Tai Chi Chuan had positive effects for persons living with osteoarthritis. Reviewed studies found that Tai Chi Chuan participants demonstrated improvement in knee extension endurance, aerobic capacity, and body balance and coordination. Due to insufficient data in the reviewed studies, there is not enough evidence to support the benefits of Tai Chi Chuan on the mental effect on patients with knee osteoarthritis.

What Additional Questions Might I Have?

Are there any adverse or harmful effects associated with Tai Chi Chuan as an intervention in persons living with osteoarthritis? What would be the effect of Tai Chi Chuan in combination with other complementary and integrative therapies in managing osteoarthritis? Are there variations in arthritis that would warrant restrictions in movement associated with Tai Chi Chuan? Are there restrictions in terms of intensity, duration, and frequency of Tai Chi Chuan that should be considered in managing osteoarthritis? Are there plans for future longitudinal studies that focus on the mental effects of Tai Chi Chuan?

What Is the Clinical Significance of This Study?

This systematic review has considerable value for nurses caring for our expanding aging population frequently living with osteoarthritis. Nurses should be cognizant that this intervention may add to the quality of life for those with osteoarthritis as it has the potential to enhance mobility and may influence the ability to engage in social events. Participants in Tai Chi Chuan may also experience a delay of medical interventions such as planned surgeries to address the pain and limitations associated with living with osteoarthritis.

Source: Contributed by Dolores M. Huffman, RN, PhD.

References

Brennan, R. (2012). *Change Your Posture, Change Your Life.* London, UK: Watkins.

Cohen, M. R. (2015). *The New Chinese Medicine Handbook.* Beverly, MA: Quarto Publishing.

Delany, J. (2015). Massage, bodywork, and touch therapies. In M. S. Micozzi (Ed.), *Fundamentals of Complementary and Alternative Medicine* (7th ed., pp. 247–274). St. Louis, MO: Elsevier, Saunders.

Hippocrates. (1983). *Hippocratic Writings* (Vol. 451). Edited by G. E. R. Lloyd, J. Chadwick, & W. N. Mann. Penguin Books Limited.

Hsu, C. Y., Moyle, W., Cooke, M., & Jones, C. (2016). Seated tai chi versus usual activities in older people using wheelchairs: A randomized controlled trial. *Complementary Therapies in Medicine,* 24: 1–6. doi: 10.1016/j.ctim.2015.11.006

Hwang, H. F., Chen, S. J., Lee-Hsieh, J., Chien, D. K., Chen, C. Y., & Lin, M. R. (2016). Effects of home-based tai chi and lower extremity training and self-practice on falls and functional outcomes in older fallers from the emergency department: A randomized controlled trial. *Journal of the American Geriatric Society,* 3: 518–125. doi: 10.1111/jgs.13952

Jahnke, R. (2002). *The Healing Promise of Qi.* New York, NY: Contemporary Books.

Keeney, B., & Keeney, H. (2014). *Seiki Jutsu: The Practice of Non-Subtle Energy Medicine.* Rochester, VT: Healing Arts Press.

Kunde, L. (2012). Feldenkrais Method. Joanna Briggs Institute Evidence Summary. Retrieved from http://connect. jbiconnectplus.org/ViewDocument. aspx?0=6331

Lauche, R., Schuth, M., Schwickert, M., Ludtke, R., Musial, F., Michalsen, A., . . . Choi, K. E. (2016). Efficacy of the Alexander Technique in treating chronic non-specific neck pain: A randomized controlled trial. *Clinical Rehabilitation,* 3: 247–258. doi: 10.1177/0269215515578699

Liao, W. (2012). *Restoring Your Life Energy.* Boston, MA: Shambhala.

Lynn, G. (2016). *Awakening Somatic Intelligence: Understanding, Learning & Activating the Alexander Technique, Feldenkrais Method & Hatha Yoga.* London: Singing Dragon.

Ni, X., Liu, S., Lu, F., Shi, X., & Guo, X. (2014). Efficacy and safety of tai chi for Parkinson's disease: A systematic review and meta-analysis of randomized controlled trials. *PLoS One,* 9(6): e99377. doi: 10.1371/journal.pone .0099377

Rathnayake, T. (2011). Sleep problems (adults 60+): Physical exercise. Joanna Briggs Institute Evidence Summary. Retrieved from http://connect .jbiconnectplus.org/ViewDocument .aspx?0=5639

Teixeira-Machado, L., Araujo, F. M., Cunha, F. A., Menezes, M., Menezes, T., & Melo DeSantana, J. (2015). Feldenkrais method-based exercise improves quality of life in individuals with Parkinson's disease: A controlled, randomized clinical trial. *Alternative Therapies in Health and Medicine*, 21(1): 8–14.

Wang, X.-Q., Pi, Y.-L., Chen, P.-J., Liu, Y., Wang, R., Li, X., . . . Niu, Z.-B. (2016). Traditional Chinese exercise for cardiovascular diseases: A systematic review and meta-analysis of randomized controlled trials. *Journal of the American Heart Association*, 3: e002562. doi: 10.1161/JAHA.115.002562

Yang, Y., Qiu, W. Q., Hao, Y. L., Lv, Z. Y., Jiao, S. J., & Teng, J. F. (2015). The efficacy of traditional Chinese medical exercise for Parkinson's disease: A systematic review and meta-analysis. *PLoS One*, 10(4): e0122469. doi: 10.1371/journal.pone.0122469

Zhang, T. C. (2008). *Earth Qi Gong for Women*. Berkeley, CA: Blue Snake Books.

Resources

American Society for the Alexander Technique
11 West Monument Ave., Suite 510
Dayton, OH 45402-0620
800.473.0620
www.amsatonline.org

East West Academy of Healing Arts
www.eastwestqi.com

Feldenkrais Method® of Somatic Education
401 Edgewater Place, Suite 600
Wakefield, MA 01880
781.645.8935
www.feldenkrais.com

Tai Chi Australia
www.taichiaustralia.com

International College of Medical Qigong
73145 Guadalupe Ave.
Palm Desert, CA 92260
www.medicalqigong.org

Qigong Institute
www.qigonginstitute.org

Spiritual Therapies

Regard heaven as your father,
Earth as your mother,
And all things as your brothers
and sisters.

NATIVE AMERICAN PROVERB

24

Shamans

Few people even scratch the surface,
much less exhaust the contemplation
of their own experience.

RANDOLPH BOURNE

Shaman (pronounced "SHAH-min") is a word from the Tungus people of Siberia. This term has been adopted widely by anthropologists to refer to those known in the West as "medicine men," "witch doctors," "witches," "magicians," and "seers." Not every kind of medicine person or witch doctor, however, is a shaman. A shaman is a woman or man who enters an altered state of consciousness, at will, to contact and utilize another type of reality to acquire knowledge and power and to help other people. Shamans use ancient techniques to achieve and maintain well-being and healing for themselves and members of their communities, serving as a link between the worlds of matter and spirit. Shamanism is not a belief system. Rather, it is a broad umbrella covering ancient, indigenous, and holistic healing practices worldwide. Shamanism is a living spiritual system and as such continues to evolve as culture and knowledge change over time (Matthews, 2014). For further information on Native American healers, see Chapter 6.

BACKGROUND

The origins of shamanism date to at least 40,000 to 50,000 years ago, to Stone Age times, making it the oldest of all healing therapies. Worldwide, evidence from ancient cave drawings and similar records supports the conclusions that indigenous peoples shared a similar understanding of how the universe works, how to maintain health and strength, how to cope with serious illness, and how to deal with the trauma of death. One of the most remarkable aspects of shamanism is that concepts and treatment methods are similar in widely separated and remote parts of the planet among peoples isolated from one another. Anthropologists have studied shamanism in North, Central, and South America, Africa, Australia, Indonesia, Malaysia, Bali, Tibet, Korea, Siberia, and across Europe and have found that shamans functioned fundamentally in much the same way and with similar techniques worldwide. The basic uniformity suggests that, through trial and error, people arrived at the same conclusions (Hewson, 2015; Rysdyk, 2016).

Today, shamanism survives in many regions of the world in spite of the advent of Western scientific medicine. There is no equivalent health professional in Western medicine, and the scope of the shaman as a healer extends beyond the capacities and expertise of physicians. The field of holistic medicine is reclaiming many techniques long practiced in shamanism, such as visualization, altered state of consciousness, hypnotherapy, meditation, positive attitude, and stress reduction. Shamanic healing is rapidly gaining popularity among urban Americans as people turn back to the old cultures for help and guidance in finding a better balance with nature and with themselves. Shamanic practice and biomedical treatment are not in conflict. Contemporary shamans are perfectly willing to have their patients see a conventional physician, because the primary goal is wellness. Any kind of technological treatment or medication that will contribute to the strength of the patient is welcomed (Hewson, 2015).

PREPARATION

People discover in a wide variety of ways that their purpose in life is to become a shaman. Often, potential healers have prophetic dreams about their future calling. The dream may even include details about locating a teacher and how long the training period will be. In some cases, individuals are led to shamanism through personal and private mystical experiences, while others come from the ranks of cured patients.

The journey from apprentice to shaman is illustrated in the following example of Native American shamans. The first step is "embracing personal history." This process includes working through old traumas, fears, anger, hate, abandonment, betrayals, and wounds. The purpose is to heal the emotions so that one is no longer controlled by them but, rather, is consciously guided by feelings. The second step is "facing death and making death an ally." This step means examining one's attitudes and beliefs to "put to death" any that are inaccurate or outdated. It includes remembering that bodies are temporary and will one day be claimed by death. It also means moving beyond personal history and recognizing that all people are part of a family, village, tribe, city, country, and ultimately all humanity. The third step is "stopping the world," which involves clearing the mind of its mental garbage. The fourth step is "controlling the dream and finding new vision and purpose." It is the time to quest for vision and seek direct connection with the dream world and its spiritual teachers. The **vision quest** is part of many old-world cultures and is a time when one fasts and prays in a sacred place, often on a mountaintop, for up to 4 days and nights. The person prays for a vision and thus a reconnection with the Creator and Creation. Following the vision quest, the person is expected to make life changes that were called for. The fifth and final step is taking full responsibility for all one's actions without guilt or shame. Apprentice shamans follow this path of transformation as they become healers and helpers in service to other people (Mackinnon, 2016).

Those who would be healers in Africa must first suffer a mysterious illness that does not respond to treatment. This is followed by dreams where ancestral spirits call the person to become a healer. The person is then both treated and taken on an as apprentice by an established traditional healer. The apprenticeship is long and strenuous and often lasts a number of years.

Shamanic initiation is experiential and often gradual. Shamans must learn how to achieve the shamanic state of consciousness, must become familiar with their own guardian spirits, and must successfully help others as a shaman. After learning the basic principles and methods, new shamans extend their knowledge and power by shamanic journeying. The few shamans who become true masters of knowledge, power, and healing must have many years of shamanic experience.

CONCEPTS

Environment

For the shaman, everything exists as part of an infinite web of life. Plants, stones, and the earth are all perceptive beings; they are all consciously aware and have a story to tell. In the shamanistic tradition, people communicate intimately and lovingly with "all their relations," as the Lakota would say, talking not just with other people but also with animals, plants, and all the elements of the environment, including rocks and water. From the shaman's viewpoint, one's surroundings are not "environment" but family. The shaman has a deep respect for all forms of life and a great awareness of dependence on the environment. Shamans believe their powers are the powers of the animals, of the plants, of the sun, and of the basic energies of the universe. They are expected to live in harmony with nature and to provide strength in daily life and help save others from illness and death (Mackinnon, 2016).

Power

In shamanism, the preservation of one's personal power is fundamental to well-being. Specific shamanic methods restore and maintain personal power and use it to help others who are weak, ill, or injured. In shamanism, the word *medicine* means "vital force" or "energy." People's medicine is their power, their knowledge, and their expression of their life energy.

Many shamans keep power objects—their medicine—in a medicine bundle. This bundle is normally kept wrapped up and is unrolled publicly only on ritual occasions. The objects inside are highly personal, and, as with other matters of power, one does not boast of them because to do so might result in loss of power. Almost any small object can be included, but the quartz crystal is highly prized among the shamans of North and South America, Australia, Southeast Asia, and elsewhere. Quartz crystals are six-sided stones that are usually transparent to milky white and, in a sense, appear to be "solidified light." The quartz crystal is considered the strongest power object and is viewed as a spirit helper. For thousands of years, shamans have used their quartz crystals for power in seeing and divination. Interestingly, in modern physics, the quartz crystal is also involved in the manipulation of power. Its remarkable electronic properties made it a basic component in early radio transmitters and receivers. Later, quartz crystals became basic components for modern electronic hardware such as computers and timepieces (Rysdyk, 2013).

State of Consciousness

The **ordinary state of consciousness (OSC)** is a consensus of what reality is. This OSC, also called "ordinary reality" or simply "reality," is determined by every society and learned by individuals from childhood. Reality, then, is composed of predetermined expectations. For example, in Western societies, people are not surprised when they insert a card in a machine and money comes out. Another characteristic of Western ordinary reality is that it can be measured and quantified. As Candace Pert (1997) stated, "Measurement! It is the very foundation of the modern scientific method, the means by which the material world is admitted into existence. Unless we can measure something, science won't concede it exists, which is why science refuses to deal with such 'nonthings' as the emotions, the mind, the soul, or the spirit" (p. 21).

Nonordinary realities are other levels of consciousness. They can be experienced during dreaming or induced by drugs, fasting, sleep deprivation, or environmental factors. In Western society, this level of consciousness is often viewed as psychosis rather than another legitimate reality.

Shamans move, at will and with serious intention, between an ordinary state of consciousness and a **shamanic state of consciousness (SSC)**. The SSC is an altered state of consciousness that may vary from a light to a deep trance. Shamans journey back and forth between these realities for the specific purpose of healing or aiding the community in some manner. Shamans operate in nonordinary reality or SSC for only a small portion of the time and then only as needed to perform shamanic tasks. During this trance state, shamans' souls are believed to leave their bodies and either ascend to the upper world or descend to the lower world. Unlike the altered state of consciousness during dreaming, the SSC is a conscious waking state, and at any time, shamans can will themselves out of it, back into the OSC. The experience is like a waking dream in which shamans can control their actions and direct their adventures. Unlike a mind-altering drug experience, the SSC experience is not dependent on a chemically determined length of time, nor does it risk the possibility of being locked into a "bad trip" (Rysdyk, 2016).

Shamanic Cosmology

Shamanic cultures throughout the world have a three-tiered cosmology or way of viewing the universe. The *middle world* is the world of OSC or ordinary reality. It is the world of matter and the world in which people live their daily lives. The lower world and the upper world are SSC worlds, nonordinary reality, or worlds of the spirit, not to be confused with heaven and hell. These worlds are just as real as the ordinary reality of the middle world.

The *lower world* is the world of **power animals.** These archetypical energies take the form of animal guides who have knowledge and wisdom to share and help people navigate through life. Power animals tend to provide practical help and guidance. The capability of power animals to speak to humans is an indication of their power. The belief that shamans can shape-shift into the form of their power animal is common to many cultures. Sharing the identity of one's power animal varies among shamans. Some speak publicly about them, while others fear that disclosing the animal's identity may cause it to leave the person. Many cultures believe that every person is born with a particular animal spirit that is to be their guide throughout life. A similar belief in Western cultures is that of guardian angels watching over people, especially children (Matthews, 2014; Rysdyk, 2016).

The *upper world* is the world of **spirit guides,** who are beings that look more like people and are more familiar to most individuals. It is in the upper world that people meet their guardian angels. The help from spirit guides tends to be more general and philosophical in comparison with the practical help from the lower world. These worlds are complementary and equal, and neither is superior to the other.

Power animals and spirit guides teach people how to empower themselves, improve their lives, and even heal themselves. One does not have to be a shaman to make contact with one's personal power animal and spirit guide. The most traditional method of accessing this nonordinary reality is the shamanic journey.

Imagination

Most indigenous people make little distinction between what Westerners call *imagination* and reality. Imagination is just as real and just as concrete as ordinary reality. In fact, most of the material things of the "real" world were someone's imagination first. Automobiles, televisions, and computers originated in the imaginary realm. In fact, logic and reason have always been preceded by imagination. Western people often ask whether the power animals and guardian spirits are real or imagined. If the information that is received from power animals and guardian spirits empowers people, improves their lives, and helps them heal, the question does not apply. Power animals and guardian spirits are real because people's lives are changed (Sandore, 1997).

VIEW OF HEALTH AND ILLNESS

In the shamanic worldview, the ability to maintain good health is a matter of power. If the body is "power-full," it resists the intrusion of external, harmful forces. No room is available for disease and illness in a power-filled body. Being power-full is like having a protective force field surrounding the body. Possession of guardian spirit power is also fundamental to health. From a shamanic point of view, illnesses usually are intrusions that break the force field of power-fullness. In some ways, this concept is not too different from the biomedical concept of infection. Serious illness and other misfortunes are usually only possible when people are "dis-spirited," meaning they have lost their power and their guardian spirits. This loss results in an inability to fight off unwanted intrusions. Illness is viewed as a separation—from one's power, from one's guardians, from nature, from community, and from the Great Spirit. Even Western everyday language reflects this view when people say, "I'm having a low-energy day," or "I wasn't myself last night."

Severe trauma can result in soul loss, a natural survival mechanism. It is believed that a part of one's self or soul goes into hiding to ensure that the individual will survive the extreme stress. Western psychiatrists refer to this phenomenon as *dissociation*. Some people believe that soul loss occurs when people stop being generous and become selfish and dishonest. Sometimes, people's souls remain lost until they go through a process of soul retrieval. Symptoms of soul loss are an inability to focus and concentrate, a lack of connection to one's emotions, a feeling of being "spaced out" and not really present, a feeling of being an observer of life, or chronic depression. Soul retrieval, much like the process of psychotherapy, brings buried memories and emotions back to the surface (Tobert, 2017).

The Hmong believe there are two treatments of illness. Natural causes of illness are treated with herbs and massage. Supernatural causes of illness are more serious, and treatment consists of a shaman journeying to the spirit world. Hmong people living in the West are often willing to use Western medicine for acute illnesses (Baker, Dang, Ly, & Diaz, 2010).

In Africa, illness is believed to be caused by emotional or spiritual conflicts or by conflicts with other people, living or dead. Treatment may be herbal, a purification process, and/or appeasing bad spirits. Spirituality and psychosocial relationships are an important aspect of the healing process (Hewson, 2015).

Tribal peoples of the Amazon believe that some diseases are the result of natural processes and some are the consequence of social or cosmic problems. Diseases are further classified as spiritual or nonspiritual in origin (Herndon et al., 2009).

TREATMENT

The goal of treatment is integration and wholeness. Shamans use a wide variety of interventions, including ceremonies, stories, rhythms, sounds, movements, meditation, and herbs and plant medicine. It is a complex "dance" of examination, communication, ritual, and interventions. More detailed information on treatment modalities utilized by Native American shamans is found in Chapter 6.

Shamans may be called on to help those who have become ill or those who have lost their power, their spirit guides, or even their souls. In such cases, shamans use the shamanic journey to recover that which was lost. Shamans also journey to gather information to help and guide individuals or groups, to solve problems, and to answer questions. Shamans, by offering their total commitment to a patient for as long as several days, develop intense relationships that underscore the importance of caring as well as curing in the shamanic healing tradition. In old cultures, shamans would do the journeying for patients, but in today's world, anyone can experience a shamanic journey. Through this process people meet and talk with their power animals and spirit guides and restore their own power and self-healing (Mackinnon, 2016).

Basic tools for entering the shamanic state of consciousness prior to the shamanic journey are the drum, which provides lower vibrations, and the rattle, which provides higher vibrations. A drumbeat at a steady 200 to 280 beats per minute serves as a focus for concentration and quiets the chattering mind. The tempo of the drumbeat corresponds to theta brain waves associated with the hypnotic state, facilitating the move into nonordinary reality. It is a remarkably safe practice for most people because one can return to an ordinary state of consciousness at any time. Some people add dancing or chanting to the drumbeat as another way to reach this altered state of consciousness (Hove et al., 2016).

Some shamans use teacher plants as a catalyst to the shamanic journey. Among the many teacher plants worldwide are peyote, San Pedro cactus, ayahuasca, psilocybin, and red-and-white mushrooms. Shamans consider these plants to be gifts to be used with care and awareness. Their use is never intended to be recreational but rather as part of a sacred ceremony (Cohen, 2007).

Sometimes, communities share in a group healing ceremony. It is believed that each individual's contribution will benefit the group as a whole. The pow-wow is a group ceremony that may be familiar to many. The participants sit in a circle and pass a talking stick around. The person who holds the talking stick speaks her or his heart while others listen carefully. This process continues until all have said everything they needed to say (Mackinnon, 2016).

Another example of a group healing ceremony is found among the indigenous people of Hawaii, who come together and experience a forgiveness ritual before the shaman begins the healing work. Family and community members convey concern for the patient by their participation in the ritual. This process underscores the belief that no one lives in isolation but is connected to and affected by other people. When people join in a show of community support, new levels of healing are possible (Wesselman, 2011).

Hawaiian medical practices are experiencing a resurgence, and researchers are studying the healing modalities, training patterns, cultural attributes, and the use of Hawaiian medicines. The three significant modalities are massage (ho'olomilomi), herbal medicine (la'au lapa'au), and conflict resolution (ho'oponopono). The majority of the practitioners are skilled in more than one healing modality. All treatment sessions begin and end with spiritual blessings to initiate the healing process. Health is considered to be a state of harmony between people, nature, and the gods (Wesselman, 2011).

RESEARCH

Clinical evidence of results from shamanic healing is anecdotal, and most published studies have been done by social scientists, folklorists, and historians. In another sense, the ancient methods of shamanism have been tested immeasurably longer than those of biomedicine. The similarities between shamans and scientists include an awareness of the complexity of the universe and the vast array of knowledge still to be uncovered and understood. As Harner (1990) described the similarity:

> Both shamans and scientists personally pursue research into the mysteries of the universe, and both believe that the underlying causal processes of that universe are hidden from ordinary view. And neither master shamans nor master scientists allow the dogma of ecclesiastical and political authorities to interfere with their explorations. It was no accident that Galileo was accused of witchcraft [shamanism]. (p. 45)

Research has demonstrated that drumming produces changes in the brain. The beat of the drum contains many sound frequencies that transmit impulses along the nerve pathways in the central nervous system. As mentioned previously, the rhythmic auditory stimulation of drumming increases the production of theta waves, the brain waves of the trance state. Studies have found that shamanic drumming produces frequencies in the theta wave range of 4 to 7 cycles per second (Hove et al., 2016).

INTEGRATED NURSING PRACTICE

Albert Schweitzer reportedly once observed, "The witch doctor succeeds for the same reason all the rest of us [doctors] succeed. Each patient carries his own doctor inside him. They come to us not knowing this truth. We are at our best when we give the doctor who resides within each patient a chance to go to work" (Harner, 1990, p. 135). This belief is almost identical with Florence Nightingale's basic premise that healing is a function of nature that comes from within the individual.

Currently, Dr. O. Carl Simonton and Stephanie Matthews-Simonton combine the techniques of shamanism with biomedicine in their well-known work treating people with cancer. As part of their treatment, clients are taught to relax and visualize themselves on a walking journey until they meet an "inner guide," which is a person or animal. The client then asks the guide for help in getting well. The process is similar to a shamanic journey and the meeting of a power animal.

Contemporary shamans work among today's Native American, Hmong, and other indigenous cultures. Their repertoire of curative powers now includes some modern and biomedical practices, and they may collaborate with conventional health-care practitioners. Today, many shamans share their knowledge about healing with others, which has contributed to a recent renewal of interest in this oldest of healing therapies. Lectures, retreats, and weekend meetings, where shamans teach the principles of living in balance with nature, are now available to the general public (Mackinnon, 2016).

As nurses, we must remember that we all have our own worldview. Until we recognize this ethnocentrism (our way is the best way), we are likely to impose this view on our clients. We must not only raise our awareness of other worldviews but also respect and honor worldviews that are different from ours.

In sharing information with clients, you can explain that shamanism offers a chance for contemplation. Guides offer more in the way of introspection and insight than physical cure. A shamanic journey may increase self-understanding, provide guidance for living, and produce a spiritual rejuvenation—all of which are important for the healing process.

In old cultures, shamans would do the journeying while an apprentice or helper drummed. In today's world, it is more appropriate to learn to journey for oneself and restore one's own power. Personal power is believed to be basic to health and well-being. Some clients may wish to meet in drumming circles every 1 or 2 weeks, while others will prefer to work alone. Drumming tapes have been designed and produced for shamanic journeying. As in any other field of learning, it may be more effective initially to work with a professional during a workshop or retreat.

The shamanic journey begins with the drum. Among all the instruments used in healing, the drum produces some of the most powerful effects. Human bodies are multidimensional rhythm machines with everything pulsing in synchrony. Drumming can influence how strongly and harmoniously life moves within and around every person. Drumming has been used in organizations ranging from therapy groups and 12-step programs to rehabilitation centers. The exercise in the "Try This" feature presents an overview of the shamanic journey that you may want to experience for yourself.

In the shamanic tradition, healing is not just for the individual but also for the community. In shamanism, ultimately no distinction is made between helping others and helping oneself. By helping others, one becomes more powerful, self-fulfilled, and joyful. The broader purpose is the helping of humankind. The desire to help others is what draws many people into the profession of nursing.

The North American Nursing Diagnosis Association identifies the diagnoses' "ineffective community coping" and "readiness for enhanced community coping." It is expected that nurses will apply the nursing process with individual clients, families, groups, and communities. Perhaps someday a modern version of the shaman will work side by side with nurses. Such cooperation is already starting to take place where native shamans live, as on some North American Indian reservations and in some places in Australia and Indonesia. Equally exciting is the idea that nurses will be trained in shamanic techniques and health maintenance so that they can combine both approaches in their practice.

TRY THIS
Shamanic Journey

- Find a private, secure place where you will not be disturbed.
- Assume a comfortable position, either sitting or lying down. You may want to cover your eyes to block out room light.
- Set the intent of your journey: Decide if you want to go to the upper world or lower, and form the intent to meet your guardian spirit or your power animal.
- Turn on a drumming tape. Let your body relax; let it sink down into Mother Earth. Take a few deep, slow breaths. Let the drumbeat become part of you; feel it resonate through your body.
- In your mind, bring yourself to a place in nature that is special for you, one that holds personal meaning. It might be a tree you climbed as a child, the lake you swam in on summer vacations, or the place you now walk your dog. Imagine that place and go there in your mind. Feel the energy of that place.
- If you are going to the lower world, find a place where you can enter the earth, such as a hollowed out tree stump, an animal den, a cave, or whatever else you want to imagine. When you enter the earth, you will be in a long cave. Take your time and follow it. Eventually it will open up into the lower world. Walk around and enjoy the beauty of the lower world. Explore. Soon you will come in contact with power animals. Introduce yourself. Dialogue with the animal, and ask what information the animal has for you.
- If you are going to the upper world, find a way to get up into the sky. You may climb a mountain or a tall beanstalk, use a hot-air balloon, or even shape-shift into the form of an eagle, and fly up. Eventually, you will come to the interface between the middle world and the upper world. Find a way through this interface, which is something like a membrane. The upper world is an ethereal, light, crystalline place. Explore. Soon you will meet your guardian spirit. Introduce yourself. Dialogue with the spirit, and ask what information the spirit has for you.
- Eventually, the journey has to end. It can end when you decide to end it, when no more information remains to be gained, or when the drumbeat changes, signaling an end. Return home by the same path you took to get there.
- Allow the information to sink into your consciousness. It is best if you write the information in a notebook, in a concrete form you will remember. The shamanic journey is much like a dream—it will leave you quickly. Writing it down is a method to keep the information you gained during the journey.

Source: Richard Sandore, MD (personal communication, 1998).

References

Baker, D. L., Dang, M. T., Ly, M. Y., & Diaz, R. (2010). Perceptions of barriers to immunization among parents of Hmong origin in California. *American Journal of Public Health*, 100(5): 839–845. doi: 10.2105/AJPH.2009.175935

Bourne, R. S. (1913). *Youth and Life*. Library of American Civilization. Houghton Mifflin. Originally from the University of Michigan.

Cohen, K. (2007). *Honoring the Medicine: The Essential Guide to Native American Healing*. New York, NY: Random House.

Harner, M. (1990). *The Way of the Shaman*. San Francisco, CA: Harper.

Herndon, C. N., Uiterloo, M., Uremaru, A., Plotkin, M. J., Emanuels-Smith, G., & Jitan, J. (2009). Disease concepts and treatment by tribal healers of an Amazonian forest culture. *Journal of Ethnobiology and Ethnomedicine*. doi: 10.1186/1746-4269-5-27

Hewson, M. G. (2015). African healing and becoming a traditional healer. In M. S. Micozzi (Ed.), *Fundamentals of Complementary and Alternative Medicine* (5th ed., pp. 660–666). St. Louis, MO: Elsevier/Saunders.

Hove, M. J., Stelzer, J., Nierhaus, T., Thiel, S. D., Gundlach, C., Margulies, D. S., . . . Merker, B. (2016). Brain network reconfiguration and perceptual decoupling during an absorptive state of consciousness. *Cerebral Cortex*. doi: 10.1093/cercor/bhv137

Mackinnon, C. (2016). *Shamanism*. Carlsbad, CA: Hay House.

Matthews, J. (2014). *The Shamanism Bible*. London: Octopus Publishing Group Ltd.

McLuhan, T. C. (1995). *Way of the Earth*. Simon and Schuster.

Pert, C. (1997). *Molecules of Emotion*. New York, NY: Scribner.

Rysdyk, E. C. (2013). *Spirit Walking: A Course in Shamanic Power*. San Francisco, CA: Weiser Books.

Rysdyk, E. C. (2016). *The Norse Shaman*. Rochester, VT: Destiny Books.

Sandore, R. (1997). *Introduction to the Shamanic Journey*. Prone Stone Recording. Soaring Spirit.

Tobert, N. (2017). *Cultural Perspectives on Mental Wellbeing*. London: Jessica Kingsley Publishers.

Wesselman, H. (2011). *The Bowl of Light: Ancestral Wisdom from a Hawaiian Shaman* (16th ed.). Boulder, CO: Sounds True.

Resources

Dance of the Deer Foundation Center for Shamanic Studies
P.O. Box 699
Soquel, CA 95073
888.455.3337
www.shamanism.com

Eagle's Wing Center for Contemporary Shamanism
BM Box 7475
London WCIN 3XX
http://eagleswing.co.uk

The Foundation for Shamanic Studies
P.O. Box 1939
Mill Valley, CA 94942
415.897.6416
www.shamanism.org

Four Winds Society
877.892.9247
www.thefourwinds.com

Institute for Contemporary Shamanic Studies
125-720 King St. W.
416.603.4912
www.icss.org

25

Faith and Prayer

Prayer indeed is good, but while calling on the gods a man should himself lend a hand.

HIPPOCRATES

The most powerful . . . prayer is the one that does not seek its own interest.

MEISTER ECKHART

Health-care sciences have begun to demonstrate that spirituality, faith, and religious commitment may play a role in promoting health and reducing illness. Nurse clinicians and researchers, as well as others, are becoming more interested in the connection between religious faith and survival. Increasingly, people are beginning to recognize that faith is good medicine.

Spirituality is that part of individuals that deals with relationships and values and addresses questions of purpose and meaning in life. Spirituality unites people and is inclusive in nature, not exclusive. It is not loyal to one group, continent, or religion. Although spirituality is not a religion, being involved in a particular religion is a way some people enhance their spirituality. Yet, people can be very spiritual and not religious. Spirituality involves individuals, family, friends, and community. *Individual* aspects are the development of moral values and beliefs about the meaning and purpose of life and death. The development of spirituality provides a grounding sense of identity and contributes to self-esteem. Spiritual aspects relating to *family* and *friends* include the search for meaning through relationships and the feeling of being connected with others and with an external power, often identified as God or a Supreme Being. *Community* aspects of spirituality can be understood as a common humanity and a belief in the fundamental sacredness and unity of all life. It is that which motivates people toward truth and a sense of fairness and justice toward all members of society. Spiritual health is expressed through humor, compassion, faith, forgiveness, courage, and creativity. Spirituality enables people to develop healthy relationships based on acceptance, respect, and compassion.

Religion can be described in a number of ways. The definition chosen for this text is one developed by Mickley, Carson, and Soeken (1995), three nursing researchers. They believe that religion develops and changes over time and is composed of people's beliefs, attitudes, and patterns of behavior that relate to the supernatural—God, the Divine One, the Great Spirit, Creator, and so forth. Religion usually includes a group of people who hold similar beliefs, have sacred texts, share religious symbols, and participate in shared traditions or rituals. Many people may say they are spiritual but not religious, while most religious people also identify themselves as spiritual (Burkhardt & Nagai-Jacobson, 2016).

Faith refers to one's beliefs and expectations about life, oneself, and others. In a religious context, faith refers to a belief in a Supreme Being who listens and responds to people and who cares about their well-being. In a spiritual context, faith is thought of as the power to accept the nature of life as it is and live in the present moment. It is a sense of letting go of the need to control while trusting and waiting for the moment when answers come.

Prayer is most often defined simply as a form of communication and fellowship with the Deity or Creator. The universality of prayer is evidenced in all cultures' having some form of prayer. The Hindus speak of the thousand names of God, and surely there are a hundred ways to pray. Imagine a circle or wheel with many spokes leading to the center or Supreme Being. Each spoke is a different religion with different prayers, but they all lead to the center. Prayer has been and continues to be used in times of difficulty and illness, even in the most secular societies. Prayer for self and prayer for others are the most frequently used forms of alternative therapies (Burkhardt & Nagai-Jacobson, 2016).

A common image of prayer in the United States is something like this: "Prayer is talking aloud to yourself, to a white, male, cosmic parent figure, who prefers to be addressed in English" (Dossey, 1997, p. 10). This cultural view of prayer fails to encompass how prayer is regarded by many other people throughout the world. For some, prayer is more a state of being than of doing; for others, prayer is silence rather than words; for some, prayer is a thought or a desire of the heart; and others pray to a female Goddess or a Divine Being who looks like they do. Buddhists do not believe in a personal God as creator and ruler of the world, yet prayers offered to the universe are central to the Buddhist tradition. Prayer may be simply being still and knowing that God is God. Prayer is part of many religious traditions and rituals and may be individual or communal, public or private (Westera, 2016).

Larry Dossey (1997) provides a broad definition of prayer: "Prayer is communication with the Absolute. This definition is inclusive, not exclusive; it affirms religious tolerance; and it invites people to define for themselves what 'communication' is, and who or what 'the Absolute' may be" (p. 11). According to a Sufi saying, prayer is when you talk to God, and meditation is when God talks to you. In this definition, meditation is thought of as passive and receptive, and prayer as active and engaging. The boundaries between meditation and prayer, however, are often blurred.

BACKGROUND

Until approximately 200 years ago, medicine and religion were so thoroughly united that healers and priests were often the same individuals. The first hospitals were founded in monasteries by physicians who were usually monks. Today, many cultures throughout the world continue to regard their healers as a source for guidance in matters of faith and wellness. In the West, religion and medicine were fused until the end of the Middle Ages in the mid-1400s. Philosophers such as Descartes (1596–1650), Locke (1632–1704), and Hume (1711–1776) promoted the scientific basis of knowledge, believing that truth could be realized only through the examination of empirical data and the rational, scientific method. Centuries later, Western societies continue to experience the consequences of this split between religion and medicine. Western physicians are educated to think primarily in terms of what can be empirically proven in the laboratory. Discussions of spirituality and religion are considered by many physicians to be "off limits," with such discussion relegated to spiritual or religious leaders. In the past, when arguments arose between religion and medicine, religion usually did not fare well. As nurses such as M. Dossey, Carson, Burkhardt, Nagai-Jacobson, Taylor, Winslow, Treloar, Koerner, Goertz, Westera, and Holt-Ashley and physicians such as B. M. Dossey, Matthews, Koenig, and Benson research and write more about the blending of religion and health care, the practice of their professions will evolve to, once again, include the forgotten "faith factor" in health care.

In end-of-life situations, many individuals find comfort and peace through faith in a loving God. In other situations, some people believe in divine healing and may let God decide how to manage their health problems, giving up personal control and responsibility. Studies have found that this group may have negative medical consequences but at the same time report greater life satisfaction (Hayward, Krause, Ironson, & Pargament, 2016).

In some situations, religion may have a negative impact on people's lives. Religious participation can lead to more, not fewer, problems when unscrupulous leaders coerce or manipulate others to give up all personal autonomy. Problems also occur when religion fosters excessive guilt or shame or encourages people to avoid dealing with life's problems. Some religious groups urge their members to avoid all conventional medical care, which can lead to life-threatening situations (Micozzi & Larson, 2015).

CONCEPTS

Universality of Faith

Throughout history and around the world, people have called on a Divine Being to sustain them. People are nourished by life-affirming beliefs and philosophies. They meditate and say prayers that elicit physiological calm and a sense of peacefulness, both of which contribute to longer survival. Benson (1997) believes that a genetic blueprint makes believing in the Great Mystery part of people's nature. Through the process of natural selection, mutating genes retain the impulses of faith, hope, and love, and faith is a natural physiological reaction to the threats of mortality that everyone faces. Benson (1997) went on to say that "according to my investigations, it does not matter which God you worship, nor which theology you adopt as your own. Spiritual life, in general, is very healthy" (p. 212).

Spiritual Crises

Serious illness presents a spiritual crisis. As long as people are well, they maintain their autonomy and their ability to function at home, work, or school. Their feelings of self-worth are supported as they find meaning and purpose in their many activities. Once serious illness occurs, some of these things change. Ill people may have to depend on others for personal care, and they may experience other radical lifestyle changes. Body concept changes may threaten self-esteem. In these situations, most people are forced to re-evaluate life's meaning and purpose. Religious people draw heavily on their resources of faith to see them through difficult situations like serious illness. Positive religious coping involves such beliefs as "God will care for me." One research study asked 345 patients with advanced cancer which of the two interventions they would prefer: (1) interventions to extend life even though that would mean more pain or (2) interventions to relieve pain even though it would mean they would not live as long. There was a positive correlation between greater use of positive religious coping and wanting more aggressive end-of-life care near the time of death (Phelps et al., 2009).

Twelve Remedies

Numerous studies demonstrate that religious involvement promotes health. It appears at this time that a number of religious "ingredients" promote health and well-being. Although some may be found in nonreligious settings, they are more commonly found operating together in religious organizations. Matthews and Clark (1998) termed these "religious remedies," a listing of which appears in Box 25.1.

The first remedy is the **relaxation response,** which can be evoked with meditation and prayer (Matthews & Clark, 1998). The relaxation response buffers stress by clearing the mind and freeing the body from everyday tension. Practiced regularly, the relaxation response decreases heart rate, lowers

BOX 25.1
Religious Remedies

1. Relaxation response
2. Healthful living
3. Aesthetics of worship
4. Whole-being worship
5. Confession and absolution
6. Support network
7. Shared beliefs
8. Ritual
9. Purpose in life
10. Turning over to a Higher Power
11. Positive expectations
12. Love for self and others

Source: Matthews and Clark (1998).

metabolic rate, decreases respirations, and slows brain waves. In addition, it enhances measures of immunity. Benson (1997) found that when religious beliefs were added to relaxation response activities, worries and fears were significantly reduced compared with the relaxation response alone. Most worship services provide time for silent prayer or meditation and help people take time out from busy schedules. With regular practice of the relaxation response, people report experiencing an increase in spirituality. They often describe the presence of an energy, a power, or God, which is beyond themselves. Those who feel this presence often experience the greatest medical benefits (Benson, 1997).

The second remedy is one of **healthful living** (Matthews & Clark, 1998). Some religious groups actively promote a healthy lifestyle as part of their doctrine. Religious prescriptions may include dietary moderation, rules about sexual behavior, and regulations regarding hygiene as well as avoidance of tobacco, alcohol, and drugs.

The third remedy is the **aesthetics of worship,** which taps into a universal appreciation for beauty. Visual symbols of faith are reassuring and calming images. Stained-glass windows, beautiful architecture, and floral arrangements all provide an experience of harmony and balance. Sacred music uses audible beauty to communicate the splendor of God. The smell of incense may evoke a deep sense of peace and quietude (Matthews & Clark, 1998).

The fourth remedy is **whole-being worship.** Christians who sing familiar hymns, Jews who sing "Torah Ora" when the Torah scroll is presented,

Muslims who recite Quran, and Buddhists who chant their prayers all participate in whole-being worship through music or words. This combination of physical activity (singing, reciting), cognitive activity (reading the words), and spiritual activity (prayer through songs or words) evokes a sense of peace. Movements such as kneeling, standing, bowing heads, folding hands, or even dancing engage people on all levels of being. As people worship with body, mind, and spirit, they undergo a unifying experience that is as good for them as it feels (Matthews & Clark, 1998).

The fifth remedy is **confession and absolution.** Harboring guilty feelings can literally make people sick. In many religions, people are encouraged to confess their sins and repent, after which they are given assurance of forgiveness and absolution. This process allows individuals to review their mistakes, share their personal pain, learn from their errors, and move on rather than becoming preoccupied with personal shortcomings (Matthews & Clark, 1998).

The sixth remedy is one's **support network**—those family members and friends who offer practical help, emotional support, and spiritual encouragement in times of need. People are social beings whose health often deteriorates when they become isolated and lonely. Lack of human companionship has been linked to depression of the immune system and a lowered production of endorphins, the neurotransmitter that produces feeling of well-being. Religious organizations often provide many opportunities for social interaction, from religious services to sacred study groups; to youth, women's, and men's groups; and to community outreach groups. Koenig (2008) describes some of the benefits of group interaction: it offers a sense of partnership, helps with coping, creates a sense of community and safety, encourages a cooperative approach to problem solving, helps change behaviors and thoughts, supports taking control, and encourages personal action.

The seventh remedy is **shared beliefs.** Most people prefer to associate with individuals who share similar beliefs and points of view. Great things can be achieved when groups are unified around common values. Religious traditions are opportunities for people to share common beliefs. Individuals who feel they are part of a group find they are not alone and gain strength from the power of shared beliefs. Participation in regular worship not only helps people feel connected and rise above their differences, but also is an antidote to the alienation often prevalent in Western society (Matthews & Clark, 1998).

The eighth remedy is **ritual.** Ceremony and ritual are ways of creating sacred space and time, when normal ways of relating are put aside, and people can listen and pray with an open heart to their Divine Being. Religious ritual is a powerful healing mechanism that has soothing and calming effects. Rituals provide people a link with tradition and give them a sense of security (Matthews & Clark, 1998). As Benson (1997) stated:

> There is something very influential about invoking a ritual that you may first have practiced in childhood, about regenerating the neural pathways that were formed in your youthful experience of

faith. . . . Even if you experience the ritual from an entirely different perspective of maturity and life history, the words you read, the songs you sing, and the prayers you invoke will soothe you in the same way they did in what was perhaps a simpler time in your life. (p. 177)

The ninth remedy is that of finding a **purpose in life** (Matthews & Clark, 1998). Viktor Frankl (1984) described people's search for meaning as being the primary motivation in their lives. This search for meaning becomes more intense during periods of illness as people struggle with age-old questions such as Why me? Why now? Did I do something to deserve this? Religion and worship attendance provide a framework of meaning, a sense of purpose in life, and a meaningful interpretation for difficult times. People who are dying often seem to arrive at a sense of life's purpose. As they tell it, the purpose of life is to grow in wisdom and to learn to love better. They discover that health is not an end but rather a means. In other words, health enables people to serve a purpose in life, but health is not the purpose of life.

The 10th remedy is **turning one's life over** to the Great Mystery or God. It is an acknowledgment that no one has total control over her or his life. Religion provides an avenue for asking for guidance, intervention, and strength. Faith in a God who is loving and caring provides comfort for those going through difficult times. Worship services often leave people feeling less burdened and anxious, as well as more peaceful (Matthews & Clark, 1998).

The 11th remedy is that of **positive expectations.** During a time of illness or distress, religion often provides a sense of hope and the strength to endure that which has happened. The expectancy of help from the Divine Source works in the same way as does the expectancy of help from a medication, procedure, or caregiver. Various holy writings promise health and healing to the faithful, and researchers are beginning to document the effect of this expectation on the outcome of disease (Matthews & Clark, 1998). Gregg Braden (2008) wrote about the role of belief in both creating illness and healing from illness on personal, community, and worldwide levels.

The 12th, and last, remedy is **love for self and others.** All religions focus on loving God and other people. This love includes helping others—strangers as well as family and friends (Matthews & Clark, 1998). When people love and help others, they often experience better health than those who do not.

These 12 religious remedies can be found outside of religious organizations. Frequent religious participation, however, provides many of these remedies in one context. Research is demonstrating that religious participation is an important factor in the prevention of disease, achievement of well-being, healing from illness, and extension of life span. One mystery that remains, however, is why some people are cured and others are not. One can be very spiritual and still get sick and die. It must be remembered that religious participation and spirituality are no guarantee for physical health. Failure to recognize this basic reality can result in inappropriate self-blame (Matthews & Clark, 1998).

How Prayer Works

No one knows how praying for others works. Skeptics say it cannot happen because no accepted scientific theory explains it. In the development of theories, however, empirical facts often lead to the development of an explanatory theory. For example, it was well known that penicillin worked before anyone discovered how it worked. The debate has now shifted from *whether* prayer works to *how* prayer works.

Larry Dossey (1993), JoEllen Goertz Koerner (2011), and Gregg Braden (2008) have proposed that prayer is "nonlocal," an idea derived from the field of quantum physics. The word *local* means that something is present in the here and now; each of us exists here and not somewhere else, and now and not at some other time. The word *nonlocal* means that something is not confined by place or time. All the major theistic (belief in a personal God as creator) religions agree on the nonlocal nature of God; that He or She is everywhere, is not confined by space and location, and exists throughout time. According to the concept of nonlocality, consciousness cannot be localized or confined to one's brain or body, nor can it be confined to the present moment. Consciousness is basic to the universe, perhaps similar to matter and energy. According to this theory, neither energy nor information travels from one mind to another, because the two minds are not separate but rather interconnected and omniscient. Dossey, Koerner, and Braden have proposed that consciousness-mediated events such as prayer, telepathy, precognition, and clairvoyance may become explainable with continuing developments in quantum physics. Like any other new theory, the nonlocal theory raises more questions than it answers. Evidence exists that prayer works, even though the exact mechanism is unknown at this time. What is known is that prayer is the most common complementary therapy added to biomedicine (Tobert, 2017).

TREATMENT

Some people seek nurses, doctors, counselors, and therapists who focus on spiritual concerns as well as physical and emotional concerns. This focus is especially helpful for those who are dealing with issues related to meaning and purpose in life. Alternatively, people may seek the help of religious leaders who include healing practices in their religious practice. Faith healing has not been scientifically proven but remains a popular option for many. Some people go to specific places for healing. The Catholic Church has documented 36 "miracles" at Lourdes, for example. A variety of spiritually focused healing groups are also available. People with addictive disorders benefit from 12-step programs, which rely on both the group support and the specific invocation of a Higher Power.

Two different types of prayer are directed and nondirected prayer. In **directed prayer,** the praying person asks for a specific outcome, such as for the cancer to go away or for the baby to be born healthy. In contrast, in **nondirected prayer,** no specific outcome is asked. The praying person simply asks for the best thing to occur in a given situation. Studies show that both approaches are effective in promoting health.

Prayer can also be described according to form. **Colloquial prayer** is an informal talk with God, as if one were talking to a good friend. **Petitional prayer** or intercessory prayer is asking God for things for oneself or others. The focus is on what God can provide. **Intercessory prayer** is simply praying for someone else. **Ritual prayer** is the use of formal prayers or rituals such as prayers from a prayer book or Quran or from the Jewish Siddur, or the Catholic practice of saying the rosary. **Meditative prayer,** also known as contemplative prayer, is similar to meditation and is a process of focusing the mind on an aspect of God for a period of time.

RESEARCH

It is difficult to compare studies on faith and prayer when researchers do not agree on conceptual models with operational definitions. Different opinions exist on what should be included in the research studies. This is a hurdle that must be overcome before a systematic review is possible.

The following is a small sample of studies related to spirituality, religious practice, and prayer:

- A systematic review and meta-analysis regarding religious and spiritual interventions in mental health care found that these interventions demonstrated significant levels of decreases in anxiety, stress, alcohol abuse, and depression (Goncalves, Lucchetti, Menezes, & Vallada, 2015).
- A study of intercessory prayer added to normal cancer treatment randomized 999 participants to either an intervention group or a control group. An external group was asked to offer Christian intercessory prayer for those in the study group. The people praying were given nonidentifying details about the recipients. The intervention group showed significantly greater improvements in spiritual, emotional, and functional well-being compared with the control group (Olver & Dutney, 2012).
- An analytical review of clinical studies considered the relationship between people who prayed for their own health and depression, optimism, coping, anxiety, and confusion. There was significantly less depression, anxiety, and confusion and more optimism and improved coping. There was no significant effect of prayer on physical health (Anderson & Nunnelley, 2016).
- A qualitative study looked at the role of spirituality in Arab Muslims who survived a stem cell transplant. Three themes were noted that helped the survivors cope with their illness experiences: illness viewed in the light of belief in God; use of religious/spiritual resources; and support from family and community. Health-care providers in Western cultures need to respect and support these needs (Alaloul, Schreiber, Al Nusairat, & Andrykowski, 2016).

- Adults with chronic health issues have increased prevalence of depression. The study of 1,696 subjects looked at involvement in religious activities, religious meaning, religious hope, prayer, peace, and view of God. Greater religiousness/spirituality contributed to significant protection against depression (Lucette, Ironson, Pargament, & Krause, 2016).
- A qualitative study of U.S. physicians found that the majority believe that spiritual suffering intensifies physical pain. They also believe that spiritual suffering should be treated with the same intensity as physical pain (Smyre, Yoon, Rasinski, & Curlin, 2015).

INTEGRATED NURSING PRACTICE

Every serious illness is a spiritual crisis because it is a confrontation with one's own mortality. Every nurse, regardless of personal belief, must recognize that religion or spirituality or both are often an essential part of the lives of those entrusted to her or his care. To avoid these issues is to fail to truly be a nurse healer because the nurse's task is to address the physical, psychological, and spiritual needs of clients.

As a nurse, you can incorporate faith and prayer issues in your care of clients, regardless of your own personal religious beliefs or worldviews. When you remember that people are spiritual beings, you will be more alert to spiritual concerns. It is important that you promote an atmosphere that accepts and encourages many forms of spiritual expression.

The International Code of Ethics for Nurses, the ANA Code of Ethics, and the Joint Commission on Accreditation of Healthcare Organizations all state that nurses must assess clients' spiritual needs. The North American Nursing Diagnosis Association includes the following nursing diagnoses: impaired religiosity; readiness for enhanced religiosity; spiritual distress; and readiness for enhanced spiritual well-being.

Why is it, then, that some nurses do not incorporate faith and prayer into their professional practice? Some nurses are unaware of the research data regarding the faith factor. That situation is beginning to change as schools of nursing develop courses to teach students about the faith–health connection. Some nurses have been told specifically that they are not to mix nursing and faith. This recommendation was made out of a concern that nurses might blur the professional–personal boundaries and cause harm to their clients. Some nurses believe they do not have enough time, while others are unfamiliar with spiritual assessment tools. As research continues to be documented, nurses are re-examining the relationship between nursing and faith (O'Brien, 2014; Yilmaz & Gurler, 2014).

Faith and prayer can be explored effectively with people of most age groups. The depth and focus of the conversation will vary based on the cognitive and developmental ability of the individual or family. Health maintenance visits provide an opportunity to explore spiritual beliefs and practices in the context of an overall assessment of lifestyle, risks, and resources. Doors

BOX 25.2

Faith and Prayer Assessment

Do you consider yourself a spiritual or religious person?

What does your faith mean to you? Has it changed during your illness?

What is the importance of this faith in your daily life?

Do your beliefs influence the way you think about your health or look at your illness?

How important is your religious identification? Do you belong to an organized group?

Tell me about your religious practices, such as worship, prayer, or meditation.

How important is prayer for you now?

What type of prayer would feel comfortable to you now?

What aspects of your faith would you like me to keep in mind as I care for you?

Would you like to discuss religious implications of your care?

Sources: Burkhardt and Nagai-Jacobson (2016); O'Brien (2014); Westera (2016).

can be opened in a nonthreatening, nonurgent fashion, and the topic can be validated for future discussion. See Chapter 2 for a list of nursing spirituality assessment tools. In the face of major illness, terminal disease, or dying, the discussion of faith and prayer is even more relevant. Clearly though, discussion of this topic should not be restricted to these types of client encounters. Box 25.2 provides an example of a nursing assessment regarding faith and prayer.

Respecting people's beliefs and experiences also means that nurses do not force spiritual issues on clients, push religion on them, or attempt to convert them to a particular faith. Prayer should never be imposed on patients or used as a substitute for high-quality nursing care. Nor should prayer be used as an invocation of magic. Doing so violates the trust that is basic to the nurse–client relationship. Promoting the benefits of faith and prayer includes respecting clients' choices about doctrine, denomination, beliefs, and traditions (Minton, Isaacson, & Banik, 2016; O'Brien, 2014; Westera, 2016).

Of course, some nurses and physicians do incorporate faith and prayer into their care. Dr. Alijani, a faculty member at Georgetown University Medical School and a well-known surgeon, believes that faith plays a significant role in his patient's well-being. He sees prayer as the literal lifeline between health and spirituality: "Just as my body needs water, carbohydrates, protein, and lipids, my mind needs Allah, and the only way to receive Allah is to pray" (Matthews & Clark, 1998, p. 73).

Health-care practitioners are not meant to replace clergy; the roles are distinct. Although many clients may want their spiritual needs addressed by nurses and physicians, others do not, preferring to have these issues addressed by clergy. The practitioner needs to take into account, however, where and how the client's belief enters into the healing process. Nor should health-care practitioners be forced against their wishes into participating in clients' religious practices. In the best of worlds, health-care professionals and clergy work closely together to provide meaningful holistic care.

Although intercessory prayer is guided by beliefs, experiences, and faith traditions, you can provide clients with some basic guidelines on how to incorporate the benefits of intercessory prayer into their lives (Matthews & Clark, 1998):

- If you are ill, ask specifically for people's prayers for healing. It may involve clergy, members of a congregation, adding your name to a prayer list, or asking family and friends to pray for you on a regular basis.
- Pray for your own healing.
- Seek out healing services. Many churches, mosques, and synagogues offer opportunities to participate in a prayer service or healing service.
- Pray persistently. Keep praying regardless of apparent results. Continuing prayer is an expression of faith and hope.
- Pray for others who are suffering.

As a nurse, you can also teach yourself and others to take time out to count blessings and say "thanks" for the good things in life. Paying attention to what you already have and what is going right helps alleviate stress, anxiety, and depression. An act of gratitude often restores a sense of balance and perspective. You can make the following suggestions:

- Remember to say "thank you." Make it a habit whenever someone helps you out, gives you a compliment, or gives you a gift.
- Create rituals of thanks, for example, saying grace before meals or daily prayers. Practice them until they become a habit.
- Every night before you go to bed, make a list of five things for which you are grateful. It will help take the focus off the stresses in your life.
- Take the time to give back. Look for opportunities to help others and recycle the good fortune you have in your life.
- Once a day, strike a grateful pose, for example, kneeling in prayer or standing with your arms extended joyfully to the sky.
- Take 10 minutes each day to be grateful. Go outside into nature, meditate, or pray. Whatever you do, take the time to appreciate all that you have right now.

As nurses, you must educate yourselves about the clinical relevance of faith and prayer for your clients. The time has come to give more than lip service to the spiritual aspects of nursing care. It is important that you let your clients know that you will do everything you can do scientifically but that science and technology have their limitations. Perhaps it is appropriate also to let them know that you may pray for guidance in providing competent and compassionate care.

References

Alaloul, F., Schreiber, J. A., Al Nusairat, T. S., & Andrykowski, M. A. (2016). Spirituality in Arab Muslim hematopoietic stem cell transplantation survivors: A qualitative approach. *Cancer Nursing.* doi: 10.1097/NCC .0000000000000312

Anderson, J. W., & Nunnelley, P. A. (2016). Private prayer associations with depression, anxiety and other health conditions: An analytical review of clinical studies. *Postgraduate Medicine.* doi: 10.1080/00325481.2016.1209962

Benson, H. (1997). *Timeless Healing.* New York, NY: Fireside Books.

Braden, G. (2008). *The Spontaneous Healing of Belief.* Carlsbad, CA: Hay House.

Burkhardt, M. A., & Nagai-Jacobson, M. G. (2016). Spirituality and health. In B. M. Dossey & L. Keegan (Eds.), *Holistic Nursing: A Handbook for Practice* (7th ed., pp. 135–164). Burlington, MA: Jones & Bartlett Learning.

Dossey, L. (1993). *Healing Words: The Power of Prayer and the Practice of Medicine.* San Francisco, CA: Harper.

Dossey, L. (1997). The return of prayer. *Alternative Therapies,* 3(6): 10–17, 113–120.

Eckhart, M. (1994). *Selected Writings.* Translated by Oliver Davies. United Kingdom: Penguin.

Frankl, V. (1984). *Man's Search for Meaning.* New York, NY: Simon & Schuster.

Goncalves, J. P. B., Lucchetti, G., Menezes, P. R., & Vallada, H. (2015). Religious and spiritual interventions in mental health care: A systematic review and meta-analysis of randomized controlled clinical trials. *Psychological Medicine.* doi: 10.1017/S0033291715001166

Hayward, R. D., Krause, N., Ironson, G., & Pargament, K. I. (2016). Externalizing religious health beliefs and health and well-being outcomes. *Journal of Behavioral Medicine.* doi: 10.1007/ s10865-016-9761-7

Hippocrates. (1983). *Hippocratic Writings* (Vol. 451). Edited by G. E. R. Lloyd, J. Chadwick, & W. N. Mann. Penguin Books Limited.

Koenig, H. G. (2008). *Medicine, Religion, and Health.* West Conshohocken, PA: Templeton Foundation Press.

Koerner, J. G. (2011). *Healing Presence: The Essence of Nursing* (2nd ed.). New York, NY: Springer.

Lucette, A., Ironson, G., Pargament, K. I., & Krause, N. (2016). Spirituality and religiousness are associated with fewer depressive symptoms in individuals with medical conditions. *Psychosomatics.* doi: 10.1016/j.psym.2016.03.005

Matthews, D. A., & Clark, C. (1998). *The Faith Factor: Proof of the Healing Power of Prayer.* New York, NY: Viking.

Mickley, J. R., Carson, V., & Soeken, K. L. (1995). Religion and adult mental health. *Issues in Mental Health Nursing,* 16: 345–360.

Micozzi, M. S., & Larson, D. (2015). Prayer, religion, and spirituality. In M. S. Micozzi (Ed.), *Fundamentals of Complementary and Alternative Medicine* (5th ed., pp. 141–156). St. Louis, MO: Elsevier/Saunders.

Minton, M. E., Isaacson, M., & Banik, D. (2016). Prayer and the registered nurse (PRN): Nurses' reports of ease and disease with patient-initiated prayer request. *Journal of Advanced Nursing.* doi: 10.1111.jan.12990

O'Brien, M. E. (2014). *Spirituality in Nursing: Standing on Holy Ground* (5th ed.). Burlington, MA: Jones & Bartlett Learning.

Olver, I. N., & Dutney, A. (2012). A randomized, blinded study of the impact of intercessory prayer on spiritual well-being in patients with cancer. *Alternative Therapies in Health & Medicine*, 18(5): 18–27.

Phelps, A. C., Maciejewski, P. K., Nilsson, M., Balboni, T. A., Wright, A. A., Paulk, M. E., . . . Prigerson, H. G. (2009). Religious coping and use of intensive life-prolonging care near death in patients with advanced cancer. *Journal of the American Medical Association*, 301(11): 1140–1147.

Smyre, C. L., Yoon, J. D., Rasinski, K. A., & Curlin, F. A. (2015). Limits and responsibilities of physicians addressing spiritual suffering in terminally ill patients. doi: 10.1016/j.jpainsymman .2014.06.016

Tobert, N. (2017). *Cultural Perspectives on Mental Well-being*. London: Jessica Kingsley Publishers.

Westera, D. A. (2016). *Spirituality in Nursing Practice*. New York: Springer Publishing Company.

Yilmaz, M., & Gurler, H. (2014). The efficacy of integrating spirituality into undergraduate nursing curricula. *Nursing Ethics*. doi: 10.1177/ 0969733014521096

Resources

Anglican Fellowship of Prayer
1106 Mansfield Ave.
Indiana, PA 15701
724.463.6436
www.afp.org

Australian Islamic College of Sydney
33 Headcom St.
Mount Druitt, NSW 2770
61.2.9677.2613
www.aics.nsw.edu.au

Buddhist Association of Canada
1330 Bloor St. W
Toronto ON M6H 1P2
416.910.4858
www.buddhismcanada.com

The Healing Trust
21 York Rd.
Northampton, UK NN1 5QG
www.thehealingtrust.org.uk

The Interface Between Medicine
  and Religion
John Templeton Foundation
300 Conshohocken State Rd., Suite 500
West Conshohocken, PA 19428
610.941.2828
www.templeton.org

Institute for Jewish Spirituality
135 W 29 St., Suite 1103
New York, NY 10001-5224
646.461.6499
www.jewishspirituality.org/
  resources/related-organizations/

Shalem Institute for Spiritual
  Formation
3025 Fourth St. NE, Suite 22
Washington, DC 20017
301.897.7334
www.shalem.org

Other Therapies

*Respect means listening until everyone
has been heard and understood; only
then is there a possibility of
"Balance and Harmony," the goal
of Indian Spirituality.*

DAVE CHIEF, GRANDFATHER OF RED DOG

26

Bioelectromagnetics

You, yourself, as much as anybody in the entire universe, deserve your love and affection.

BUDDHA

Bioelectromagnetics is the emerging science that studies how living organisms interact with electromagnetic fields. *Electromagnetism*, a form of energy, underlies all biochemistry. Quantum physics has demonstrated that what people see as solid matter—be that a person or an object—is actually 99.9999% empty space filled with energy. Everything is, in fact, energy vibrating at different rates.

BACKGROUND

In the 18th century, Luigi Galvani, an Italian physician, conducted experiments on frog muscle to demonstrate that bioelectricity exists within living tissue. Shortly thereafter, Alessandro Volta, a physicist, found that animal tissue was not needed to produce a current and went on to invent the electric battery in 1800. Michael Faraday, a British chemist, became the greatest experimentalist in electricity and magnetism of the 19th century; he produced the first electric motor and succeeded in showing that a magnet could induce electricity. This early work led to several devices for the diagnosis and treatment of disease, including many that are in use today.

In the late 1950s in Japan, doctors began to see a new syndrome of low energy, insomnia, and generalized aches and pains. After extensive research, it was discovered that these complaints came from people who spent large amounts of time in metal buildings and were thus shielded from the earth's natural magnetic field. The disorder was labeled "magnetic field deficiency syndrome," and symptoms were alleviated by the external application of magnetic fields to the patient's body. Today, magnetic healing continues to be a significant part of mainstream medicine in Japan. Similarly, early Russian cosmonauts who spent more than a year in space were amazed to find that they had lost nearly 80% of their bone density. As a result, spacecrafts were designed to include strong artificial magnetic fields on board to avoid this problem. Both these examples illustrate that magnetic fields are essential to good health and well-being (Micozzi, Weintraub, & Gehl, 2015).

CONCEPTS

Geomagnetic Field

Every atom and cell of the body is a small magnetic field that radiates into space, decreasing in strength with distance and ultimately becoming lost in the jumble of other magnetic fields. Like the human body, the earth radiates an energy field, called the **geomagnetic field.** This field originates in convection currents in the earth's liquid outer core and radiates beyond the atmosphere, stimulating and protecting all life on earth. Migrating birds or fish returning to their spawning grounds navigate great distances with the help of magnetic field receptors in their brain. It is believed that they tune in to the magnetic field of the earth to determine location and direction. Animals are attuned to the geomagnetic field and can sense subtle changes in it. For example, dogs, horses, and cattle often become agitated just before an earthquake (Oschman, 2016).

The lines of force of a magnetic field can penetrate the body as if it were air. A strong magnet held on one side of the hand can easily deflect a compass needle on the other side of the same hand. As the magnetic field penetrates the body, it can interact with electric and electromagnetic fields within the body.

Endogenous Magnetic Fields

Endogenous magnetic fields are those produced within the body. This electrical activity demonstrates patterns that provide medically useful information. For example, electrocardiography (ECG or EKG) and electroencephalography (EEG) measure heart and brain activity, respectively, by measuring electric potentials on the surface of living tissue. New technologies in instruments under development that are extremely sensitive have opened new lines of research.

Like other kinds of magnetic fields, the human energy field is the strongest at its source and fades with distance. Another name for this energy field is **aura,** and it is the field that surrounds the body as far as the outstretched arms and from head to toe. See Chapter 2 for more detailed information on auras. The human energy field is both an information center and a highly sensitive perceptual system that transmits and receives messages as people interact with their surrounding environment. Patterns of circulation of energy within the body include the meridian system and the chakras. Virtually every complementary healing therapy has a way of interpreting these subtle energy fields (Oschman, 2016; Shields & Wilson, 2016).

Recent research has uncovered a form of endogenous radiation, an extremely low-level light known as **biophoton emission**. It is believed that biophoton emission may be important in gene expression, membrane transport, and bioregulation. Externally applied energy fields may alter biophoton emission to the benefit or detriment of the organism. This, as well as other endogenous fields of the body, may prove to be involved in energetic therapies such as Therapeutic Touch (Oschman, 2016).

Exogenous Magnetic Fields

Exogenous magnetic fields are those produced by sources outside the body and can be classified as either artificial or natural. **Artificial exogenous fields** are created by such things as power lines, transformers, appliances, radio transmitters, and medical devices. The frequencies of some of these exogenous fields can also create problems for people. For example, the frequency of household current in the United States is 60 cycles per second, or 60 hertz, compared with brain frequencies of 8 to 22 cycles per second while awake and as low as 2 cycles per second while sleeping. The more the electrical devices in the bedroom, the more likely the interference with the brain's natural frequencies, resulting in disturbed sleep and fatigue. As long as televisions and computers are plugged in, they produce electromagnetic fields, even when turned off. It would be best, therefore, to unplug all electrical devices in the bedroom prior to sleep (Oschman, 2016).

The earth's geomagnetic field is one example of a **natural exogenous field**. Another example is the field produced by moving water. When people are at beaches, on riverbanks, beside waterfalls, or even walking outside after a powerful rainstorm, they often experience feelings of relaxation and peace. While these feelings may be attributed to the psychological cues from these environments, they also have an energetic basis. When water moves or flows, it releases negative ions into the air. When people are surrounded by negative ions, they seem to balance their energy fields. As Collinge (1998) stated, "It is as if the metaphors of 'cleansing' and 'washing away' that we associate with moving waters have a real basis in their impact on the field of emotional energy that surrounds and penetrates our body" (p. 93).

Ionizing and Nonionizing Fields

Electromagnetic fields can also be classified as ionizing or nonionizing. A field is an **ionizing electromagnetic field** if its energy is high enough to dislodge electrons from an atom or molecule. Gamma rays and X-rays are two types of ionizing radiation that can penetrate the body and cause damage on prolonged exposure. **Nonionizing electromagnetic fields** may have nonharmful and even beneficial effects on biological tissue. This effect is the basis for bioelectromagnetic (BEM) field application and research.

The actual mechanism by which BEM produces biological effects is under intense study. It is likely that BEM affects the cell membrane, perhaps at the receptors where neurotransmitters and neurohormones bind. Alteration in the binding process then alters internal cellular processes. Interestingly, some specific frequencies of BEM affect specific target tissues, just as drugs affect specific tissues. Magnetic fields are also believed to stimulate cellular metabolism and oxygenate tissues, which relieves inflammation and facilitates cellular repair.

TREATMENT

Magnetic field therapy works on the principle that every animal, plant, and mineral has an electromagnetic field that enables organic beings and inorganic objects to communicate and interact as part of a single, unified energy system. **Static magnetic fields** are produced by natural or artificial magnets, and **pulsating magnetic fields** are produced by electrical devices. These magnetic fields are able to penetrate the body and affect the functioning of cells, tissues, organs, and systems (Figure 26.1). These therapies work best in combination with other healing modalities and are considered to be adjunct treatments to conventional medicine. They should not be used by themselves for any major disease or medical condition (Micozzi et al., 2015).

Nonionizing bioelectromagnetic medical applications are classified into two types: thermal or nonthermal. *Thermal,* or heat, applications include radio-frequency (RF) hyperthermia, laser and RF surgery, and RF diathermy. The most important BEM modalities in complementary and integrative medicine are the nonthermal applications. *Nonthermal* means that the application

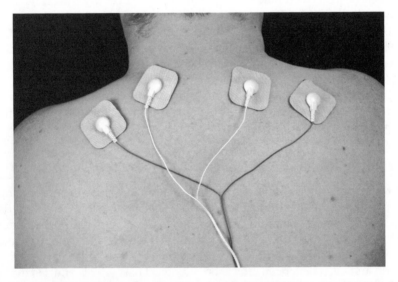

FIGURE 26.1 Transcutaneous Electrical Nerve Stimulation (TENS) Provides Pain Relief to a Male with Neck Pain—Electrodes Plugged to TENS Unit

Source: UTBP/Shutterstock.

does not cause any significant gross heating of tissue. An example is microwave resonance therapy, in which the mechanism of action is thought to be modification of the cell membrane. The major alternative healing applications of nonthermal, nonionizing electromagnetic fields are bone repair, nerve stimulation, wound healing, the treatment of osteoarthritis, electroacupuncture, tissue regeneration, immune system stimulation, and neuroendocrine modulations (Oschman, 2016). Box 26.1 describes these applications.

BOX 26.1

Applications of Nonthermal, Nonionizing Electromagnetic Fields

Transcutaneous electrical nerve stimulation (TENS)	Used for pain relief
Transcranial electrostimulation (TCES)	Used to reduce symptoms of depression, anxiety, and insomnia; may be effective in drug dependence
Repetitive transcranial magnetic stimulation (rTMS)	Used in place of electroconvulsive therapy in certain types of mood disorders; used in diagnostic nerve conduction studies
Pulsed electromagnetic fields (PEMFs)	Used to stimulate bone growth; fractures
Electromyography	Used to diagnose and treat carpal tunnel syndrome and other movement disorders
Magnetoencephalography (MEG)	Measures brain waves and thinking activity; more accurate and precise than EEG
Electroretinography	Used to noninvasively monitor rapid eye movement (REM) sleep
Magnetic resonance imaging (MRI)	Used to identify structural abnormalities in three dimensions
Magnetic resonance spectroscopy (MRS)	Used to identify biochemical information in tissues; used to detect changes in neurophysiology after concussion.
Magnetic molecular energizing (MME)	Used to improve oxygen carrying capacity, assimilation of nutrients, manufacture of enzymes, metabolic waste removal, and reduction of free radicals
Vagus nerve stimulation (VNS)	Used for hard-to-treat seizure disorders; depression
Power spectral analysis (PSA)	Used to monitor the amplitude and latency of brain electrical discharges

(continued)

Low-level laser therapy (LLLT)	Used to improve healing, pain, bone growth, and immune response
Radio shock waves (rESW)	Used to improved wrist and finger flexors spasticity in stroke patients
Optune® tumor-treating field device	Used as a continuous treatment for glioblastoma

Magnetic resonance imaging (MRI) provides close-up views of tissues and their biological processes. MRI helps researchers better understand disease prevention, detection, and treatment. Continued success with MRI has led to more individualized treatment choices (Shields & Wilson, 2016).

Magnetic resonance spectroscopy (MRS) detects chemicals underlying metabolic processes. The MRI provides information on the location of a tumor while the MRS provides information on the aggressiveness of the tumor. Together they provide detailed information about pathology and potential treatment choices (Hone-Blanchet et al., 2015).

Low-level laser (light) therapy (LLLT), sometimes called cold laser therapy, uses infrared light to affect mitochondria, which then stimulate healing responses at the molecular, cellular, and tissue levels. It is used to reduce pain inflammation, promote nerve and tissue regeneration, and restore bodily functions. Protective glasses must be worn during the application to protect the retinas of participants. Low-level laser therapy is contraindicated for people who have photosensitive skin or who are taking photosensitizing medications. It is also contraindicated for people who have recently had steroid injections (Avci et al., 2013; Oschman, 2016).

A tumor-treating electrical field device has recently been developed for the treatment of glioblastoma (brain tumor). The FDA approved device Optune®, which is in its EF-14 phase 3 trials, emits low-intensity, intermediate-frequency, alternating electric fields that block the division of the rapidly dividing cancer cells. This is a noninvasive, continuous treatment utilizing 36 electrodes placed on the shaved scalp. There are minimal side effects such as scalp irritation or headache (Mehta, Wen, Nishikawa, Reardon, & Peters, 2017; Murphy, Bowers, & Barron, 2016; Schwartz & Onuselogu, 2016).

A low-energy neurofeedback system (LENS) has been developed to treat a number of conditions ranging from autism spectrum disorder to headaches to traumatic brain injuries. The purpose of the system is to help the brain adapt to imbalances caused by physical or emotional trauma. A low-power electromagnetic field is used to provide feedback and to stimulate brain-wave activity (Oschman, 2016).

Being immersed in a field of negative ions seems to balance people's energy and relieve pain. Physicians specializing in orthopedics and sports medicine have been recommending *magnets* since 1993. Athletic performance is enhanced and risk of serious injury is decreased when magnets are used to warm up muscles and joints. People wear magnets on their wrists, elbows, and knees for joint pain or on their heads for headaches. Magnets are used to speed the healing of wounds. Though not recognized as medical devices by the U.S. Food and Drug Administration, magnets have been widely used in Asia for years. The magnets used are about 5 to 10 times as strong as refrigerator door magnets and cost between $15 and $35 a pair depending on the size.

A few *contraindications* for magnetic therapy need to be observed. Until further research is conducted, pregnant women should not wear magnets over the abdominal area. Magnets should not be used by persons wearing pacemakers, defibrillators, aneurysm clips in the brain, cochlear (inner ear) implants, insulin pumps, or other implanted electrical devices. Magnets decrease the stickiness of platelets, which contributes to increased bleeding. For that reason, they should not be used by people on anticoagulants or who have an actively bleeding or open wound. Magnets should not be used on a freshly torn muscle that is still bleeding internally. In this situation, it is best to wait 3 to 5 days after the injury, or 10 to 14 days if the tear is severe, before using magnets to aid the healing process.

RESEARCH

Little research has been conducted in the United States regarding the clinical effects of magnets. In Europe and Russia, however, where magnetism is well regarded, hundreds of scientific studies have been documented. However, bioelectric magnetic therapy has been studied in the United States and the following is a small sample of the studies:

- The following electrotherapy modalities were investigated for treatment of rotator cuff disease: therapeutic ultrasound, LLLT, transcutaneous electrical nerve stimulation (TENS), and pulsed electromagnetic field therapy (PEMFT) as components of physical therapy treatment. A Cochrane systematic review found that therapeutic ultrasound and LLLT had short-term benefits on pain and function over placebo. Since the evidence was low quality, further trials are necessary (Page et al., 2016).
- A systematic review of the effectiveness of neurofeedback for posttraumatic stress disorder (PTSD) found that protocols and methods varied widely. Out of five studies, three found a significant effect, but more consistent and higher quality studies are needed (Reiter, Andersen, & Carlsson, 2016).
- A systematic review of 17 trials evaluated the use of LLLT in the treatment of people with shoulder tendinopathy. LLLT demonstrated a significant level of pain relief and a more rapid course of improvement when compared with control groups (Haslerud, Magnussen, Joensen, Lopes-Martins, & Bjordal, 2015).
- A randomized, double-blind, parallel group studied the effect of a magnetic pulsing field on paresthesia in people with multiple sclerosis. Thirty-five people had the magnetic treatment two times a week for 8 weeks while 28 people had a magnetically inactive treatment for the same length of time. People with the magnetic field treatment had significant improvement in the severity of paresthesia compared to the control group (Afshari et al., 2016).

- A systematic review of several pilot studies and clinical trials has demonstrated the potential benefit of tumor-treating fields for people with glioblastoma. Additional studies are needed to determine cost effectiveness and the impact on quality of life (Mittal et al., 2017).

INTEGRATED NURSING PRACTICE

Pulsed magnetic fields are used to stimulate osteoblast cells in osteoporosis and in fractured bones as well as in osteoarthritis and musculoskeletal pain. Some of the devices are wearable, which makes the intervention more convenient. Low-level laser therapy is used to increase the pace of wound healing, pain relief, stimulation of endorphin release, repair of bone, and modulation of the immune system. A variety of health-care professions provide low-level laser therapy, such as nurse practitioners, physical therapists, chiropractors, and integrative health physicians.

Awareness of healing with magnets is gaining credibility in the United States and is being applied by increasing numbers of conventional as well as integrative health-care practitioners as an adjunct therapy. Increasing numbers of people are wearing small magnets during the day for pain relief, greater energy, and healing. Treatments can last from just a few minutes to overnight and, depending on the situation and severity, may be applied several times a day for days or weeks at a time.

Explain to clients that the effectiveness of magnetic treatment depends on the number of magnets used and their strength, thickness, and spacing. Magnets vary in strength, and the magnetic flux density or field strength of those used for healing purposes is generally between 1,000 and 5,000 gauss (G). (The tesla is the preferred international unit of measurement: 1 tesla (T) equals 10,000 G.) In comparison, the magnetic field strength at the surface of the earth is approximately 0.5 G. The thicker the magnet, the greater the depth of penetration, but increasing thickness makes the magnet more uncomfortable to wear. Most people wear magnets that are between 1/4 and 3/8 inch thick. In general, the magnet should be larger than the size of the area being treated. Clients who are treating finger joints for arthritis will use a small magnet, while those who are treating the lower back will apply a much larger magnet.

When teaching clients about magnetic therapy, you can explain that the most common use is in the treatment of pain, with reports of successful treatment in arthritis, rheumatism, fibromyalgia, back pain, headaches, muscle sprains and strains, joint pain, tendonitis, shoulder pain, carpal tunnel syndrome, and torn ligaments.

Magnetic therapy may be one of the most effective methods for achieving relief from arthritis, especially in the hands and feet. People with carpal tunnel syndrome can apply magnets to the front and back of the wrist to help control symptoms. Individuals diagnosed with fibromyalgia can sleep on a magnetic mattress pad and use a magnetic pillow. They may also use magnets over the painful areas during the day. Magnetic insoles increase circulation and help conditions such as numbness, burning, aches, restlessness, and leg cramps. A client with phantom pain following an amputation may be able to use magnets to improve the flow of blood in the stump and cause the phantom pain to disappear. People with asthma and bronchitis may find that wearing a strong neodymium magnet over the chest and at an equal level on the back will help return breathing to a normal state. For minor burns, people can place a magnet over the site of injury to speed the healing and reduce the pain (Micozzi et al., 2015).

It is currently unclear whether you should suggest that clients wear the magnets full time or intermittently. This recommendation will need to be determined through further research. At this time, you can encourage clients to experiment with time periods that seem most effective. As scientific and clinical understanding increases, you will be able to provide more information about how to manipulate magnets for the best effects.

TRY THIS

Absorbing Earth Energy

Find a grassy, open area that is in its relatively natural state. You may or may not choose to use a blanket. Lie face down with your arms and legs extended in a spread-eagle fashion. Notice that all your chakras are in direct contact with the earth. Visualize an exchange of energy as you release to the earth, with each out-breath, any stress or negativity you have been carrying. With each in-breath, imagine that your chakras are receiving fresh, balanced, healing energy from the earth. Do this relaxation breathing for at least 20 minutes. You should feel yourself in a pleasant and refreshed state.

TRY THIS

Going to the Mountains

If you live near hills or mountains, go to the highest natural point you can reach. High places are concentrations of energy and seem to lift one above normal conflicting energies. Looking below, get a sense of the differences in the two energetic environments. You may feel clear, focused energy on the higher point while sensing a mixture of many different energies in the area below. After a while, you should experience clearer thinking and a sense of inspiration.

Source: Collinge (1998).

References

Afshari, D., Moradian, N., Khalili, M., Razazian, N., Bostani, S., Hoseini, J., . . . Ghiasian, M. (2016). Evaluation of pulsing magnetic field effects on paresthesia in multiple sclerosis patients: A randomized, double-blind, parallel-group clinical trial. *Clinical Neurology and Neurosurgery*. doi: 10.1016/j.clineuro.2016.08.015

Avci, P., Gupta, A., Sadasivam, M., Vecchio, D., Pam, Z., Pam, N., & Hamblin, M. R. (2013). Low-level laser (light) therapy (LLLT) in skin: Stimulating, healing, restoring. *Seminars in Cutaneous Medicine and Surgery*, 32(1): 41–52.

Bukkyo Dendo Kyokai. (1900). *The Teachings of Buddha*. Sterling Publishers.

Collinge, W. (1998). *Subtle Energy*. New York, NY: Warner Books.

Haslerud, S., Magnussen, L. H., Joensen, J., Lopes-Martins, R. A., & Bjordal, J. M. (2015). The efficacy of low-level laser therapy for shoulder tendinopathy: A systematic review and meta-analysis of randomized controlled trials. *Physiotherapy Research International*. doi: 10.1002/pri.1606

Hone-Blanchet, A., Salas, R. E., Celnik, P., Kalloo, A., Schar, M., Puts, N. A. J., . . . Edden, R. A. (2015). Co-registration of magnetic resonance spectroscopy and transcranial magnetic stimulation. *Journal of Neuroscience Methods*. doi: 10.1016/j.jneumeth.2014.12.018

Mehta, M., Wen, P., Nishikawa, R., Reardon, D., & Peters, K. (2017). Critical review of the addition of tumor treating fields (TTFields) to the existing standard of care for newly diagnosed glioblastoma patients. *Critical Reviews in Oncology Hematology*. doi: 10.1016/j.critrevonc .2017.01.005

Micozzi, M. S., Weintraub, M. I., & Gehl, J. (2015). Biophysics: Electricity, light, magnetism, and sound. In M. S. Micozzi (Ed.), *Fundamentals of Complementary and Alternative Medicine* (5th ed., pp. 213–239). St. Louis, MO: Elsevier/Saunders.

Mittal, S., Klinger, N. V., Michelhaugh, S. K., Barger, G. R., Pannullo, S. C., & Juhasz, C. (2017). Alternating electric tumor treating fields for treatment of glioblastoma: Rationale, preclinical, and clinical studies. *Journal of Neurosurgery*. doi: 10.3171/2016.9.JNS16452

Murphy, J., Bowers, M. E., & Barron, L. (2016). Optune®: Practical nursing applications. *Clinical Journal of Oncology Nursing*. doi: 10.1188/16.CJON./ S1.14-19

Oschman, J. I. (2016). *Energy Medicine: The Scientific Basis* (2nd ed.). St. Louis, MO: Elsevier/Saunders.

Page, M. J., Green, S., Mrocki, M. A., Surace, S. J., Deitch, J., McBain, B., . . . Buchbinder, R. (2016). Electrotherapy modalities for rotator cuff disease. *Cochrane Database of Systematic Reviews*. doi: 10.1002/14651858.CD012225

Reiter, K., Andersen, S. B., & Carlsson, J. (2016). Neurofeedback treatment and posttraumatic stress disorder: Effectiveness of neurofeedback on posttraumatic stress disorder and the optimal choice of protocol. *Journal of Nervous and Mental Disease*. doi: 10.1097/NMD.0000000000000418

Schwartz, M. A., & Onuselogu, L. (2016). Rationale and background on tumor-treating fields for glioblastoma. *Clinical Journal of Oncology Nursing*, doi: 10.1188/16.CJON.S1.20-24

Shields, D. A., & Wilson, D. R. (2016). Energy healing. In B. M. Dossey & L. Keegan (Eds.), *Holistic Nursing: A Handbook for Practice* (7th ed., pp. 187–220). Burlington, MA: Jones & Bartlett Learning.

Twin Light Trail. (1999). *American Indian Review*, Issues 19–29. Originally from the University of Wisconsin—Madison.

Resources

Advanced Magnetic Research Institute
International
6230 E. Tropical Pkwy
Las Vegas, NV 89115
1.800.265.1119
www.amri-intl.com

The Magnetic Resonance Imaging
Institute for Biomedical Research
440 East Ferry St.
Detroit, MI 48202
313.758.0065

27

Animal-Facilitated Therapy

Treat the earth well: it was not given to you by your parents, it was loaned to you by your children. We do not inherit the Earth from our Ancestors, we borrow it from our Children.

ANCIENT INDIAN PROVERB

A nimal-facilitated therapy (AFT) is the umbrella term for a variety of therapies involving animals in health and human service settings. The use of animals has been steadily gaining in popularity in the United States and has been shown to be a successful intervention for people with a variety of physical or psychological conditions. Despite reluctance and skepticism on the part of many administrators of health-care facilities, nurses have often advocated the use of animals as a therapeutic intervention. One of the earliest recorded observations of a connection between animals and health was made by Florence Nightingale (1969) in 1860 when she noted, "a small pet is often an excellent companion for the sick, for long chronic cases especially" (p. 103). She further suggested that when possible, patients should participate in the care of the animal, because this activity was helpful to their recovery. Long banned from health-care facilities, dogs, cats, and other pets are gradually being welcomed with open arms.

BACKGROUND

In 900 B.C., Homer wrote about Asklepios, the Greek god of healing, whose healing power was transmitted through sacred dogs.

In the ninth century, people in Geel, Belgium, began using animals to care for people with disabilities. Theirs was the first recorded therapeutic farm animal program for patients. The York Retreat in England, founded in 1792 for the treatment of people with mental illness, used small animals such as rabbits and poultry in their treatment plan. The goal was to decrease the use of restraints and medications by helping residents learn self-control through animals that relied on them for care. Bethel, a residential treatment center for people with epilepsy, founded in 1867 in Germany, utilized pets as an important part of the treatment program. This pet program is still in place today and has expanded to include farm animals and a wild game park. In the United States in the 1940s, injured World War II soldiers were encouraged to work with the hogs, cattle, and horses on the farm of the Army Air Corps Convalescent Hospital in New York. Since that time, animals have been used in many medical specialties, from pediatrics to geriatrics; in varied U.S. clinical settings, from acute care facilities, chronic care homes, group accommodations, private homes; to schools and correctional facilities; and in prevention and healing, nationwide (Fine, 2015).

PREPARATION

In the 1990s, Pet Partners (formerly the Delta Society) developed the first program for animal-assisted therapy. Rainbow Animal Assisted Therapy focuses on children with special needs. The goals include improving physical skills such as reaching for or grasping objects or brushing a dog, and cognitive skills such as reading aloud to or giving commands to a dog.

Therapy dogs and cats are specifically selected for temperament, companionability, and interaction. *Temperament* is the animal's natural or instinctive behavior and is important in terms of the way the animal will react when stressed. A good therapy pet is calm, tolerant, and friendly. The second major criterion is that the animal has a person who is willing to volunteer time and energy to share the pet with others. Dogs must be obedience trained prior to participating in the program. A dog or cat must be at least 1-year old before enrolling in the training and visiting program to ensure that the pet has been effectively socialized and is comfortable interacting with numerous people in a crowded setting. In addition, the animal's immune system is more stabilized by this age. A veterinarian must verify the animal's health, and all inoculations must be current. Animal-assisted therapy registering organizations require that a dog and its handler pass several tests prior to registration. In general, dogs have to demonstrate basic obedience skills and must be indifferent to crowds and distractions and unfazed by exuberant or clumsy handling, including ear tugging and "bear hugging." In addition, they must have a high tolerance for unfamiliar or loud noises and peculiar smells. In addition to the familiar dogs and cats in pet therapy, other animals may include parrots, cockatoos, guinea pigs, rabbits, pot-bellied pigs, dwarf goats, llamas, donkeys, and horses. Therapeutic riding horses must have a gentle, tolerant temperament; be well balanced and well muscled; and move with even strides. In recent years, dolphin-assisted therapy has become very popular, and a number of these programs exist worldwide. The cost is significantly higher for dolphins than for other animal-assisted therapy programs.

CONCEPTS

Companion Animals

Many people think of their animals as surrogate children. And these are children who rarely, if ever, disappoint their parents. Pets, especially dogs, often seem to understand what their owners are feeling. For some people, a pet is a reason to get up in the morning. It is something to nurture, touch, and stroke. For stress relief, it apparently does not matter much whether the pet is a Great Dane, a tomcat, or a canary. What is most important is the person's relationship with the pet.

The contributions companion animals make to the emotional well-being of people include providing unconditional love and opportunities for affection; functioning as a confidant, playmate, and companion; and assisting in the establishment of trust, responsibility, and empathy toward others. Studies of children with pets indicate that the unconditional love and acceptance conveyed in the child–animal relationship may validate a child's sense of self-worth. In addition, older school-age children often turn to companion animals in times of stress for reassurance. Children often perceive their companion animals as play partners, most often during middle childhood than during adolescence or early childhood (Dietz, Davis, & Pennings, 2012).

Children with interactive pets such as dogs and cats are more attached to their companion animals than are children with other types of pets such as hamsters, fish, and turtles. Emotional bonds are more likely to be formed with animals that are able to respond in an outwardly loving and affectionate way. Behaviors such as tail wagging, barking, and purring often elicit affectionate responses in human caregivers. In North America and Europe, families with children, especially school-age children, are more likely to own companion animals than are families without children. Multiple-pet ownership is also common. Pet ownership remains higher in rural versus urban areas, and in houses versus apartments. Still, across a variety of settings, the majority of children in Western countries are living with companion animals.

Therapy Animals

The characteristics that make many pets cherished family members—unconditional affection, responsiveness, and companionability—also make pets effective in therapy. In this age of high technological health care, it is sometimes easy to forget the importance of unconditional affection. Animals pay little attention to age or physical ability but accept people as they are. It is insignificant if the person has no hair, is in a wheelchair, or is hallucinating. The underlying concept that supports the use of animals for therapeutic reasons is the bonding experience it provides. Frail or depressed older adults often brighten up and adopt a more positive outlook when they are in the presence of an animal "therapist."

Many health-care professionals are finding that loneliness may be as serious as cancer and heart disease for older adults. Older people who stay active, find substitutes for work, and build new relationships when partners and friends die have been found to be the most satisfied with life. Not all older adults, however, have options for remaining active and forming new friendships. Visiting with animals can help people feel less lonely and less depressed. Animals can provide a welcome change from routine or a distraction from disability or pain. People often talk to the animals and share with them their thoughts, feelings, and memories (Figure 27.1). When people talk to people, their blood pressure tends to go up because of concern about how one is being evaluated or judged. With animals, who are always eager to please and unconditionally accepting, people's blood pressure levels tend to go down (Reed, Ferrer, & Villegas, 2012).

Animals also make it easier for two strangers to talk. They give people a common interest, provide a focus for conversation, and broaden the circle of friends. When animals visit long-term care facilities, residents laugh and mingle more than when the animals are not around. Animals also help stimulate socialization by providing an opportunity to share stories of animals the residents may have had in the past. Many people like to stroke the animal while talking about the pets that shared their lives.

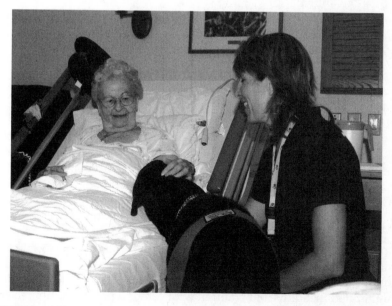

FIGURE 27.1   A Therapy Dog Provides Interaction and Comfort—A Hospice Patient with a Therapy Dog and Her Careworker

Source: Dennis Sabo/Shutterstock.

TREATMENT

Animal-Assisted Therapy

Animal-assisted therapy (AAT) is the use of specifically selected animals as a treatment modality in a variety of settings. In AAT, an accredited professional guides the human–animal interaction toward specific, individualized therapeutic goals. In one treatment session, a variety of goals can be addressed: *physical goals* such as range of motion, balance, and mobility; *cognitive goals* such as improved memory or verbal expression; *emotional goals* such as increased self-esteem and motivation; and *social goals* such as building rapport and improved socialization skills. Linda Hume, LPN, AAT specialist, has developed a program of animal facilitation in occupational and physical therapy at Northeast Rehabilitation Hospital in Salem, New Hampshire (www.noretheastrehab.com/features/animal-facilitated-therapy). The following are a few of the goals and activities she has identified for AAT in her clinical setting:

- *Increased upper extremity range of motion:* Throw an object for dog to retrieve; use leash to maneuver dog; pet, stroke, brush animal
- *Mobility:* Ambulate with dog
- *Improved coordination:* Throw an object for dog to retrieve (releasing); reach for object dog has retrieved
- *Improved memory:* Ask client to recall dog's name, breed, age, and so forth; command dog to sit and remember to release dog from command
- *Increased language production:* Use commands with dog; simply talk to or about animal
- *Object identification:* Direct dog to retrieve specific familiar items by appropriate name—ball, spoon, pen, or cup
- *Attention/concentration:* Attend to dog, task, and therapist

Therapeutic horseback riding, or *hippotherapy,* is defined as all rehabilitative uses of horses. The term derives from the Greek word *hippo,* meaning "horse." In *hippopsychotherapy,* the riding is designed to support the psychotherapeutic treatment plan. Goals include increased self-confidence, improved self-esteem, refined social competence, the experience of pleasure, and the ability to establish a relationship with the horse. *Remedial educational riding* is used to further the educational and behavioral goals for school-age children with learning problems. The horse is used as a strong motivator for accomplishing specific treatment goals. *Physical hippotherapy* is the use of the rhythmic movement of the horse to increase sensory processing and improve posture, balance, and mobility in people with movement dysfunctions. The transfer of movement from the horse to the client is designed primarily to achieve physical goals but may also affect psychological, cognitive, behavioral, and communication outcomes. Clients benefiting from hippotherapy include, but are not limited to, adults and children with cerebral palsy, multiple sclerosis, orthopedic problems, posttraumatic spasticity, strokes, scoliosis, genetic syndromes, autism spectrum disorder, and developmental delays (Wilson, Buultjens, Monfries, & Karimi, 2015).

Dolphin-assisted therapy (DAT) programs worldwide are used to lessen symptoms of a wide range of conditions such as depression, Down syndrome, autistic spectrum disorders, speech disorders, cerebral palsy, and traumatic brain injury. However, there is currently no evidence that DAT provides greater benefit than other animal-assisted therapies. Recently, a virtual reality program has been developed for children with autistic spectrum disorders. Rather than swimming with the dolphins, the children act as trainers and learn nonverbal communication skills with the virtual dolphins (Cai et al., 2013; Salgueiro et al., 2012).

The National Animal Assisted Crisis Response and the Hope Animal-Assisted Crisis Response organizations provide dog and handler teams to help victims of crisis situations or disasters, such as the Sandy Hook Elementary School shooting, the Orlando mass shooting, and natural disasters such as tornados, floods, and fires. Some victims talk to the comfort dogs, while others just want to pet or hug the dogs.

Animal-Assisted Activities

A less formal approach, **animal-assisted activities (AAAs)**, includes motivational, educational, and recreational approaches. The goal is to provide "meeting and greeting" human–animal interactions to enhance the quality of life, rather than a specific treatment plan. AAA is used in many types of facilities with a wide variety of animals. AAA visits to sheltered homeless families have been effective. Most shelters do not allow families to bring their pets, and seeing the visiting animal can be therapeutic, especially for children. AAA visits give homeless children a chance to participate in everyday experiences they may not have had recently, such as walking a dog or playing fetch.

Pet Visits

A family **pet visit** is an arrangement for a pet to visit the owner in a health-care setting. The concept of pet visits as therapy for hospitalized people is not new, especially in facilities with rehabilitation, oncology, and mental health units. The pet that visits may belong to a pet therapy program or may be the client's own pet. It is believed that allowing a pet to visit can be a healing experience for patients, family members, and even the pet. Pets are even allowed to visit in ICU settings, with the approval of the nurses, provided there are no medical contraindications.

Resident Animals

Resident animals live at health-care facilities. Species include fish, birds, hamsters, gerbils, guinea pigs, rabbits, cats, and dogs. The staff is responsible for the complete health and well-being of the animals, and residents are included in providing routine daily care. Grooming and brushing a resident dog, for example, are good therapies for the hands. Some staff report that full-time pets become so perceptive that they gravitate to the rooms of people who are the most isolated or depressed. Those residents who have regular visits are more receptive to treatment, have a greater incentive to recover, and have an increased will to live.

Green Care

Green care is a total environmental approach using plants, gardens, and animals as therapeutic tools for individuals with physical or emotional problems. The intervention takes place on farms where clients assist in the care of animals and participate in other types of farm work. The program has been implemented in several European countries with positive results (Berget, Ekeberg, & Braastad, 2008).

Green Chimneys is a therapeutic residential program in New York. The participants are children with special needs or children who have been unsuccessful in a traditional school setting. The program has a global reputation in the use of animals in helping children succeed academically, socially, and emotionally.

Service Animals

Service animals are individually trained to do work or perform tasks for a person with a physical or emotional disability. Because they are not considered a "pet," they may legally go anywhere that a person with disabilities goes. Some service animals are trained to "alert" the person that a specific event is going to occur in the near future and is able to notify the human partner of this impending event. Other service animals are trained to "respond," that is, to act in a predetermined manner when a specific event occurs (Gilmer, Baudino, Tielsch Goddard, Vickers, & Akard, 2016).

Most people are familiar with *guide dogs* for those with visual impairment. Other *disability service animals* can be trained to pull a wheelchair, open doors, retrieve dropped objects as small as a dime, turn light switches on and off, carry items in a backpack, and bark to alert for help. *Hearing animals* alert owners to important sounds that need a response such as smoke, fire, and clock alarms, telephones, baby crying, sirens, and knocks at the door. *Seizure response animals*, usually dogs or cats, are able to alert people to the onset of their owner's seizures and can be trained to stay with the person or get help. They also help the person become reoriented and mobile after the seizures. *Diabetic service animals* alert their owners to episodes of hypoglycemia before there are symptoms, giving those persons time to monitor and correct their glucose level. When breathing machines malfunction, *respiratory service dogs* can be trained to nose the phone receiver out of its cradle and hit the speed-dial buttons, all of which are programmed to 911. *Psychiatric service animals* alert and/or respond to human partners experiencing panic attacks, social phobias, agoraphobia, posttraumatic stress disorder, dissociative amnesia, and depersonalization disorder. Any person who has a physical or mental impairment that substantially limits a major life activity might be a candidate for a service dog (Fine, 2015).

Training service dogs is an expensive and time-consuming project. The dog spends the first year of life with a foster family who is responsible for socialization and basic obedience training. Next, 5 to 6 months of intensive training is followed by 6 months of in-home training with the new owner. The expense of training an animal is usually more than $10,000. The benefit, of course, is that people can lead more independent and fulfilling lives.

Screening Animals

Early detection of cancer improves both quality of life and life expectancy. Research is focusing on a dog's sense of smell that might provide a better early warning system for some cancers than modern science. While people have about 5 million smell-sensing cells, dogs have about 220 million such cells. It is estimated that dogs are 1,000 to 100,000 times more sensitive to smells than humans. **Screening dogs** are being trained to detect prostate cancer by smelling urine, lung cancer by smelling breath, and skin cancer by smelling the entire body. It is thought that cancer patients have a different odor that is detectable to trained sniffer dogs. Dogs have also been taught to detect hypoglycemia and epileptic seizures before they occur (Amundsen, Sundstrom, Buvik, Gederaas, & Haaverstad, 2014; Wells, 2012).

Past research has demonstrated that pigeons can identify letters of the alphabet, basic categories such as cars, chairs, or cats, and identify whether facial photos are female or male. Based on this information, studies are emerging on the ability of pigeons in the detection of breast cancer in humans. Pigeons have been trained to distinguish benign from malignant breast cancer, both histopathological (slides of breast tissue samples) and radiological (mammograms), with an 80–85% accuracy rate. While it is unlikely that pigeons will become active in diagnosing cancer, what is hoped is that pigeons will be a model for the development of more sophisticated technology in the future (Levenson, Krupinski, Navarro, & Wasserman, 2015).

Dogs in the Correctional Setting

Canine Assistants, an organization that trains service dogs, has an at-risk youth program for juvenile male offenders, aged 13 to 18 years. The program is jointly sponsored with the West Florida Wilderness Institute and Camp Sierra Blanca in New Mexico. It is a residential program with an average stay of 6 months. The young men work with service puppies and dogs under the supervision of experienced trainers. The goal is to learn responsibility, patience, and goal setting. Statistics demonstrate increased self-esteem, improved school grades, and a decreased recidivism rate for those involved in the program.

In correctional institutes all across Ohio, puppies and prisoners are teaming up in an unusual program. A nonprofit organization called Pilot

Dogs, Inc., places service puppies under the care of prisoners until the pups are ready for formal training as service dogs. Since the inception of the program in 1992, hundreds of dogs have been placed in prisons. Inmates are chosen based on their records of good behavior and experience with dogs. No violent offenders are permitted to raise the dogs. The puppies sleep in crates in the cells with their partners and accompany them on their daily activities, including trips to the dining hall, where the puppies learn to be well behaved around people and become accustomed to the noise and crowds they will be faced with later. The prisoner is responsible for the care and well-being of the dog and for housebreaking, leash-training, and putting the dog through a basic obedience course. After spending about 12 months at the correctional facility, the puppies are moved and placed in an intensive training program for service dogs.

Other prison programs train dogs for adoption by the general public. While the training sessions are only 2 months, the process is similar to that for service dogs. A major advantage for the dogs is having human contact 24 hours a day, which is less likely to occur in regular foster homes. The chosen prisoners have the pleasure and delight of having a puppy to give love to and receive love in return. Prisoners learn to manage anger issues, calm down, and improve social skills. They also have the satisfaction of seeing the benefits of their training as the puppy progresses. Another benefit is that prisoners learn marketable skills that help them find jobs after they are released (Allison & Ramaswamy, 2016).

RESEARCH

To date, much of the literature on the therapeutic use of animals in health care is anecdotal, but scientific research is beginning to appear. Most of the studies recommend further investigations because they show associations but not causal relationships. The following is a small sample of the literature:

- A systematic review of animal-assisted therapy for children and adolescents with intellectual disabilities found a positive improvement in psychosocial skills. Some skills, but not all, reached statistical significance (Maber-Aleksandrowicz, Avent, & Hassiotis, 2016).
- A systematic review of hippotherapy found improvement in motor function, spasticity, posture, balance, and gait. The improvements were most noticeable in those individuals who had at least one session per week for multiple weeks (Rigby & Grandjean, 2016).
- A small-scale randomized controlled trial found that people with schizophrenia who experienced animal-assisted therapy showed a significant improvement in negative symptoms of the disorder compared to the control group (Calvo et al., 2016).
- Children with Down syndrome were randomized into a control group and an experimental group that received Thai elephant-assisted therapy twice a week for 2 months. There was no significant difference between

the two groups in balance or postural control. The experimental group had a significant improvement in visual motor integration (Satiansuk-pong, Pongsaksri, & Sasat, 2016).
• Thirty-seven patients with the diagnosis of hepatocellular carcinomas (HCC) and 111 people as control sample were involved in a study of using smell detection by a dog trained to detect the cancer. Breaths were collected using facemasks and sent to the study test site. The dog had a statistically significant accuracy of 78% (p:0.001). Further studies will be needed before clinical application can occur (Kitiyakara et al., 2017).

One of the largest organizations devoted to animal-assisted therapy is Pet Partners, with 1,500 members, 20% of whom are health-care professionals. The objectives of Pet Partners are to promote study and research relating to human–animal interactions, to increase the awareness of the significance of these interactions among health-care professionals, and to assess the role of the effect of human–pet bonds on the mental and physical well-being of people. Warrior Canine Connection utilizes veterans to train service dogs. The training process helps veterans heal themselves of post-traumatic stress disorder. At the end of the training period, the service dogs are placed with disabled veterans. Rainbow Animal Assisted Therapy focuses primarily on children with special needs and is active in hospitals and health-care facilities, residential centers, schools and libraries, parks, and camps.

INTEGRATED NURSING PRACTICE

An important nursing role is that of advocate. Nurse advocates serve as links between clients and other health-care professionals of the community. In that role, nurses in a wide variety of clinical settings can explore and encourage the therapeutic use of animals. The many benefits of human–animal interaction include attachment, bonding, caring, pain management, stress management, motivation, communication, improved self-esteem, cardiovascular benefits, and improved coordination and balance. Disinterest on the part of health-care professionals has been the major obstacle to growth in the field of animal-assisted therapy.

To set up an AAT program, you must begin by approaching the facility's administration with a well-organized plan. This plan should include the following aspects:

• Theory and research background
• Goals and outcomes
• Clearly written policy and procedures
• Staff education about the proposed program
• A plan for volunteer recruitment and training
• A plan for testing and training of potential therapy animals
• A plan for implementing the program
• A plan for evaluating the program

You can anticipate some opposition to the initiation of an AAT program. One of the biggest concerns is the potential for transmission of infectious diseases. Although the risk is low, several *zoonoses,* or animal-transmitted infections, can occur. Seek the assistance of a veterinarian to identify the risks for specific types of infections and measures to prevent them. Infection risk can be reduced by making sure each animal is clean, vaccinated, and healthy; keeping the animal out of the areas where food is prepared and served; and having residents wash their hands after the animal visits. Products can be sprayed on the animal's fur to reduce the risk of an allergic reaction (Friedmann & Son, 2009).

Robotic animals, as opposed to living animals, are used in some institutions caring for people with dementia. The PARO robotic pet looks like a baby harp seal that is covered in artificial fur. Internal software allows the PARO pet to imitate seal behavior and respond to environmental stimuli. For many individuals, the PARO pet improved mood, reduced the need for medication, and improved socialization (Birks, Bodak, Barlas, Harwood, & Pether, 2016; Petersen, Houston, Qin, Tague, & Studley, 2017).

"No pets" policies may not be applied to service animals. Hospitals, medical offices, laboratories, imaging services, day care centers, schools, restaurants, and others are covered under the Americans with Disabilities Act. The ADA requires that places of public accommodation modify their policies and practices to permit the use of a service animal by a person with a disability, unless doing so would create a direct threat to the safety of others or the facility. There is no legal requirement that a service animal wear special equipment or tags. Facilities are advised to accept the verbal reassurance of the person that he or she has a disability and that the animal is a service animal. Requiring "proof" is prohibited by the ADA.

If you are a pet owner, you can consider becoming a pet therapy volunteer. Many long-term care facilities encourage regular visits from people with trained and screened animals. Increasingly, these pets are also welcome at hospitals, cancer clinics, and hospices. This type of personal involvement in animal-assisted therapy can be wonderfully rewarding.

Very new to the use of animals in health care are the Mexican hairless breed known as Xolos (pronounced "show-low"). These dogs cuddle up to their owners and radiate the same amount of heat as a heating pad, which seems to work wonders for people with arthritis or fibromyalgia. The body temperature of Xolos is the same as that of all dogs, 102°F, but the lack of hair means that body heat is transferred directly to the surface the dog is touching. A nonprofit group, Xolos for Chronic Pain Relief, matches dogs with pain sufferers.

As a nurse, you have wonderful opportunities to incorporate AAT in your work with people infected with HIV/AIDS. In the past, these individuals were told to give up their pets for fear that their compromised immune system would place them at high risk for zoonotic infections. The reality is that people are more likely to contract zoonotic infections from contaminated food, water, soil, or even other people than from pets. You may need to explain to some clients that HIV infects only humans and other primates and therefore cannot be spread from or to dogs, cats, birds, or even fish. With this understanding, you can become an advocate for the physical, emotional, and psychological benefits of pet companionship for those with HIV/AIDS.

With proper care and understanding and a healthy pet, the potential health risks of pet companionship are minimal and the benefits may far outweigh the risks. People living with HIV often deal with feelings of isolation, rejection, and lack of purpose. Companion animals offer such individuals purpose, a feeling of being needed, a way to increase socialization, and a constant source of unconditional affection. Clients selecting a new pet should consider one whose temperament, energy levels, and environmental needs match their own. An older pet may be more appropriate than a young one. Box 27.1 describes the teaching you should do with any clients who are ill or immunosuppressed as a result of a disorder, chemotherapy, or organ transplants. The precautions are designed to protect people from acquiring secondary infections.

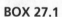

BOX 27.1

Client Teaching: Pet Owners Experiencing Illness

Veterinary Care

- Have your veterinarian examine your pet initially and then at least once a year.
- Keep your pet up to date on annual shots and rabies vaccination.
- Seek veterinary care immediately for sick pets.
- Have your veterinarian check street animals that are "adopted" before bringing them into your home.

Pet Care

- Keep your pet clean and well groomed with short, blunt toenails.
- Keep the pet's living and feeding areas clean.
- Keep your cat's litter box out of the kitchen; use a litter box liner and change it daily.
- Always walk your pet on a leash, and minimize the pet's contact with other animals and garbage.
- Keep cats indoors and prevent them from hunting birds and rodents.
- Feed your pet only commercially prepared pet foods; never feed raw meat or unpasteurized milk.
- Do not allow birds to fly free in your home; avoid their droppings.

General Hygiene

- Wash your hands frequently, especially before eating, smoking, or attending to open wounds.

(continued)

- Keep your cat off all kitchen surfaces. If that is not possible, be sure to wipe down, with a gentle disinfectant, any surface on which food may be placed.
- Do not allow your dog or cat to drink out of the toilet, because it is a place of many germs.
- Try to avoid contact with your pet's bodily fluids. Wear gloves and a face mask for cleaning a litter box, aquarium, or birdcage.

Sources: POWARS, New York, NY; PAWS, San Francisco, CA; Pet Partners, Bellevue, WA; Action AIDS, Philadelphia, PA.

A number of communities provide services to enable people who are ill to keep their pets. Volunteers provide dog-walking services for people physically unable to walk their dogs, deliver pet food and supplies, clean litter boxes and birdcages, provide in-home care for cats whose owners must go to the hospital, and foster care for dogs in the same situation. You could volunteer your time and energy to this type of program, or if your community has no such program, you could establish one.

TRY THIS

Interacting with Your Pet

When you are feeling tense or anxious and if you have a dog or a cat to which you are attached, try the following:

- Note your physical and emotional signs of tension: Are your hands clenched? Body trembling? Are you restless? Unable to relax? Mouth dry? Stomach upset? Breathing rapidly? Unable to concentrate? Worrying?
- Do something with your pet for at least 20 minutes: play, groom, or talk.
- Conduct another self-assessment. What, if anything, has changed?

If you have a dog or a cat to which you are attached, try this:

- Have a friend take your pulse and blood pressure.
- Gently play with your pet, stroke, pet, and talk to your animal for 15 minutes.
- Have your friend take your pulse and blood pressure again and compare the results with those taken prior to the interaction.

Animal contact contributes to self-concept, social interaction, a decrease in loneliness and anxiety, and in general contributes to physical, psychological, and spiritual well-being. Nurses can and should be at the forefront of designing and supporting more humane approaches to those in their care.

Considering the Evidence

Kamioka, H., Okada, S., Tsutani, K., Park, H., Okuizumi, H., Handa, S., . . . Mutoh, Y. (2014). Effectiveness of animal-assisted therapy: A systematic review of randomized controlled trials. *Complementary Therapies in Medicine, 22*(2): 371–390.

What Was the Approach of the Research?

Systematic review of randomized clinical trials (RCTs).

What Was the Aim/Purpose/Objective(s) of the Research as Related to Complementary and Integrative Therapies?

The objective of this systematic review was to evaluate and summarize the evidence from randomized controlled trials on the effects of animal-assisted therapy as related to specific targeted illnesses.

How Was the Study Done?

The protocol used for this systematic review included the following database searches for studies meeting the inclusion criteria: Cochrane, MEDLINE via PubMed, CINAHL, Web of Science, Ichushi Web (in Japanese), Global Health Library, Western Pacific Region Index Medicus, and PsycINFO. In addition, the researchers incorporated the following databases in their search: the Database of Abstracts of Reviews of Effects (DARE), the Health Technology Assessment Database (Technology Assessments), the NHS Economic Evaluation Database (NHS EED), and the Campbell Systematic Reviews. The results of the review identified 11 RCTs with seven studies focusing on "mental and behavioral disorders" and AAT meeting inclusion criteria. Type of animal was not a restriction of this review except for the exclusion of "robotic animals." A variety of animals (dogs, cats, dolphins, birds, cows, rabbits, ferrets, and guinea pigs) used in animal-assisted therapy intervention studies were included in this study.

What Were the Significant Findings of the Research?

The selected RCTs conducted did not meet the expectations of the researchers for quality using standardized tools for evaluation. However, one of the exceptions for a good quality study was the research involving dolphins. The researchers found that dolphin therapy may be effective for treating persons living with mild to moderate depression. This was based on a holistic approach through interaction with animals in their natural environment. In addition, animal-assisted therapy may have an effect on improvement in specific target diseases and mental health (anxiety and mood), decrease feeling of isolation, and enhance quality of life. The reviewed studies suggested that AAT may have a positive impact on the lives of those living with schizophrenia and/or serious mental health concerns. AAT has the potential to enhance conventional therapy in psychiatric rehabilitation.

What Additional Questions Might I Have?

What would be the benefit of AAT in persons with other "target" diseases? Are some pets found to be more beneficial in animal-assisted therapy than others? Would robotic animals work for persons who have an aversion to live animals or reside in an animal-restricted environment? What is the long-term benefit of animal-assisted therapy? What community/insurance resources may reimburse costs associated with animal-assisted therapy? What other animals may be considered in implementing AAT? How does one obtain access to animals/mammals that are not typically found in urban environments? Is AAT cost effective compared to conventional therapies? What risk/adverse factors should be considered prior to suggesting AAT for select persons living with specific target diseases?

What Is the Clinical Significance of This Study?

This systematic review has clinical value for nurses caring for persons living with depression, addiction behaviors, and other mental health/behavioral concerns. AAT should be considered as a possible intervention to enhance well-being and quality of life. Animal-assisted therapy may lessen the feelings of loneliness and isolation experienced by persons living with psychiatric/addiction disorders. In addition, nurses should be aware of the need for additional studies of methodological quality in providing stronger evidence to inform nursing practice.

Source: Contributed by Dolores M. Huffman, RN, PhD.

References

Allison, M., & Ramaswamy, M. (2016). Adapting animal-assisted therapy trials to prison-based animal programs. *Public Health Nursing.* doi: 10.1111/phn.12276

Amundsen, T., Sundstrom, S., Buvik, T., Gederaas, O. A., & Haaverstad, R. (2014). Can dogs smell lung cancer? First study using exhaled breath and urine screening in unselected patients with suspected lung cancer. *Acta Oncologica.* doi: 10.3109/0284186X.2013.819996

Berget, B., Ekeberg, O., & Braastad, B. O. (2008). Attitudes to animal-assisted therapy with farm animals among health staff and farmers. *Journal of Psychiatric and Mental Health Nursing,* 15: 576–581.

Birks, M., Bodak, M., Barlas, J., Harwood, J., & Pether, M. (2016). Robotic seals as therapeutic tools in an aged care facility: A qualitative study. *Journal of Aging Research.* doi: 10.1155/2016/8569602

Cai, Y., Chia, N. K., Thalmann, D., Kee, N. K., Zheng, J., & Thalmann, N. M. (2013). Design and development of a virtual dolphinarium for children with autism. *IEEE Transactions on Neural Systems and Rehabilitation Engineering.* doi: 10.1109/TNSRE.2013.2240700

Calvo, P., Fortuny, J. R., Guzman, S., Macias, C., Bowen, J., Garcia, M. L., . . . Fatjo, J. (2016). Animal assisted therapy (AAT) program as a useful adjunct to conventional psychosocial rehabilitation for patients with schizophrenia: Results of a small-scale randomized controlled trial. *Frontiers in Psychology.* doi: 10.3389/fpsyg.2016.00631

Dietz, T. J., Davis, D., & Pennings, J. (2012). Evaluating animal-assisted therapy in group treatment for child sexual abuse. *Journal of Child Sexual Abuse,* 21(6): 665–683. doi: 10.1080/10538712.2012.726700

Fine, A. H. (2015). *Handbook on Animal-Assisted Therapy* (4th ed.). London, UK: Academic Press.

Friedmann, E., & Son, H. (2009). The human–companion animal bond. *Veterinary Clinics of North America: Small Animal Practice*, 39(2): 293–326.

Gilmer, M. J., Baudino, M. N., Tielsch Goddard, A., Vickers, D. C., & Akard, T. F. (2016). Animal-assisted therapy in pediatric palliative care. *Nursing Clinics of North America* doi: 10.1016/j.cnur.2016.05.007

Hume, L. (2002). Animal facilitation in occupational and physical therapy sessions. Retrieved from www.northeastrehab.com/features/animal-facilitated-therapy

Kitiyakara, T., Redmond, S., Unwanatham, N., Rattanasiri, S., Thakkinstian, A., Tangtawee, P. . . . Kositchaiwat, C. (2017). The detection of hepatocellular carcinoma (HCC) from patients' breath using canine scent detection: Proof of concept study. *Journal of Breath Research.* doi: 10.1088/1752-7163/aa7b8e

Levenson, R. M., Krupinski, E., A., Navarro, V. M., & Wasserman, E. A. (2015). Pigeons (*Columba livia*) as trainable observers of pathology and radiology breast cancer images. *PLoS One.* doi: 10.1371/journal.pone.0141357

Maber-Aleksandrowicz, S., Avent, C., & Hassiotis, A. (2016). A systematic review of animal-assisted therapy on psychosocial outcomes in people with intellectual disability. *Research in Developmental Disabilities.* doi: 10.1016/j.ridd.2015.12.005

Nightingale, F. (1860). *Notes on Nursing: What It Is, and What It Is Not.* Adelaide Nutting Historical Nursing Collection. Harrison. Original from Oxford University.

Nightingale, F. (1969). *Notes on Nursing.* New York, NY: Dover.

Petersen, S., Houston, S., Qin, H., Tague, C., & Studley, J. (2017). The utilization of robotic pets in dementia care. *Journal of Alzheimer's Disease.* doi: 10.3233/JAD-160703

Reed, R., Ferrer, L., & Villegas, N. (2012). Natural healers: A review of animal assisted therapy and activities as complementary treatment for chronic conditions. *Revista Latino-Americana de Enfermagem*, 20(3): 612–618. doi: org.S0104-11692012000300025

Rigby, B. R., & Grandjean, P. W. (2016). The efficacy of equine-assisted activities and therapies on improving physical function. *Journal of Alternative and Complementary Medicine.* doi: 10.1089/acm.2015.0171

Salgueiro, E., Nunes, L., Barros, A., Maroco, J., Salgueiro, A. I., & Santos, M. E. (2012). Effects of a dolphin interaction program on children with autism spectrum disorders: An exploratory research. *BMC Research Notes*, 5:199. doi: 10.1186/1756-0500-5-199

Satiansukpong, N., Pongsaksri, M., & Sasat, D. (2016). Thai elephant-assisted therapy programme in children with Down syndrome. *Occupational Therapy International.* doi: 10.1002/oti.1417

Ward, J. E. (2006). *Earth Spirit: A Few of My Favorite Quotes and Native American Quotes Presented with My Poetry and Prose.* iUniverse.

Wells, D. L. (2012). Dogs as a diagnostic tool for ill health in humans. *Alternative Therapies in Health and Medicine*, 18(2): 12–17.

Wilson, K., Buultjens, M., Monfries, M., & Karimi, L. (2015). Equine-assisted psychotherapy for adolescents experiencing depression and/or anxiety: A therapist's perspective. *Clinical Child Psychology and Psychiatry.* doi: 10.1177/1359104515572379

Resources

Canine Assistants
3160 Francis Rd.
Milton, GA 30004
800.771.7221
www.canineassistants.org

Equine Assisted Growth and Learning
Association (EAGALA)
P.O. Box 993
Santaquin, UT 84655
877.858.4600
www.eagala.org

Federation of Horses in Education and
Therapy International
P.O. Box 134
Damariscotta, ME 04543
www.frdi.net

Green Chimneys
400 Doansburg Rd.
Brewster, NY 10509
845.279.2995
info@greenchimneys.org

Invisible Disabilities Association
P.O. Box 4067
Parker, CO 80134
www.invisibledisabilities.org

Pet Partners
875 124th Ave., NE, Suite 101
Bellevue, WA 98005
425.679.5500
www.petpartners.org

Puppies Behind Bars
263 West 38th St., 4th Floor
New York, NY 10018
212.680.9562
www.puppiesbehindbars.com

Rainbow Animal Assisted Therapy
6042 West Oakton St.
Morton Grove, IL 60053
773.283.1129
www.rainbowaat.org

DAWGS in Prison
1007 10th St.
Port St. Joes, FL 32456
www.dawgsinprison.com

Therapet
P.O. Box 130118
Tyler, TX 75713
903.535.2125
www.therapet.com

Therapy Dogs International
88 Bartley Rd.
Flanders, NJ 07836
973.252.9800
www.tdi-dog.org

Warrior Canine Connection
14934 Schaeffer Road
Boyds, MD 20841
301.260.1111
www.warriorcanineconnection.org

APPENDIX

Complementary Therapies for Common Health Problems

This appendix provides information related to the management of minor health problems. These types of problems often respond well to alternative therapies and lifestyle modification. If in doubt about the seriousness of symptoms, see your health-care practitioner. A number of suggestions are given for various problems. Select one that seems to be the most appropriate for your situation, and keep notes on what seems to work and what does not. Modify these suggestions according to your individual needs.

ABRASIONS, SCRAPES

- Aromatherapy: After washing with soap and water, apply 1–3 drops of lavender or tea tree oil to the wound; reapply oil twice a day until healed.
- To disinfect, pour 3% hydrogen peroxide into the wound and let it foam up.
- Apply the skin of a freshly peeled banana to the affected area, or cut a thin slice of raw potato and tape it over the affected area.
- Herbs: Sprinkle goldenseal powder on the wound. Crushed garlic mixed with honey makes a soothing salve: spread on a piece of clean gauze and cover the injured area.

ACNE

- Aromatherapy: Bergamot, cedarwood, chamomile, clary sage, lemon grass, melissa, patchouli, rosemary, sandalwood, tea tree oil, thyme, and ylang-ylang can be made into a facial mask, compress, or topical cream. Tea tree and lavender oils can be applied directly to blemishes.
- Herbs: arnica, borage, calendula skin products, tea tree oil
- Supplements: vitamin A, vitamin B_6, zinc, or evening primrose oil

AIDS

- Acupuncture
- Herbs: curcumin, extract of boxwood plant, echinacea, licorice, goldenseal, garlic, Chinese bitter melon
- Hyperbaric oxygen
- Massage
- Supplements: iron; vitamins C, E, and B; beta-carotene; glutamine; selenium

ALCOHOL ABUSE

- Acupuncture
- Antioxidants: selenium, zinc, vitamins C and E
- Bach flower essence, chrysanthemum, milkweed
- Herbs: milk thistle, kudzu, oatstraw, skullcap; evening primrose oil for withdrawal
- Meditation
- Megavitamin therapy: B vitamins
- Therapeutic Touch, Healing Touch
- Yoga

ALLERGIES

- Applied kinesiology
- Herbs: Stinging nettles to alleviate runny nose and sneezing. Teas made from chamomile, elder, or yarrow flowers can reduce reactions.
- Homeopathy: *Allium cepa* (onion); windflower; for swelling in the face: 1 tablet of apis every 15 minutes—maximum 6 doses
- Supplements: Vitamin C to decrease histamine production
- Water: Important to keep well hydrated; 64–96 ounces of water a day

ALZHEIMER'S DISEASE (DEMENTIA)

- Oils: rosemary, lemon, orange, chamomile, lavender, clary sage
- Reflexology
- Supplements: zinc, selenium, evening primrose oil, fish oil, coenzyme Q10; vitamins B_6, C, and E; Chinese herbal medicine
- Music

AMPUTATIONS: PHANTOM PAIN

- Magnets: Improve blood flow to stump and cause phantom pain to disappear
- Massage

ANXIETY

- Acupressure: Press center of inside wrist 1 inch above crease toward elbow. Use Sea-Bands: acupressure elastic wrist bands placed between 2 tendons, 3 finger-widths from wrist crease.
- Animal-assisted therapy
- Aromatherapy: basil, bergamot, chamomile; frankincense deepens breathing to induce calm-ness; green apple, juniper, lemon balm, orange, neroli for panic attacks

- Biofeedback
- Flower essences: aspen, mimulus, red chestnut
- Herbs: valerian, passionflower, lemon balm, chamomile, ylang-ylang
- Homeopathy: St. Ignatius bean, arsenic, Rescue Remedy
- Massage
- Meditation
- Reiki
- Relaxation techniques
- Therapeutic Touch, Healing Touch
- Watsu®
- Yoga
- Performance anxiety: hypnosis, guided imagery, Alexander Technique

ARTHRITIS

- Aromatherapy: cedarwood, coriander, cypress massage or cold compress, compress of rosemary to swollen joints, ginger, and orange oil massage
- Acupuncture
- Alexander Technique: To relieve muscular tension and uneven weight bearing
- Bioelectromagnetics
- Chiropractic
- Exercise (non-weight-bearing) in water or moderate exercise as tolerated
- Feldenkrais Method®
- Guided imagery
- Herbs: devil's claw, boswellia, SAMe, evening primrose oil; ginger; feverfew, capsaicin cream applied topically, glucosamine (1500 mg), and chondroitin (1200 mg) to help restore joint integrity; natural anti-inflammatories such as willowbark, turmeric, and ginger; drink: ¼ tsp. cinnamon and ½ tsp. honey in hot water
- Homeopathy: poison ivy
- Ice joints and then rub in analgesic oils.
- Low-level laser therapy
- Local application of magnesium gel
- Magnets: Place over an inflamed area on a regular basis.
- Massage
- Reflexology: Work all joints of the hands and feet for pain relief and mobility of corresponding body joints.
- Rolfing
- Supplements: thiamine, vitamins B_6 and B_{12}, calcium, magnesium, glucosamine, chondroitin, green tea, avocado-soybean unsaponifiables
- Therapeutic Touch
- Watsu®
- Yoga or t'ai chi: Practice slowly, seeing how far the affected joints can be moved without pain. Do not exercise joints when they are inflamed.

ASTHMA

- Acupuncture
- Alexander Technique: Teaches a more relaxed way of breathing and enables an individual to manage an asthma attack
- Aromatherapy: Put several drops of cypress on a handkerchief and inhale deeply. Put frankincense on a pillow at night to slow and deepen the breathing.
- Biofeedback
- Breathing exercises
- Hypnosis
- Herbs: holy basil, elecampine, country mallow, malabar nut, bayberry. Mix 3 parts tincture of lobelia with 1 part tincture of capsicum. Take 20 drops in water at the start of an asthmatic attack. Repeat every 30 minutes for a total of 3 or 4 doses.
- Homeopathy: arsenicum album, 1 tablet 3 times daily for maximum of 1 week
- Meditation
- Reflexology: During an asthma attack, work the reflexes for the diaphragm and lungs on the balls of the feet.
- Water: Drink plenty of water to keep the respiratory tract secretions fluid.
- Yoga: Focus on expansive postures and breathing practices designed to increase the length of the exhalation.

ATHLETE'S FOOT

- Acupressure: Do full foot or hand acupressure massage sessions twice a week to stimulate the immune and endocrine systems. Do not press on areas of broken, sore, or cracked skin.
- Aromatherapy: cedarwood, lemon balm, rosemary. Mix 2 drops of lavender oil and 1 drop of tea tree oil, and apply between toes.
- Herbs: bitter orange oil—external use only. Apply black walnut tincture directly to fungus patches, and drink a tea of green crushed walnut hulls for fungus anywhere in body.
- Naturopathy: kyolic garlic tablets. Dust your feet and shoes with garlic powder.
- Supplements: Take B-complex vitamins, 50–100 mg, 3 times a day, with meals. Dust vitamin C powder directly onto affected area. Zinc may help clear the skin and boost the immune system.

ATTENTION DEFICIT HYPERACTIVITY DISORDER

- Aromatherapy: lavender, rosemary, valerian
- Change diet from "junk foods" high in artificial flavors, preservatives, and sucrose to nutrient-dense foods

- Herbs: chamomile
- Homeopathy
- Massage
- Meditation
- Neurofeedback
- Supplements: B vitamins, iron, magnesium, omega-3 fatty acids
- Yoga

AUTISM

- Animal-assisted therapy
- Service animal
- Biofeedback
- Massage
- Melatonin for sleep

BACK PAIN

- Acupuncture
- Alexander Technique: Teaches a more balanced use of body, since muscular imbalance often contributes to back pain
- Applied kinesiology
- Ayurvedic massage
- Biofeedback
- Chiropractic
- Equine-assisted therapy
- Herbs: valerian, nutmeg, gotu kola. To ease local discomfort, soak a compress in ½ cup hot water containing 1 tsp. camp bark and 1 tsp. cinnamon tinctures.
- Homeopathy: arnica, 4 tablets as soon as possible after an injury, repeated every hour for the first day while awake; second day: 4 tablets every 2 hours; third day: 4 tablets 4 times a day
- Hydrotherapy: For acute back pain, use an ice pack on affected area for 20 minutes every 1–2 hours.
- Magnets: Place small magnets over area of muscle spasm in back.
- Massage with warm oil.
- Reflexology: Work the spinal reflexes, especially the tender points, on the medial longitudinal arches of the feet (the bony ridges on the inside).
- Sleep on back with pillows under knees or on side with pillow between bent knees.
- Watsu®
- Yoga: Lie down with legs bent, feet flat on floor, exhale fully and slowly for at least 12 breaths. Long-term yoga practice can strengthen back muscles.

BALANCE PROBLEMS

- Alexander Technique
- Equine-assisted therapy
- Qigong
- T'ai chi
- Watsu®
- Yoga

BEE STINGS/INSECT BITES

- Aromatherapy: tea tree oil, basil, bergamot, lavender, thyme, ylang-ylang
- Add enough water to baking soda or meat tenderizer to make a paste and apply it to the sting.
- Cover affected area with a small amount of mashed fresh papaya.
- Herbs: Apply fresh aloe vera sap directly to the bite. If bite becomes infected, bathe with marigold or echinacea tea. Apply a fresh slice of onion to both bee and wasp stings. A mixture of honey and crushed garlic makes a soothing ointment.
- Homeopathy: apis, 1 tablet every 30 minutes; maximum of 6 doses for burning and swelling

BONES (BROKEN)

- Aromatherapy: Massage in elemi oil prior to casting.
- Bioelectromagnetics: Place magnets into the dressings over fractures.
- Healing Touch
- Low-level laser therapy
- Reiki
- Therapeutic Touch

BRUISES

- Aromatherapy: cypress. Combine 1 drop of chamomile with 2 tsp. of ice-cold water. Soak a cotton pad in this mixture and apply to the affected area.
- Herbs: witch hazel (topical), arnica tablets, or massage tincture of arnica into bruised area; 200–400 mg of bromelain 3 times a day on an empty stomach
- Homeopathy: aconite, 1 or 2 doses only over 15 minutes immediately for the "shock" of the injury
- Hydrotherapy: Cold compresses for first 12 hours with occasional breaks to prevent excessive chilling.
- Supplements: 2,000 mg vitamin C, 3 times a day, for people who bruise easily. Drink pineapple juice, because enzymes speed the rate at which the blood causing the bruise is resorbed.

BURNS (MINOR)

- Aromatherapy: For pain relief: chamomile, eucalyptus, geranium, lavender. To reduce inflammation: chamomile, clary sage, geranium, lavender, myrrh, tea tree oil. To regenerate skin: chamomile, clary sage, eucalyptus, geranium, myrrh, rose, tea tree oil
- Herbs: aloe vera sap, calendula lotion, or raw honey
- Hydrotherapy: Immediately immerse the affected part in cool water for 5–10 minutes with a brief break during the first 20 minutes after the injury.
- Magnets: Place over site of injury to control pain and speed healing.

CANCER

- Acupuncture to treat side effects and symptoms
- Antioxidants: vitamins A, C, and E; coenzyme Q10
- Faith and prayer
- Herbs: betulinic acid from birch trees, thuja tincture, bromelain, gotu kola, essiac, green or black tea, maitake mushroom, selenium
- Imagery
- Massage
- Meditation
- Qigong
- Shark cartilage: works best against solid tumors, especially ovarian and prostate tumors
- Shark liver oil may help people tolerate chemotherapy and radiation.
- Supplements: reishi mushroom
- Yoga

CANKER SORES

- Herbs: licorice root gel, echinacea tincture, butternut, comfrey. Gargle with a mixture of 1 cup of warm water with ¼ tsp. of salt and ½ tsp. of goldenseal powder.
- Supplements: vitamin A (25,000–50,000 IU daily) prevents infection from spreading. B-complex (50–100 IU 3 times a day); vitamin E (400–800 IU daily); selenium (200 mcg daily); acidophilus, 4 capsules, 4–6 times a day

CARPAL TUNNEL SYNDROME

- Acupressure: Firmly press (for 2 minutes) on point on inside surface of forearm about 1 inch up from wrist fold. Also press on point on outside surface of forearm one-third of way up between wrist fold and elbow.

- Chiropractic
- Herbs: ginger compress; topical chamomile
- Hydrotherapy: contrast applications
- Low-level laser therapy
- Magnets: Place over the front and back of the wrist to control symptoms
- Massage
- Pressure point therapies

CHEST CONGESTION

- Aromatherapy: cedarwood, steam inhalation of eucalyptus, frankincense. Massage chest with lavender. Inhale marjoram, peppermint, eucalyptus, or rosemary. Place drops of tea tree oil on handkerchief.
- Herbs: Tea made with peppermint and yarrow (½ tsp. each). Mix sage or eucalyptus leaves in a bowl of steaming water and inhale with a towel draped over the head.

CHOLESTEROL (HIGH)

- Herbs: ginger, green tea, Indian gooseberry, soy, artichoke leaf extract
- Meditation
- Supplements: ProFibe (grapefruit fiber), oatmeal, flaxseed, red yeast rice (not when pregnant or breast feeding)
- Yoga

CHRONIC FATIGUE SYNDROME

- Acupuncture
- Herbs: acute phase—echinacea, goldenseal, licorice; chronic phase— goldenseal, astragalus, Siberian ginseng
- Supplements: beta-carotene, vitamin C, zinc

CIRCULATION (POOR)

- Aromatherapy: rosemary (increases circulation to skin), vetiver
- Biofeedback: Increases circulation to specific areas of the body
- Exercise
- Herbs: ginkgo, garlic, cayenne, hawthorn, bilberry, grape seed extract, horse chestnut
- Hypnosis
- Imagery
- Magnets
- Massage
- Therapeutic Touch
- Yoga

COLD SORES

- Aromatherapy: Apply tea tree oil at onset and continue until cleared.
- Herbs: echinacea or goldenseal, L-lysine. Lemon-balm tea shows significant antiviral activity against herpes simplex.
- Hydrotherapy: For early stages, apply ice—on the sore for 10 minutes, off for 5 minutes.
- Supplements: vitamins C, B-complex, and E

COLIC

- Aromatherapy: chamomile (rubbed on abdomen), coriander, orange, peppermint
- Chiropractic
- Massage abdomen. Massage bottom of feet with warmed sesame oil.

COMMON COLD

- Acupressure: If sinuses become blocked or painful
- Aromatherapy: Inhale lavender, eucalyptus, or peppermint oil in steam vaporizer to speed recovery and lessen stuffiness. Add 3 drops lemon oil, 2 drops each of thyme and tea tree oil, and 1 drop eucalyptus into hot bath.
- Herbs: Tea from fresh ginger and brown sugar; echinacea at the first sign of a cold; astraga-lus, garlic, goldenseal, eyebright, elecampane
- Homeopathy: *Allium cepa* (onion), monkshood or aconite, or natrum muriaticum
- Reflexology: Work the fingers and thumbs, the webs between the fingers, the pads beneath the fingers, and the spaces on the back of the hands for the reflexes of the head, lungs, and upper lymphatics.
- Supplements: vitamins A and C, zinc lozenges; selenium for 3 days to help resist a cold

CONSTIPATION

- Aromatherapy: Massage abdomen in a clockwise direction with orange, black pepper, ginger, or marjoram mixed in carrier oil.
- Biofeedback of pelvic floor muscles
- Exercise, especially activities that work the abdominal muscles such as rowing, swimming, walking, or sit-ups
- Herbs: dandelion root, chicory root, angelica root, cascara sagrada, senna, flaxseed. Psyllium can be used for several days; long-term use can be damaging.
- Homeopathy: bryonia (wild hops) or nux vomica
- Reflexology: Areas for the colon on the soles of both feet

- Supplements: probiotics
- Water: Drink 6–8 glasses daily.
- Yoga: Twisting postures and forward bends are often helpful.

CORNS

- Aromatherapy: Mix 2 drops each of orange, lemon, and lavender oils in a basin of warm water and soak feet for at least 15 minutes per day.
- Hydrotherapy: Hot Epsom salts foot bath, then rub corns with fresh lemon juice
- Reflexology: Around and directly on the corns

COUGH

- Aromatherapy: cedarwood. Place several drops of cypress or tea tree oil on handkerchief and inhale deeply. Add 3 drops eucalyptus and 2 drops thyme oil to 2 tsp. vegetable oil. Massage into neck and chest. Do steam inhalation using sandalwood, benzoin, eucalyptus, frankincense, or peppermint.
- Herbs: licorice, wild cherry bark, thyme; tincture of mullein in warm water 3 times a day; horehound
- Homeopathy: bryonia (wild hops), monkshood, rumex, stannum
- Reflexology: Work the lung and diaphragm reflexes on and beneath balls of feet and webs between big toes and second toes.

DEPRESSION

- Acupuncture
- Animal-assisted therapy
- Aromatherapy: bergamot, geranium, jasmine, lemon balm, rose, ylang-ylang. Add 15 drops geranium, 10 drops of bergamot, and 5 drops of lavender to bath.
- Exercise
- Flower essences: gentian, hornbeam, mustard, gorse, sweet chestnut
- Herbs: Saint John's wort, valerian
- Homeopathy: Rescue Remedy
- Hypnotherapy
- Meditation
- Music therapy
- Neurofeedback
- Reiki
- Supplements: B vitamins, omega-3
- T'ai chi
- Therapeutic Touch
- Transcranial magnetic stimulation
- Yoga

DIABETES

- Aromatherapy: Using carrier oil, rub juniper or cedar oil over spleen and pancreas area.
- Biofeedback
- Exercise
- Herbs: blueberry leaf tea, 2 cups a day on a regular basis; 100–200 mg of coenzyme Q10 every day for at least 3 months to stabilize blood sugar; gymnesly, green tea, ginger, ginseng, goldenseal
- Supplements: vitamins B_6, C, and E; chromium; magnesium; essential fatty acids; flaxseed oil
- Yoga

DIAPER RASH

- 1.5% calendula ointment for 10 days

DIARRHEA

- Aromatherapy: Gently massage abdomen with coriander, chamomile, neroli, lavender, or peppermint in carrier oil.
- Herbs: 2 tsp. of your choice of one of the following: black pepper, chamomile, coriander, rosemary, sandalwood, or thyme per cup of boiling water to make tea
- Homeopathy: podophyllum—1 tablet hourly until improved, then every 4 hours—for a maximum of 5 days
- Supplements: zinc, probiotics
- Replace lost fluids.

DRUG ADDICTION

- Bach flower essence: California poppy, morning glory, chrysanthemum
- Biofeedback
- Herbs: chamomile and ginseng (cocaine withdrawal); valerian (benzodiazepine withdrawal)

EAR INFECTIONS

- Acupressure: Massage just behind the tip of the mastoid bone at the bottom of the back of the ear to relieve pain.
- Aromatherapy: Put a drop of lavender on cotton and put it in the ear. Use a chamomile tea bag that has been infused for a few minutes and place it on the side of the face or over the ear while the tea bag is still warm.
- Chiropractic

- Craniosacral manipulation
- Ear candles
- Herbs: warm mullein oil drops in ear
- Homeopathy: belladonna or ferrum phosphate
- Reflexology: Work all fingers and toes, paying close attention to the webs between the fingers and toes, especially between the third, fourth, and fifth digits.

ECZEMA

- Aromatherapy: bergamot, chamomile, lavender, melissa, neroli, eucalyptus, geranium, juniper
- Flower essences: Rescue Remedy, crab apple
- Herbs: evening primrose oil applied directly
- Hydrotherapy: heat compresses once a day

EMOTIONAL DISTRESS

- Aromatherapy: chamomile, frankincense (deepens breathing to induce calmness), marjoram
- Breathing exercises
- Gratitude exercises
- Positive affirmations
- Watsu®

ENERGY IMBALANCE

- Applied kinesiology
- Magnets
- Pressure point therapies
- Reiki
- Shiatsu massage
- Thai massage
- Therapeutic Touch

FATIGUE

- Aromatherapy: Peppermint, rose, rosemary, and basil stimulate the brain. Lemongrass and rosemary are best for physical fatigue. Use these oils in the bath, in massage oils, in vaporizers, or on a handkerchief. Do not use peppermint or rosemary at night because they are too stimulating. Rosemary should not be used by people with hypertension or epilepsy.
- Herbs: ginseng, especially for people over the age of 40
- Qigong

- Reflexology: A brisk complete foot treatment for more energy, or a slow complete foot treatment to induce sleep
- Supplements: zinc, coenzyme Q10
- Yoga: Start with relaxation and gentle movements on your back, progressing to kneeling, standing, and/or seated postures.

FEET (TIRED)

- Aromatherapy: Mix 2 drops each of rosemary, sage, and peppermint oils in basin of hot water and soak feet for at least 15 minutes. Rosemary (20 drops), sage (15 drops), and pepper-mint (10 drops) mixed in oil base can be applied directly to feet.
- Massage
- Reflexology: Massage entire foot.

FEVER

- Aromatherapy: tea tree oil and juniper encourage the body to sweat. Lavender and peppermint are cooling. Chamomile is soothing and calming, and can be used either in a bath or in cool water to sponge the body.
- Herbs: white willow. To a large mug of boiling water, add juice of 1 lemon, 2 tsp. honey, 1 tsp. grated ginger, ½ tsp. cinnamon, ½ tsp. nutmeg, and 1 tsp. brandy or whisky.
- Homeopathy: belladonna, aconite, ferrum phosphoricum, gelsemium

FIBROMYALGIA

- Acupuncture
- Biofeedback
- Herbs: topical capsaicin; 1 tsp. 3 times a day of equal parts of echinacea, black cohosh, devil's claw, licorice, dandelion, and celery
- Hypnotherapy
- Magnets: Magnets can be placed over painful areas during the day.
- Massage
- Supplements: magnesium, malic acid, vitamins E and C, fish oil, selenium, zinc, SAMe
- T'ai chi
- Watsu®

FLUID RETENTION (EDEMA)

- Herbs: dandelion leaf (diuretic and replaces potassium)
- Massage feet and ankles.
- Reflexology: lymph system, kidneys, adrenals points on the feet
- Elevate legs.

HEADACHE (TENSION)

- Acupressure: Press pressure points between eyebrows or at bottom of web between thumb and first finger.
- Alexander Technique: Helps improve posture to avoid buildup of tension in neck and shoulders
- Aromatherapy: basil, chamomile; massage lavender, peppermint, or eucalyptus around temples; rose compress to eyes
- Chiropractic
- Herbs: ginseng, chamomile, turmeric, valerian, willow bark; ½ tsp. each of betony and skullcap made into tea
- Homeopathy: bryonia (wild hops), windflower, yellow jasmine, nux vomica
- Neurofeedback
- Pulsating electromagnetic fields
- Relaxation techniques
- Therapeutic Touch
- Yoga

HEART DISEASE

- Animal-assisted therapy
- Aromatherapy: To strengthen the heart muscle—garlic, lavender, peppermint, marjoram, rose, rosemary
- Biofeedback
- Exercise
- Herbs: garlic, ginger; 1–2 capsules of hawthorn 4 times a day for mild angina
- Meditation
- Supplements: vitamins E, C, B_6, and B_{12}; L-carnitine; coenzyme Q10 to improve utilization of oxygen at cellular level, beta-carotene, selenium, magnesium, calcium, fish oil, plant sterols/stanols, and black, green, oolong, white tea
- T'ai chi, qigong

HEAT RASH

- Herbs: Sprinkle arrowroot powder on affected area. Place ½ cup of freshly grated ginger into a quart of boiling water, remove from heat immediately, and steep for 5 minutes, then cool and sponge ginger water onto affected areas and let it dry.

HEMORRHOIDS

- Aromatherapy: Massage geranium, chamomile, or lavender oil, mixed with carrier oil, into the rectal area as needed.

- Herbs: Apply aloe vera gel to relieve itching. Use compresses of witch hazel to clean area after bowel movement.
- Homeopathy: aesculus, aloe, or hamamelis
- Hydrotherapy: Sit in warm bath for 15 minutes several times a day.

HICCUPS

- Acupressure: Place your middle and index fingers behind each earlobe. Apply light to firm pressure on the neck for 2 minutes as you concentrate on breathing slowly and deeply.
- Reflexology: diaphragm and stomach points on the feet

HYPERTENSION

- Animal-assisted therapy
- Aromatherapy: ylang-ylang, clary sage, lavender, marjoram
- Biofeedback
- Chiropractic
- Exercise
- Herbs: garlic, hawthorn, olive leaf extract, maitake mushroom, reishi mushroom, evening primrose oil, ginger, goldenseal
- Hypnotherapy
- Massage
- Meditation
- Qigong
- Supplements: vitamin C, magnesium, flaxseed oil; calcium for pregnancy-induced hypertension
- T'ai chi
- Yoga

IMMUNE ENHANCEMENT

- Aromatherapy: elemi, eucalyptus
- Herbs: echinacea, goldenseal, astragalus
- Massage
- Qigong
- Supplements: vitamins E and C, beta-carotene, garlic

INDIGESTION

- Aromatherapy: Use basil, chamomile, coriander, ginger, or peppermint as a tea or in massage oil or warm compress over stomach area.
- Herbs: chamomile, peppermint, ginger as a tea; for heaviness after a meal, chew on cardamom or fennel seeds
- Homeopathy: windflower; nux vomica—1 tablet hourly for 6 doses, then 3 times a day—for a maximum of 1 week

INFECTION (BACTERIAL)

- Aromatherapy: calendula, geranium, rosemary, tea tree, lavender, eucalyptus, thyme, niaouli, bergamot. These oils work by attacking the organisms themselves, by killing airborne germs, and by strengthening the immune system.
- Herbs: echinacea at first sign of infection; echinacea may be combined with goldenseal; garlic in capsules
- Supplements: medicinal honey—manuka from New Zealand or medihoney from Australia

INFECTION (FUNGAL)

- Aromatherapy: calendula, lemon balm, rosemary
- Herbs: garlic, tea tree oil (topical)

INFECTION (VIRAL)

- Aromatherapy: eucalyptus, lemon balm
- Herbs: goldenseal, echinacea, garlic, tea tree oil (topical)
- Supplements: zinc, selenium

INFERTILITY

- Meditation for unexplained infertility
- Supplements: zinc for men
- Acupuncture immediately after in vitro fertilization

INFLAMMATION

- Aromatherapy: benzoin, birch, chamomile, clary sage, elemi, fennel, geranium, helichrysum, jasmine, myrrh, patchouli, rose, sandalwood
- Bee venom may slow down the body's inflammatory response by inhibiting the amount of free radicals or by stimulating the adrenal glands to release cortisol.
- Homeopathy: belladonna
- Hydrotherapy: applications of heat and cold
- Magnets

INSOMNIA

- Acupuncture
- Acupressure: Use Sea-Bands: acupressure elastic wrist bands placed between 2 tendons, 3 finger-widths from wrist crease.
- Aromatherapy: chamomile, which can also be used with children; clary sage, lavender, marjoram, neroli, or vetiver in bath or a pillow or as a room fragrance

- Ayurvedic oil dripping therapy
- Biofeedback
- Deep breathing exercises
- Exercise: not later than early evening
- Guided imagery
- Herbs: valerian, lemon balm, catnip, hops, passionflower, skullcap teas (If taste is unpleasant, add sugar, honey, or lemon.)
- Homeopathy: windflower, nux vomica, arsenicum album
- Hydrotherapy: warm baths
- Light therapy—full-spectrum lights for 30 minutes a day
- Magnets: Use magnetic pillow or pad for sedating effect.
- Meditation
- Neurofeedback
- Supplements: melatonin
- Watsu®

IRRITABLE BOWEL SYNDROME

- Acupuncture
- Biofeedback
- Exercise
- Herbs: enteric-coated peppermint capsules, ginger, chamomile, valerian, rosemary, lemon balm
- Hypnotherapy
- Meditation
- Supplements: probiotics
- Yoga

JET LAG

- Herbs: melatonin
- Drink fluids and avoid alcohol. Do in-flight stretches.

LEG CRAMPS (NIGHT TIME)

- Add 10 drops of rosemary, 10 drops of sweet marjoram, 5 drops of geranium, and 5 drops of lavender and blend together. Add 5 drops of the blended mixture to 1 tsp. of carrier oil. Before bed, massage entire leg up from the ankle. Massage feet.
- In the bed, place several small bars of scented soap under the bottom sheet.

LIVER DISEASE

- Herbs: milk thistle, dandelion root tea
- Hydrotherapy: Take steam baths or saunas frequently to help body eliminate toxins.

MACULAR DEGENERATION

- Herbs: gingko, bilberry, blackberry, cranberry, raspberry
- Supplements: antioxidants, zinc, fish oil
- Vitamins C and E, copper

MEMORY PROBLEMS

- Aromatherapy: basil, black pepper, coriander, ginger, peppermint, rosemary, thyme
- Exercise
- Supplements: vitamin B_6, green tea

MENOPAUSE

- Acupuncture
- Aromatherapy: geranium, rose, chamomile, yuzu, sandalwood, lavender, bergamot, fennel in bath or in body creams
- Herbs: black cohosh (estrogen enhancer, hot flashes), chasteberry (hormone balancing), Saint John's wort (mood swings), motherwort (palpitations and hot flashes), skullcap (anxiety), dong quai (estrogen enhancer), wild yam as tea; Chinese tonic of He Shou Wu, red clover, licorice
- Homeopathy: pulsatilla (mood changes), sulfur (hot flashes)
- Hypnotherapy
- Meditation
- Supplements: vitamin E, soy protein, calcium, magnesium, flaxseed, evening primrose oil

MENSTRUAL DISCOMFORT

- Aromatherapy: basil. Massage abdomen and lower back with lavender, clary sage, and rose mixed in carrier oil.
- Herbs: tea of agnus-castus with rosemary for premenstrual water retention; black haw for cramps—4 tsp. in glass of warm water, repeat after 4 hours if necessary; Chinese tonic of dong quai, dandelion leaf for water retention
- Homeopathy: viburnum, magnesium phosphate, sepia, lachesis
- Hydrotherapy: warm compresses
- Reflexology: Massage uterine reflexes below inside ankle bones and ovarian reflexes beneath outside ankle bones.
- Supplements: calcium and manganese; fish oil, parsley, celery, and dandelion leaves are all mild diuretics
- Yoga stretches; more relaxation and breathing exercises

MIGRAINE HEADACHES

- Aromatherapy: green apple (inhalant), lavender, melissa, or peppermint can be put on a facecloth with cool water and used as a compress on the forehead or back of the neck.
- Chiropractic
- Herbs: feverfew (prophylaxis), ginkgo, butterbar
- Homeopathy: iris, sanguinaria, glonoine
- Hypnotherapy
- Neurofeedback
- Pressure point therapies
- Pulsating electromagnetic fields
- Spiritual meditation

MUSCLE SORENESS

- Aromatherapy: chamomile, juniper
- Herbs: Rub in wintergreen oil or capsicum cream.
- Hydrotherapy: spa
- Massage
- Movement therapy: T'ai chi, qigong, Feldenkrais Method®
- Watsu®
- Yoga

NAUSEA

- Acupressure: Use Sea-Bands: acupressure elastic wrist bands placed between 2 tendons, 3 finger-widths from wrist crease.
- Aromatherapy: ginger, lavender, peppermint used as a compress and as teas
- Healing Touch
- Herbs: ginger
- Homeopathy: ipecacuanha, sepia, clossypium
- Imagery
- Reiki
- Therapeutic Touch

OSTEOPOROSIS

- Exercise: weight bearing unless advanced stage of disease
- Herbs: a tea of stinging nettles, alfalfa, or sage, horsetail, dandelion root, turmeric
- Supplements: calcium, vitamins D_3 and C, magnesium, natural hormone therapy, soy

PAIN

- Acupuncture
- Alexander Technique
- Biofeedback
- Chiropractic
- Herbs: feverfew, devil's claw
- Hydrotherapy: hot water packs, cold applications
- Hypnotherapy
- Guided imagery
- Low-level laser therapy
- Magnets
- Pressure point therapies
- Reiki
- Sports massage
- Therapeutic Touch
- Trager Approach®
- Trigger point massage
- Watsu®

PHYSICAL DISABILITIES

- Balance difficulties—T'ai chi, yoga, equine-assisted therapy

POISON IVY AND POISON OAK

- Rinse the exposed area with soap and cold water. Mix baking soda with water to form a paste and apply it to skin. Once the paste has hardened, remove with cool water and apply a thin layer of honey to the area.
- Aloe. For itching and discomfort, grind 1 cup raw, whole oats to a fine powder and add to tepid bath—soak for 20–30 minutes.
- Homeopathy: Rhus tox

POSTTRAUMATIC STRESS DISORDER

- Acupuncture
- Biofeedback
- Guided imagery
- Massage
- Meditation
- Watsu®
- Yoga

PREGNANCY

Although not a health care problem, it is included here for relief of some of the discomfort.

Morning Sickness

- Acupressure: Use Sea-Bands: acupressure elastic wrist bands placed between 2 tendons, 3 finger-widths from wrist crease.
- Herbs: peppermint, catnip, ginger, chamomile, cinnamon, red raspberry leaf teas

Labor

- Acupuncture and moxibustion for breech presentation
- Aromatherapy: Blend of clary sage, rose, and ylang-ylang can be used for massage. Deep massage of lower back and hips during contractions— between contractions, massage shoulders, back, hands, and feet; if contractions are lagging, a light massage of the breasts may stimulate activity.
- Herbs: red raspberry tea, black cohosh tea, blue cohosh, bethroot
- Hydrotherapy: water birth
- Hypnotherapy

Postpartum

- Herbs: lavender oil or aloe for perineal discomfort; cabbage leaves, mother's milk, alfalfa to encourage lactation
- Reflexology to encourage lactation

PREMENSTRUAL SYNDROME

- Acupuncture
- Aromatherapy: Massage or warm bath with rose oil, clary sage, ylang-ylang, lavender, lemongrass, sandalwood, jasmine, bergamot. One will have to decide, by trial and error, which of these oils best suits the individual.
- Deep breathing exercises for a least 20 minutes a day
- Exercise
- Herbs: vitex, black cohosh extract, agnus-castus, chasteberry, helonias, evening primrose oil, Chinese tonic of dong quai
- Homeopathy: windflower, pulsatilla, lachesis
- Massage
- Meditation
- Reflexology: Massage uterine reflexes below inside ankle bones and ovarian reflexes beneath outside ankle bones.
- Supplements: vitamins A, E, B1, B_2, and B_6; 2–3 g capsules of combined fish oil and evening primrose oil, magnesium, zinc, calcium

PROSTATE ENLARGEMENT (BENIGN)

- Herbs: saw palmetto, pygeum africanum, stinging nettle root tea
- Supplements: vitamins C, E, and B_3; zinc; manganese. Add soy foods to diet.

PSORIASIS

- Aromatherapy: bergamot (heal skin plaques), lavender (itching), melissa or geranium (irritated skin), jasmine (dry skin)
- Diet: Include foods with zinc, beta-carotene, vitamin D, and omega-3 fatty acids. Avoid liver and other organ meats, which aggravate psoriasis.
- Flower essences: Rescue Remedy cream, crab apple
- Herbs: evening primrose oil, echinacea, licorice, milk thistle. Apply aloe vera extract topically 3 times a day. Do not cover.
- Homeopathy: sepai, arsenicum iodatum, petroleum
- Add 2 drops calendula oil and 1 drop lavender oil to 2 tsp. almond oil, and then massage area with mixture.
- Sunshine on the skin is helpful.

RADIATION DERMATITIS

- Calendula ointment

RESTLESS LEG SYNDROME

- Massage with lavender oil.

RINGWORM

- Aromatherapy: rosemary, tea tree oil, lavender, geranium, peppermint, thyme
- Herbs: Apply a paste made of equal parts of myrrh powder and goldenseal powder mixed with a little water. A thin slice of garlic bandaged directly over the skin lesion and left for several days has a powerful antifungal effect.
- Homeopathy: sepia, arsenicum album, graphites

SCIATICA

- Acupuncture
- Applied kinesiology
- Chiropractic
- Herbs: willow bark, black cohosh, chamomile, fenugreek, juniper berries, parsley, rosemary, skullcap
- Homeopathy: colocynth, *Viscum album*, lachesis, rhus tox, aconite, belladonna
- Hydrotherapy: warm water jets
- Low-level laser therapy
- Reflexology: hip, sciatic, knee, lower spine, shoulder points on feet

SEXUAL DYSFUNCTION

- Acupuncture
- Herbs: ginkgo or topical saffron for erectile problems; ashwagandha
- Hypnotherapy
- Imagery

SHINGLES

- Aromatherapy: eucalyptus, tea tree oil, lavender, chamomile, bergamot. Smooth the oil gently over the affected areas and down either side of the spine; if body is too painful to touch, add oils to a water spray or use in a bath.
- Flower essences: Rescue Remedy, crab apple
- Herbs: echinacea, Saint John's wort tea. Apply aloe vera gel to blistering area.
- Hydrotherapy: body-temperature bath for 30 minutes

SINUS PROBLEMS

- Acupuncture
- Aromatherapy: Put basil, marjoram, or eucalyptus on handkerchief, or use with a vaporizer.
- Herbs: ephedra, goldenseal, yarrow, coltsfoot. Make a tea using 2 tsp. of herb per cup. Use herbs in cream or oil, and massage the sinus areas.
- Homeopathy: hydrastis, kali bichromicum, arsenicum album, silicea
- Hydrotherapy: hot and cold compresses, steam inhalation, nasal lavage
- Reflexology: Massage the sinus reflexes on the tips of the fingers and toes.

SKIN (DRY)

- Aromatherapy: Mix 2 drops each of sandalwood, rose, and geranium oil with 1 tsp. of almond oil. Use as a topical evening moisturizer. Other oils good for dry skin include jasmine, orange, and ylang-ylang used in a moisturizer or in a bath.

SORE THROAT

- Aromatherapy: Take several drops of sandalwood on handkerchief, or mix with carrier oil and massage into throat area. Then, wrap something warm around the throat.
- Herbs: Gargle with 1 cup of warm water with ¼ to 1 tsp. of salt and ½ tsp. of goldenseal powder.
- Homeopathy: monkshood, poison ivy, belladonna

- Hydrotherapy: contrast applications to neck and throat; heat compresses
- Reflexology: Massage the throat reflexes around the "neck" of the big toes and thumbs.

SPRAIN AND STRAINS

- Aromatherapy: chamomile, ginger, lavender as massage to area
- Herbs: Mix ¼ cup each of dry mustard powder and flour with warm water to make a thick paste, spread the paste onto cheesecloth or gauze, roll it up, and apply to the strained area.
- Homeopathy: poison ivy
- Hydrotherapy: cold compresses to reduce swelling first 24 hours; then warm compresses to increase circulation
- Low-level laser therapy
- Magnets: Cover area with magnetic pad and secure with an Ace bandage. Put it on for 12 hours, then take it off for 12 hours.
- Myofascial release
- Pressure point therapies
- Reiki
- Therapeutic Touch

STRESS

- Acupuncture
- Aromatherapy: juniper, lavender, vetiver, ylang-ylang. Use jasmine in massage oil or put in bath.
- Breathing exercises; alternate nostril breathing (pranayama)
- Exercise
- Herbs: chamomile tea, passionflower, valerian, ginseng
- Humor and laughter
- Massage
- Meditation
- Music therapy
- Progressive relaxation
- T'ai chi
- Qigong
- Watsu®
- Yoga: Focus on slow movements and long exhalations.

SUNBURN

- Aromatherapy: Spray or rub with lavender and chamomile.
- Herbs: Soak a soft cloth in cooled black or green tea and spread over the burned area. Leave on 15–30 minutes. Apply aloe vera sap to area.

- Hydrotherapy: cold compresses. Soak in a bath of tepid water and baking soda (1 pound) for 20–30 minutes; later that day or next, take a tepid bath with 1 or 2 cups of milk added.
- Grated potato applied directly to the skin will decrease pain and prevent blistering; wrap in place with a clean cloth.

SURGERY

- Hypnotherapy and visualization before surgery
- Magnets: Place magnets over the incision site for 24 to 48 hours before surgery to improve postoperative recovery. Place magnets over wound after surgery.
- Meditation before and after surgery

TENSION

- Aromatherapy: hot bath or massage using one of the following oils— bergamot, rose, cedarwood, chamomile, geranium, lavender, melissa, orange, or sandalwood
- Feldenkrais Method®
- Herbs: valerian, passionflower, chamomile, ginseng as teas
- Massage
- Meditation
- Reiki
- Therapeutic Touch

TINNITUS

- Acupuncture
- Herb: gingko
- Homeopathy: salicylicum acidum, chenopodium, cinchona officinalis
- Supplement: vitamin B_{12}

URINARY INCONTINENCE

- Biofeedback of pelvic floor muscles

URINARY TRACT INFECTION

- Aromatherapy: bergamot, sandalwood, lavender, or juniper in bath water
- Herbs: uva ursi, goldenseal; saw palmetto for men
- Homeopathy: pulsatilla, sepia, nux vomica
- Hydrotherapy: contrast sitz baths

- Supplements: unsweetened cranberry juice (300 mL daily); vitamins A and C
- Urinate after sexual activity.
- Drink plenty of water.

WARTS

- Aromatherapy: 1 drop each of lemon, thyme, and tea tree oil mixed in base oil and swabbed 2 times a day.
- Duct tape: Cover the warts with duct tape and leave undisturbed for several days.
- Hypnotherapy
- Imagery
- Supplements: vitamins A, C, B-complex, and E; zinc; L-cysteine

WEIGHT CONTROL

- Aromatherapy: green apple, fennel, juniper, rosemary, bitter orange
- Exercise
- Herb: evening primrose oil
- Supplements: 2.5 g of vitamin B_5 4 times a day; calcium, chromium, conjugated linoleic acid (CLA)
- Yoga

WOUNDS

- Aromatherapy: To disinfect: bergamot, chamomile, clary sage, jasmine, juniper, lavender, rose, tea tree oil. To relieve pain: bergamot, chamomile, geranium, jasmine, lavender, rosemary. To stop bleeding: cypress, geranium, rose. To reduce inflammation: chamomile, geranium, helichrysum, jasmine, patchouli. To promote formation of scar tissue: bergamot, chamomile, helichrysum, jasmine.
- Bioelectromagnetics
- Herbs: echinacea, goldenseal
- Homeopathy: calendula, hypericum, ledum
- Hydrotherapy: warm-water irrigation
- Low-level laser therapy
- Unprocessed honey may help disinfect wounds, sores, and actively promote wound healing.

INDEX